TOP TRAILS

Yosemite

45 MUST-DO HIKES FOR EVERYONE

SECOND EDITION

Written by

Elizabeth Wenk and Jeffrey P. Schaffer

Series created by

Joseph Walowski

 WILDERNESS PRESS . . . *on the trail since 1967*

Top Trails Yosemite: 45 Must-Do Hikes for Everyone
2nd Edition

Copyright © 2018 by Elizabeth Wenk

All photos copyright © Elizabeth Wenk, except where noted

Cover photo: Vernal Fall (see Trail 32, page 292) © shaferaphoto/Shutterstock
Interior photos and maps: Elizabeth Wenk
Cover design: Frances Baca Design and Lisa Pletka
Interior design: Frances Baca Design, with updates by Annie Long
Managing Editor: Amber Kaye Henderson
Copyeditor: Kerry Smith
Proofreader: Rebecca Henderson
Indexer: Frances S. Lennie/Indexing Research

Library of Congress Cataloging-in-Publication Data

Names: Wenk, Elizabeth, author. | Schaffer, Jeffrey P., author.
Title: Top trails Yosemite : must-do hikes for everyone / written by Elizabeth Wenk and Jeffrey
   P. Schaffer ; series created by Joseph Walowski.
Description: Second Edition. | Birmingham, Alabama : Wilderness Press, An imprint of
   AdventureKEEN, [2018] | "Distributed by Publishers Group West"—T.p. verso. | Includes
   index.
Identifiers: LCCN 2017038039| ISBN 9780899977836 (paperback) | ISBN 9780899977843
   (ebook) | ISBN 9780899979519 (hardcover)
Subjects: LCSH: Hiking—California—Yosemite National Park—Guidebooks. | Trails—
   California—Yosemite National Park—Guidebooks. | Backpacking—California—Yosemite
   National Park—Guidebooks. | Camping—California—Yosemite National Park—
   Guidebooks. | Yosemite National Park (Calif.)—Guidebooks.
Classification: LCC GV199.42.C22 Y6799 2018 | DDC 796.510979447—dc23
LC record available at https://lccn.loc.gov/2017038039

Manufactured in China

Published by: **WILDERNESS PRESS**
An imprint of AdventureKEEN
2204 First Ave. S., Ste. 102
Birmingham, AL 35233
800-443-7227; fax 205-326-1012

Visit wildernesspress.com for a complete listing of our books and for ordering information. Contact us at our website, at facebook.com/wildernesspress1967, or at twitter.com/wilderness1967
with questions or comments. To find out more about who we are and what we're doing, visit
blog.wildernesspress.com.

Distributed by Publishers Group West

SAFETY NOTICE: Though Wilderness Press and the author have made every attempt to
ensure that the information in this book is accurate at press time, they are not responsible for
any loss, damage, injury, or inconvenience that may occur to anyone while using this book. You
are responsible for your own safety and health while in the wilderness. The fact that a trail is
described in this book does not mean that it will be safe for you. Be aware that trail conditions
can change from day to day. Always check local conditions and know your own limitations.

The Top Trails Series

Wilderness Press

When Wilderness Press published *Sierra North* in 1967, no other trail guide like it existed for the Sierra backcountry. The first run of 2,800 copies sold out in less than two months, and its success heralded the beginning of Wilderness Press. In the past 35 years, we have expanded our territories to cover California, Alaska, Hawaii, the US Southwest, the Pacific Northwest, New England, Canada, and Baja California.

Wilderness Press continues to publish comprehensive, accurate, and readable outdoor books. Hikers, backpackers, kayakers, skiers, snowshoers, climbers, cyclists, and trail runners rely on Wilderness Press for accurate outdoor adventure information.

Top Trails

In its Top Trails guides, Wilderness Press has paid special attention to organization so that you can find the perfect hike each and every time. Whether you're looking for a steep trail to test yourself on or a walk in the park, a romantic waterfall or a city view, Top Trails will lead you there.

Each Top Trails guide contains trails for everyone. The trails selected provide a sampling of the best that the region has to offer. These are the must-do hikes, walks, runs, and bike rides, with every feature of the area represented.

Every book in the Top Trails series offers the following:

- the Wilderness Press commitment to accuracy and reliability
- ratings and rankings for each trail
- distances and approximate times
- easy-to-follow trail notes
- maps and permit information

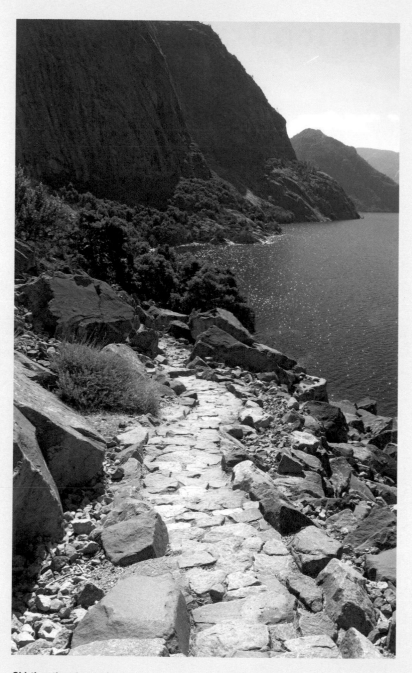

Skirting the shore *of Hetch Hetchy Reservoir (see Trail 25, page 243)*

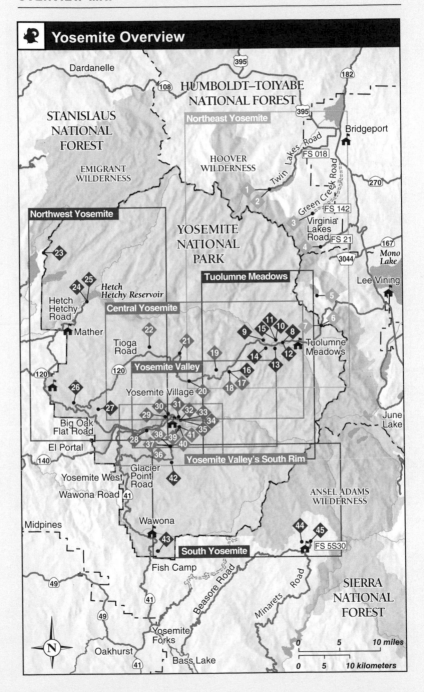

Yosemite Overview

Dardanelle

395

108 HUMBOLDT–TOIYABE
NATIONAL FOREST

182

395

STANISLAUS
NATIONAL
FOREST

Northeast Yosemite

Bridgeport

HOOVER
WILDERNESS

FS 018

EMIGRANT
WILDERNESS

Twin Lakes Road

270

1

2

Green Creek Road

3 FS 142

Northwest Yosemite

YOSEMITE
NATIONAL
PARK

Virginia
Lakes
Road FS 21

167

23

4

3044

Mono
Lake

24 25

Hetch
Hetchy Reservoir

Tuolumne Meadows

5

Lee Vining

Hetch
Hetchy
Road

Central Yosemite

6

Mather

22

21

11
15 10 8 7
9

Tioga
Road

120

Yosemite Village

12

19

14

120

Yosemite Valley

Tuolumne
Meadows

16

13

18 17

120

26

20

31
30 32 33
34
35

June
Lake

27

29

38 39 41
37 40

Big Oak
Flat Road

28

El Portal

36

Yosemite Valley's South Rim

140

Glacier
Point
Road

42

ANSEL ADAMS
WILDERNESS

Yosemite West

Wawona Road 41

Midpines

Wawona

44 45

49

43

South Yosemite

FS 5S30

Fish Camp

Beasore Road

Minarets Road

SIERRA
NATIONAL
FOREST

41

49

49

Yosemite
Forks

Oakhurst

41

Bass Lake

0   5   10 miles

0   5   10 kilometers

N

TRAIL FEATURES TABLE

Yosemite Trails

TRAIL NUMBER AND NAME	Page	Difficulty −12345+	Length in Miles	Type	Day Hiking	Backpacking	Horses	Running	Wheelchair Access	Stroller Access	Child-Friendly
1. Northeast Yosemite											
1 Benson Lake and Matterhorn Canyon Loop	36	5	50.3	Loop		Backpacking	Horses				
2 Barney Lake and Peeler Lake	56	3–4	16.2	Out-and-Back	Day Hiking	Backpacking	Horses	Running			
3 Green Creek Basin	63	2–3	6.3	Out-and-Back	Day Hiking	Backpacking					Child-Friendly
4 Virginia Lakes Basin to Green Creek	68	3	11.8	Point-to-Point	Day Hiking	Backpacking	Horses				
5 Twenty Lakes Basin	77	2	7.5	Loop	Day Hiking	Backpacking					Child-Friendly
6 Mount Dana	84	3	5.6	Out-and-Back	Day Hiking						
7 Gaylor Lakes and Great Sierra Mine	90	2	4.0	Out-and-Back	Day Hiking						Child-Friendly
2. Tuolumne Meadows											
8 Lembert Dome and Dog Lake	105	2	3.9	Out-and-Back	Day Hiking						Child-Friendly
9 Pothole Dome and the Tuolumne River	110	2	3.0	Loop	Day Hiking						Child-Friendly
10 Young Lakes	115	3	14.1	Loop	Day Hiking	Backpacking	Horses	Running			
11 Glen Aulin and Waterwheel Falls	122	4	17.6	Out-and-Back	Day Hiking	Backpacking	Horses				
12 Vogelsang High Sierra Camp and Lyell Canyon	131	4	19.3	Loop	Day Hiking	Backpacking	Horses				
13 Elizabeth Lake	139	2	4.6	Out-and-Back	Day Hiking						Child-Friendly
14 Lower Cathedral Lake	143	2	7.2	Out-and-Back	Day Hiking	Backpacking		Running			
15 High Sierra Camps Loop, Northwest Section	149	4	16.8	Point-to-Point	Day Hiking	Backpacking		Running			
16 High Sierra Camps Loop, Southeast Section	160	5	30.1	Point-to-Point		Backpacking	Horses				
3. Central Yosemite											
17 Sunrise Lakes and Sunrise High Sierra Camp	182	3	10.3	Out-and-Back	Day Hiking	Backpacking	Horses				
18 Clouds Rest	188	3–4	12.6	Out-and-Back	Day Hiking	Backpacking	Horses				
19 May Lake and Mount Hoffmann	194	3	5.7	Out-and-Back	Day Hiking	Backpacking					Child-Friendly
20 North Dome	200	3	9.2	Out-and-Back	Day Hiking	Backpacking					Child-Friendly
21 Ten Lakes Basin	207	3	12.3	Out-and-Back	Day Hiking	Backpacking	Horses				
22 Harden Lake	216	2	5.7	Out-and-Back	Day Hiking	Backpacking	Horses	Running			Child-Friendly
4. Northwest Yosemite											
23 Kibbie Lake	228	2	8.2	Out-and-Back	Day Hiking	Backpacking	Horses				Child-Friendly

TYPE
- Point-to-Point
- Loop
- Out-and-Back
- Balloon

DIFFICULTY
−12345+
less   more

USES & ACCESS
- Day Hiking
- Backpacking
- Horses
- Running
- Wheelchair Access
- Stroller Access
- Child-Friendly

TERRAIN
- Canyon
- Summit
- Lake
- Stream
- Waterfall

TRAIL FEATURES TABLE

Canyon	Summit	Lake	Stream	Waterfall	Autumn Colors	Wildflowers	Giant Sequoias	Great Views	Camping	Swimming	Secluded	Steep	Granite Slabs	Geological Interest	Historical Interest
					TERRAIN							**NATURE**			**OTHER**

Canyon	Summit	Lake	Stream	Waterfall	Autumn Colors	Wildflowers	Giant Sequoias	Great Views	Camping	Swimming	Secluded	Steep	Granite Slabs	Geological Interest	Historical Interest
✓		●	●		●	●		●	●	●	●	●	●	●	
✓		●	●		●	●		●	●	●	●		●		
		●	●		●	●		●	●	●	●				
		●	●		●	●		●	●	●	●				●
		●				●		●	●					●	
	●					●		●				●		●	
		●				●		●						●	●
	●	●						●		●			●		
	●		●					●		●			●	●	
		●				●		●	●						
✓			●	●				●	●			●	●	●	
		●	●			●		●	●	●			●		
		●				●		●							
		●						●	●	●			●		
✓		●	●	●		●		●	●				●		
✓		●	●			●		●	●	●		●	●		
		●				●		●	●	●		●			
	●					●		●	●			●	●		
	●	●				●		●	●						
	●					●		●	●				●	●	
		●				●		●	●	●	●		●		
		●			●	●			●	●				●	
		●	●						●	●	●		●		

NATURE
🍁 Autumn Colors 🌲 Giant Sequoias ✳ Wildflowers

FEATURES
🔭 Great Views 👤 Secluded 🏠 Historical Interest
⛺ Camping ⛏ Steep 🔨 Geological Interest
🏊 Swimming ⛰ Granite Slabs

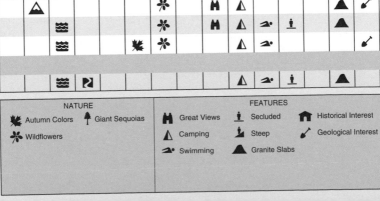

TRAIL FEATURES TABLE

Yosemite Trails

Trail Number and Name	Page	Difficulty −12345+	Length in Miles	Type	Day Hiking	Backpacking	Horses	Running	Wheelchair Access	Stroller Access	Child-Friendly
4. Northwest Yosemite (continued)											
24 Laurel Lake and Lake Vernon	235	4	21.1	Out-and-Back		Backpacking	Horses				
25 Wapama Falls and Rancheria Falls Camp	243	3	12.8	Out-and-Back	Day Hiking	Backpacking	Horses	Running			
26 Tuolumne Grove of Big Trees	250	2	2.55	Balloon	Day Hiking					Stroller Access	Child-Friendly
27 El Capitan from Tamarack Flat	255	4	16.8	Out-and-Back	Day Hiking	Backpacking	Horses	Running			
5. Yosemite Valley											
28 Bridalveil Fall	270	1	0.4	Out-and-Back	Day Hiking				Wheelchair Access	Stroller Access	Child-Friendly
29 Lower Yosemite Fall	274	1	1.2	Balloon	Day Hiking				Wheelchair Access	Stroller Access	Child-Friendly
30 Upper Yosemite Fall	280	3	6.3	Out-and-Back	Day Hiking	Backpacking					
31 Mirror Lake	287	1	1.9	Balloon	Day Hiking			Running	Wheelchair Access	Stroller Access	Child-Friendly
32 Vernal Fall Bridge	292	2	2.0	Out-and-Back	Day Hiking					Stroller Access	Child-Friendly
33 Vernal Fall–Nevada Fall Loop	297	3	6.4	Balloon	Day Hiking						
34 Half Dome	305	4	14.7	Out-and-Back	Day Hiking	Backpacking					
35 Merced Lake	315	5	26.6	Out-and-Back		Backpacking	Horses				
6. Yosemite Valley's South Rim											
36 Dewey Point	330	2	7.8	Out-and-Back	Day Hiking	Backpacking	Horses	Running			Child-Friendly
37 Taft Point	335	1–2	2.4	Out-and-Back	Day Hiking			Running			
38 Sentinel Dome	340	1–2	2.2	Out-and-Back	Day Hiking						Child-Friendly
39 Glacier Point	344	1	0.5	Balloon	Day Hiking				Wheelchair Access	Stroller Access	Child-Friendly
40 Four Mile Trail	349	2	4.7	Point-to-Point	Day Hiking						
41 Panorama Trail	355	3	8.65	Point-to-Point	Day Hiking						
7. South Yosemite											
42 Ostrander Lake	368	3	12.5	Out-and-Back	Day Hiking	Backpacking	Horses	Running			Child-Friendly
43 Mariposa Grove of Big Trees	373	2	5.8	Balloon	Day Hiking						Child-Friendly
44 Isberg–Red Peak–Fernandez Passes Loop	381	5	44.1	Point-to-Point		Backpacking	Horses				
45 Vanderburgh–Lillian Lakes Loop	402	3–4	12.2	Balloon	Day Hiking	Backpacking	Horses	Running			Child-Friendly

TYPE
- Point-to-Point
- Loop
- Out-and-Back
- Balloon

DIFFICULTY
− 1 2 3 4 5 +
less   more

USES & ACCESS
- Day Hiking
- Backpacking
- Horses
- Running
- Wheelchair Access
- Stroller Access
- Child-Friendly

TERRAIN
- Canyon
- Summit
- Lake
- Stream
- Waterfall

TRAIL FEATURES TABLE

	TERRAIN					NATURE			OTHER							
	Canyon	Summit	Lake	Stream	Waterfall	Autumn Colors	Wildflowers	Giant Sequoias	Great Views	Camping	Swimming	Secluded	Steep	Granite Slabs	Geological Interest	Historical Interest
			●	●			●		●	●	●	●		●	●	
	●		●	●	●		●		●	●				●	●	
							●	●								●
		●					●		●	●		●				
				●	●				●							
	●			●	●				●							
	●	●		●	●		●		●	●			●		●	
	●		●	●					●						●	
	●			●	●				●						●	
	●			●	●		●		●				●		●	
	●	●		●	●		●		●	●			●	●	●	
	●		●	●	●		●		●	●	●		●	●	●	
		●					●		●	●		●				
		●					●		●						●	
		●							●					●	●	
					●				●					●	●	
	●				●				●				●		●	
	●			●	●		●		●				●			
			●						●	●					●	
							●	●								●
	●		●	●			●		●	●		●	●	●	●	
			●				●		●	●	●	●		●	●	

NATURE
- Autumn Colors
- Giant Sequoias
- Wildflowers

FEATURES
- Great Views
- Camping
- Swimming
- Secluded
- Steep
- Granite Slabs
- Historical Interest
- Geological Interest

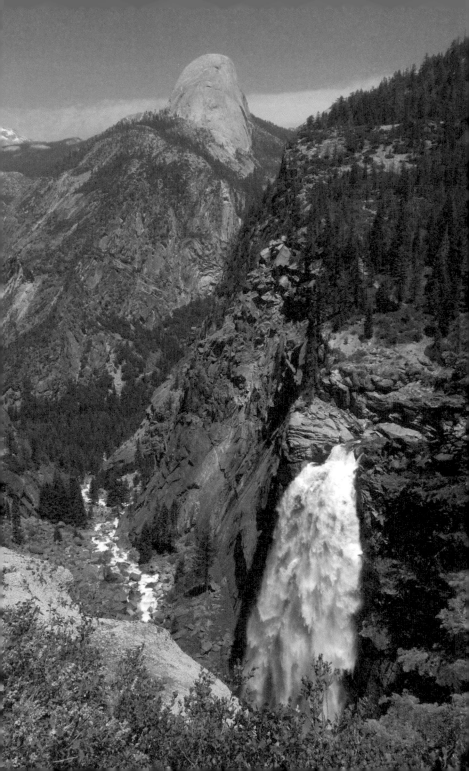

Contents

CHAPTER 1

Northeast Yosemite

Opposite: *Illilouette Fall with Half Dome behind (see Trail 41, page 355)*

CHAPTER 2

Tuolumne Meadows

CHAPTER 3

Central Yosemite

CHAPTER 4

Northwest Yosemite

Using Top Trails

Organization of Top Trails

Top Trails is designed to make identifying the perfect trail easy and enjoyable, and to make every outing a success and a pleasure. With this book you'll find it's a snap to find the right trail, whether you're planning a major hike or just a sociable stroll with friends.

The Region

Top Trails begins with the Yosemite overview map (page v), displaying the entire region covered by the guide and providing a geographic overview. The map is clearly marked to show which area is covered by which chapter.

After the overview map comes the trail features table (pages vi–ix), which is divided by area and lists every trail covered in the guide, along with attributes for each one. A quick reading of the overview map and the trail features table will give you a sense of the highlights afforded by each area within Yosemite National Park.

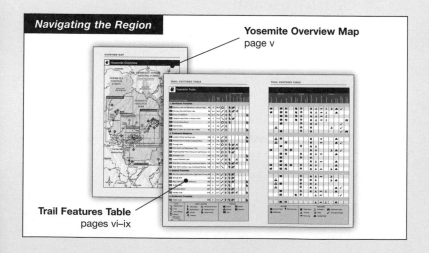

Navigating the Region

Yosemite Overview Map
page v

Trail Features Table
pages vi–ix

The Areas

For the purposes of this book, the Yosemite region is divided into seven areas, with each chapter corresponding to one area in the region.

Each area chapter starts with information to help you choose and enjoy a trail well suited to your interests. Use the table of contents or the overview map to identify the area or areas you plan to visit, and then turn to the area chapter to find the following:

- an overview of the area
- an area map with all trailheads clearly marked
- a trail features table providing trail-by-trail details
- trail summaries, written in a lively, accessible style

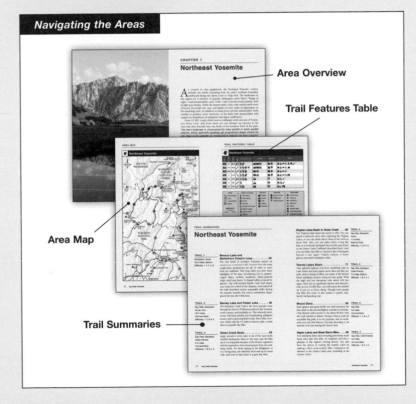

Navigating the Areas

Area Overview

Trail Features Table

Area Map

Trail Summaries

The Trails

The basic building block of the Top Trails guide is the trail entry. Each one is arranged to make finding and following the trail as simple as possible, with all pertinent information presented in an easy-to-follow format:

- a trail map
- trail descriptors covering difficulty, length, and other essential data
- a written trail description
- trail milestones, providing easy-to-follow, turn-by-turn trail directions
- an elevation profile

Some trail descriptions offer additional information:
- trail options
- trail teasers

In the margins of the trail entries, look for icons that point out notable features at specific points along the trail.

Choosing a Trail

Top Trails provides several different ways of choosing a trail, presented in easy-to-read tables and maps.

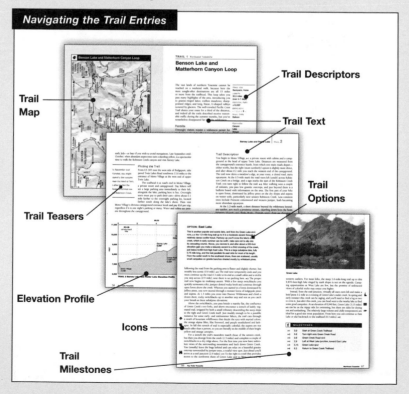

Navigating the Trail Entries

Trail Map

Trail Descriptors

Trail Text

Trail Options

Trail Teasers

Elevation Profile

Icons

Trail Milestones

Location

If you know in general where you want to go, Top Trails makes it easy to find the right trail in the right place. Each chapter begins with a large-scale map showing the starting point of every described trail in that area.

Features

This guide describes the top trails of Yosemite National Park, and each trail is chosen because it offers one or more features that make it appealing. Using the trail descriptors, summaries, and tables, you can quickly examine all the trails for the features they offer or seek a particular feature among the list of trails.

Author's note: Every trail described in this book, from the 0.4-mile round-trip to Bridalveil Fall to the 50.3-mile circuit in northern Yosemite, is worth a visit. I did not include the short walks to cater to people who, due to time or circumstance, cannot complete a longer walk. I included them because they are truly beautiful destinations that everyone should visit.

Season and Condition

Time of year and current conditions can be important factors in selecting the best trail. For example, an exposed, low-elevation trail may be a riot of color in early spring but an oven-baked taste of hell in midsummer. Wherever relevant, Top Trails identifies the best times of the day and year for the trails you plan to hike.

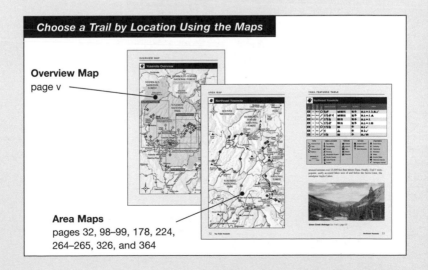

Choose a Trail by Location Using the Maps

Overview Map
page v

Area Maps
pages 32, 98–99, 178, 224, 264–265, 326, and 364

Difficulty

Each trail has an overall difficulty rating on a scale of one to five, largely based on total length and total elevation change. Also taken into consideration is elevation, because above 8,000 feet, you are likely to hike more slowly with ever-increasing elevation. Generally, the longer the trail, the more elevation gain and loss. However, some relatively short trails have a lot of elevation change, such as Trail 30 to the top of Upper Yosemite Fall. In contrast, Trail 5 through Twenty Lakes basin is slightly longer but has only about one-third of the elevation gain and loss. Some hikes have more than one destination. In this case, the difficulty rating indicates the difficulty for the full hike as described. If shortened versions or side trip options are described in the text, their ratings are given verbally as part of their description. And of course, some hikes just seem to straddle two difficulty ratings, so both are identified.

The ratings assume you are an able-bodied adult in reasonably good shape, using the trail for hiking. The ratings also assume normal weather conditions—clear and dry.

Readers should make an honest assessment of their own abilities and adjust time estimates accordingly. Also, rain, snow, heat, wind, and poor visibility can all affect the pace on even the easiest of trails.

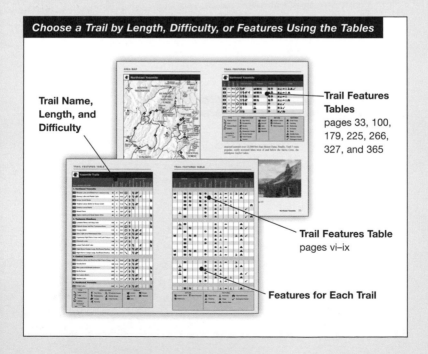

Choose a Trail by Length, Difficulty, or Features Using the Tables

Trail Name, Length, and Difficulty

Trail Features Tables
pages 33, 100, 179, 225, 266, 327, and 365

Trail Features Table
pages vi–ix

Features for Each Trail

Top Trails Difficulty Ratings

1. A route usually less than 2 miles, generally level, that can be completed in 1 hour or less. In this book, these are day hikes only.
2. A route of about 2–8 miles, usually with 500–1,500 feet of total elevation gain, that can be completed in 1–6 hours. Many of these are in day-use-only areas, but some make fine family backpacking trips.
3. A route of about 6–12 miles, usually with 1,000–2,500 feet of total elevation gain, that can be completed in 4–10 hours, spread over one to two days.
4. A route of about 12–20 miles, often with more than 2,500 feet of total elevation gain, that most will want to do as a two- to three-day backpack, but some people will choose to complete these hikes in a day.
5. A route longer than 20 miles, with more than 4,500 feet of total elevation gain, that most will want to backpack over two or more days.

Vertical Feet

Every trail description contains the approximate trail length and amount of elevation changes over the course of the trail. It's important to use all the figures when considering a hike: on average, plan 1 hour for every 2 miles, and add an hour for every 1,000 feet you climb. Formulas vary for extra time requirements for downhill walking. Most people hike a similar speed on flats and downhills excepting particularly steep, rocky downhills or stairs. Elevation change is often underestimated by hikers when looking at a topographic map because they notice the major ascents and tend to ignore the minor ups and downs, which can add up. For example, Trail 25 from O'Shaughnessy Dam east along Hetch Hetchy Reservoir to Rancheria Falls Camp has a net gain of about 700 feet, but because it roller coasters eastward to that camp, you do an extra 1,200 feet of ascending (and descending) in each direction. No wonder a traversing trail that looks like a stroll on a map seems so hard in reality!

The calculation of vertical feet in this Top Trails guide is accomplished by measuring all ups and downs along each route as mapped by the author. For routes that begin and end at the same spot—that is, loops or out-and-backs—the vertical gain exactly matches the vertical descent. With a point-to-point route, the vertical gain and loss will most likely differ because the start and endpoints most likely will be at different elevations.

Note that for *simple* out-and-back trails, both the one-way elevation gain and loss, that is, hiking in, and the round-trip elevation gain and loss are given. An example of this is Trail 2, Barney Lake and Peeler Lake, with the following numbers: one-way: +2,850', −385'/round-trip: ±3,235'. Hiking up to Peeler Lake, you will climb 2,850 feet and descend 385 feet. Returning to the trailhead, you will descend 2,850 feet and climb 385 feet. Together this leads to a total ascent of 3,235 feet and a total descent of 3,235 feet.

For branching out-and-back trails, the elevation gain and loss are to the farthest destination, including the side trips that are included in the mileages. An example of this is Trail 8, Lembert Dome and Dog Lake, with the following numbers: one-way: +890', −420'/round-trip: ±1,010'. If you visit Lembert Dome en route to Dog Lake, you will first climb a saddle, then climb Lembert Dome, then return to the main trail at the saddle, and finally drop and climb to Dog Lake. The elevation changes for all of this are +890 feet and −420 feet. But when you return, you do so directly, skipping Lembert Dome, and the elevation changes are less, +120 feet and −590 feet. Adding these numbers together gives you the round-trip value, a total gain of 1,010 feet and loss of 1,010 feet.

For loop trails, both the gains and losses continue to accumulate until you arrive back, and only round-trip elevation gain and loss are given. Because you start and end at the same point, the elevation ascent and descent will of course be the same. An example of this is Trail 5, the Twenty Lakes Basin, with the following numbers: round-trip: ±950'.

Likewise, for point-to-point trails, both the gains and losses continue to accumulate until you reach your endpoint, but because it is likely to be a different elevation than your starting point, the vertical gain and loss most likely will differ. An example of this is Trail 4, Virginia Lakes Basin to Green Creek, with the following numbers: one-way: +1,520', −3,370'. What these numbers tell you is that, on this hike, you ascend only about half as much as you descend.

Finally, the trail entries have an elevation profile, an easy means for visualizing the topography of the route. These profiles graphically depict the elevation throughout the length of the trail.

Map Legend

Featured trail		Water body
Alternate trail		River/creek
Pacific Crest Trail		Intermittent stream
John Muir Trail		Glacier/snowfield
Use trail		Forest/park boundary
Major road — (120) (395)		Wilderness boundary
Minor road		
Unpaved 2WD road		
Unpaved 4WD road		

⚠ Backcountry campsite	🅿 Parking	🛒 Store
🚲 Bike path	Parking lot	▲ Summit
≻ Bridge	)(Pass	👫 Toilet
⌂ Cabin	⋕ Picnic area	🚶 Trailhead
▲ Campground	● Point of interest	Tunnel (pedestrian)
→ Direction of travel	Ranger station	Tunnel (road)
•— Gate	Sequoia	⚡ Vista
— Log	🚌 Shuttle stop	Water faucet
Marsh	○ Spring	// Waterfall/cascade
⚒ Mine site	Stables	● Waypoint in book

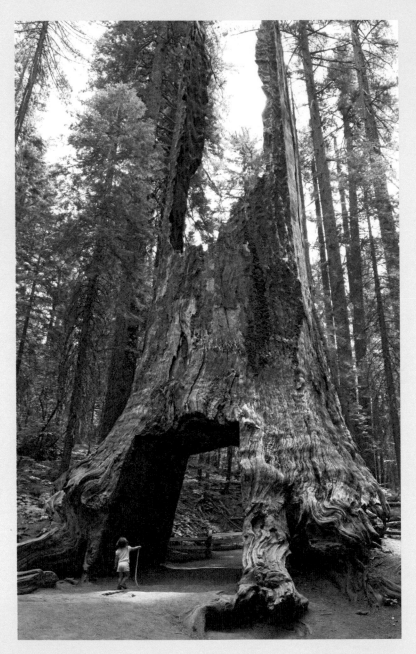

The giant Tunnel Tree (*see Trail 26, page 250*)

Introduction to Yosemite National Park

Though Yellowstone, in 1872, was the first federal land to be set aside as a national park, Yosemite, in 1864, was the first federal land to be set aside as *any* kind of park. In that year, President Abraham Lincoln signed a bill, the Yosemite Grant, that deeded Yosemite Valley and the Mariposa Grove of Big Trees to the State of California as an area to be protected for preservation and public use. Though the valley had been discovered only 13 years earlier, its sheer walls and magnificent waterfalls were rapidly attracting national fame, thanks to articles, paintings, photographs, and personal testimonials. Protecting it for future generations was a necessity.

Today, visitors from around the world still come to Yosemite National Park to experience Yosemite Valley firsthand. Who can forget his or her first visit to the valley, with its enormous granite cliffs; its leaping, dashing waterfalls; and its domes? The valley's prominent features, if not etched on the mind, are recorded by camera: the monolith of El Capitan; Bridalveil Fall backdropped by the Cathedral Rocks; the Lower and Upper Yosemite Falls and adjacent Lost Arrow Spire; and the deep, gaping Tenaya Canyon bounded on the north by Basket Dome and Mount Watkins and on the south and east by Half Dome and Clouds Rest. Finally, there is the curved Glacier Point Apron sweeping up to a vertical cliff topped by Glacier Point. These unforgettable views of Yosemite Valley rank as one of the greatest natural wonders of North America, if not the world. But they are only a small portion of the marvels that Yosemite National Park has to offer. An afternoon's jaunt away from the roadside scenery lets you absorb grand vistas, alpine lakes, endless granite slabs, and majestic trees away from distractions. Contemplate how perfectly John Muir understood why you would want to take a hike in Yosemite when he said, "It is easier to feel than to realize, or in any way explain, Yosemite grandeur."

Geography and Topography

Yosemite National Park covers an area of 1,169 square miles, all of it within two river drainages, the Tuolumne and the Merced. Despite this large area, comparable to that of the San Francisco Bay Area, most visitors converge on the few square miles of Yosemite Valley's floor and the square mile of the Mariposa Grove, never straying more than a few minutes' walk from their cars. Remarkably, few people embark on a 3-hour walk and less than 1.5% of the park's visitors backpack into the wilderness lands, which comprise nearly 95% of the park's area.

The Sierra Nevada has been called the gentle wilderness, but you may beg to differ with this definition if you're embarking on one of the trails that travels between the Yosemite Valley floor and its rim, such as the trail to the top of Upper Yosemite Fall. Indeed, few people beginning their walks at the depths of the main river canyons, the Merced and the Tuolumne, and aiming to hike to the tops of their watersheds will experience a gentle walk. However, those beginning a walk on the elevated slopes above—or better yet in the wide expansiveness of Tuolumne Meadows—will see a more rolling landscape of never-ending granite slabs, punctuated by steep granite ridges and summits.

Nestled at the base of the steeper escarpments and throughout the midelevation forests are most of Yosemite's more than 500 lakes (defined as being at least an acre in area). This means that many lakes in the Tuolumne Meadows region can be reached with less than 1,000 feet of elevation gain. Such is the advantage of the high trailheads scattered throughout the park both along Tioga and Glacier Point Roads. Of the lakes described in this Top Trails guide, there are only five hikes with lakes that require above 3,000 feet of elevation gain (one-way): Benson Lake (Trail 1), Peeler Lake (Trail 2), Lake Vernon (Trail 24), Merced Lake (Trail 35), and Lower Ottoway Lake (Trail 44). Most of Yosemite's more difficult-to-reach hikes lie in the northern third of the park, that is, north of the Tuolumne River's Hetch Hetchy Reservoir and the Grand Canyon of the Tuolumne River. The remainder lie in the Merced River drainage above Merced Lake. For these relatively remote lakes, you'd want to spend four or more days in the wilderness, and only a few lengthy hikes are included in this book. For longer hiking trips and for a description of virtually all of the park's approximately 800 miles of trails, consult *Yosemite National Park: A Complete Hiker's Guide*, with a new edition due out in 2020.

The Top Trails guide you are holding does include several stiff climbs of 3,000-plus feet of elevation gain to popular, prominent summits or viewpoints: Mount Dana (Trail 6), Upper Yosemite Fall (Trail 30), and Half Dome (Trail 34). Additionally, some trails, especially the longer ones, ramble up and down, and the elevation gain and loss can accumulate to impressive numbers.

Geology

Yosemite National Park is most famous for its renowned Yosemite Valley, arguably the world's most spectacular, which owes its origin to glacial erosion along major, nearly vertical fracture planes in its granitic rock. These have given rise to impressive cliffs such as the faces of Half Dome and Sentinel Rock. Meanwhile, the Yosemite high country is beloved for its endless glacially polished granite slabs and sharply pointed, mostly granitic peaks. A collection of geologic processes spanning more than 100 million years was required to create these landscapes.

The oldest rocks in the park's vicinity are about 540 million years old and originated as sandy sediments deposited on the ocean's floor off North America's west coast. These sedimentary rocks were later metamorphosed to schists and quartzites, which today straddle the park's lightly visited northern-boundary lands. Other significant remnants of metamorphic rocks stretch from the Saddlebag Lake environs south to Tioga Pass and into the northern Ritter Range. Those in the main Ritter Range are much younger metamorphosed volcanic rocks. These various metamorphic rocks add earth tones to our area's crest lands. Additionally, the mineral-rich soil they produce results in more plant species and greater numbers of plants than grow in adjacent granitic soil.

But like most of the Sierra Nevada, nearly all of Yosemite's lands are granitic—grayish rocks that once solidified from a melt (magma) several miles beneath the surface, but today are exposed, creating what John Muir called the Range of Light. In the Sierra Nevada there were two main periods of pluton formation, which occurred when the precursor to the Pacific Plate began to collide with the North American Plate and slid (subducted) beneath it. The subducting material was subjected to high temperatures and pressures, causing it and parts of the overlying crust from the North American Plate to melt. The hot, and therefore lower density, magma then moved upward, forcefully displacing the preexisting metamorphic rocks and subsequently cooling to form granitic rocks.

The first main period of subduction, which occurred between 165 and 148 million years ago, formed mostly darker-colored granitoid rocks that exist farther south in the Sierra but are absent from the Yosemite region. This was followed by a second window of activity between 105 and 85 million years ago, during which the lighter-colored granites and granodiorites prevalent throughout Yosemite formed. By 80 million years ago, the granites had all formed, but they were still deep underground—indeed, the high country of Yosemite and the rest of the High Sierra would not be very luminous if the ancient rocks intruded into by molten "granite" had not eroded away.

At the end of the periods of pluton formation, the granitic rocks were at a depth of 2–5 miles, covered by both the sedimentary and metamorphic rocks that formed at the edge of the North American Plate and the thick layers of volcanic rocks that had been erupting overhead. The volcanoes formed an imposing mountain range, probably as tall as—or taller than— today's Sierra, called the Ancestral Sierra Nevada. It is suspected that regional extension around the end of pluton formation fractured the range's bedrock, and the unique patterns of the local fractures gave rise to the modern range's drainages and topography. Remarkably, this meant that in the Ancestral Sierra, the major east–west-oriented river valleys already existed in approximately the same locations where they are today.

The following 50 million years, and maybe even longer, were a period where erosion dominated. Subduction halted, ending both the formation of new granite and volcanic activity. Slowly, the Ancestral Sierra was eroded away, though it is likely to still have been an imposing range. The eroded sediments were deposited in California's Central Valley, west of the park, creating sequences that tell us—in reverse—what types of rocks were being eroded, how much, and how fast. The sediments here are 2–5 miles deep. By the start of the Cenozoic era, 65 million years ago, the main difference from today was that the river canyons were shallower, perhaps half their present depths. Yosemite Valley was already a deep canyon, and the features above the canyon rims also resembled their modern equivalents and have been little reshaped.

Dating when the Central Valley sediments were deposited also tells us that accumulation rates increased around 10 million years ago, coincident with the onset of a period of rapid uplift. Data on fault movements to the east of the Sierra corroborate this interpretation. Only in the last two decades has the trigger for this uplift been proposed: delamination. This technical term describes the process whereby the bottom of the earth's crust, deep underground, is removed (by a still-uncertain mechanism). This makes the remaining crust lighter and it pops up. Think about a float in water with lead weights strapped to the bottom; when the straps are cut and the weights drop off, the float rises. Recent evidence suggests that the Sierra Nevada, from south of the Mount Whitney region to Yosemite and north toward Tahoe, is continuing to display 1–2 millimeters of uplift per year, so the mountains are still continuing to grow higher.

These tectonic events had easily observed impacts on Yosemite's landscape. The uplift and accompanying increase in erosion rates caused the overlying volcanic and sedimentary rocks to be mostly stripped away, exposing the granite. In the lower river canyons, most notably Yosemite Valley, the erosive force of water scoured the valley floor ever deeper. While the water would have deepened the canyon, the landscape-wide joints and fracture planes would simultaneously have caused whole slabs of rock to plummet downward, widening the valley and maintaining the vertical walls.

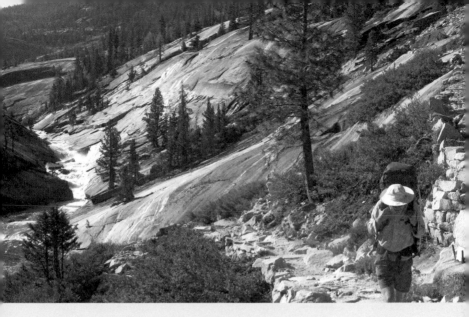

Climbing along *the Merced River (see Trail 35, page 315)*

More-recent events have fine-tuned the landscape. Repeated glaciations, beginning about 2 million years ago, carried away preexisting talus piles from the valley bottoms and fractured rock from the sides of peaks, leaving a smoother, polished landscape. Glaciations that occurred before 200,000 years ago collectively are called pre-Tahoe because they preceded the well-known Tahoe glaciation. On the east side of the range, the Sherwin glaciation, which lasted from about 900,000 to 800,000 years ago, produced the oldest known glaciers. At Yosemite's latitude, Sherwin sediments are preserved east of the Sierra Crest due in large part to burial in the mammoth Long Valley eruption of about 760,000 years ago. In contrast, on the west side there is little evidence of Sherwin glaciers. We do know that an early glaciation reached El Portal and that the glacier in the Tuolumne River drainage was much larger than the one in the Merced drainage.

In each glacial episode, cold climates would create repeated freeze-and-thaw cycles of ice, which pried rock from steep walls to collect below as talus and be carried downcanyon by the flowing ice mass. As the walls gradually retreated through rockfall, the heads of canyons became broader. The canyon heads are called cirques; the small glaciers that occupied them are called cirque glaciers. As glaciers advanced downcanyon, they excavated decomposed bedrock, leaving basins that would become lakes, which over time would accumulate sediments (on average about a foot per 1,000 years). The upper lands may have been glaciated dozens of times, and each time the glaciers would have scoured sediment across much of the landscape. Glacial landscapes are most apparent near the Sierra Crest, not down in Yosemite Valley, because mass wasting, particularly earthquake-induced rockfall, in the 15,000 years since the last glacial maxima has erased most glacial evidence. We know, however, that Yosemite Valley was filled to its brim during past glaciations, while the domes surrounding it emerged from the ice. As the glaciers melted, they left behind piles of rock, moraines. The terminal moraine of the most recent glaciation, the Tioga glaciation, is readily visible on the valley floor about halfway between Bridalveil Fall and El Capitan Meadow; it is an elongate pile of jumbled rock, rising above the otherwise flat valley floor.

Small glaciers are still present along much of the Sierra Crest, though with warming temperatures, all those in Yosemite save the Maclure Glacier have now transitioned to ice patches, a designation that indicates the ice is no longer moving. Landforms continue to evolve through other processes as well. Riverine flood events have deposited rounded boulders high beyond the normal riverbanks. Avalanches and debris flows have carved gullies down the steep mountainsides, depositing material in the valleys below. Rockfalls build up piles of talus at the bases of cliffs, sometimes in dramatic events. The pervasive joints that have led to Yosemite Valley's near-vertical walls mean that large rockfalls will continue to occur—and make the nightly news, given their impact on people sightseeing, hiking, rock climbing, or otherwise exploring the base of Yosemite Valley's walls.

Flora

Plants are the most conspicuous living organisms in Yosemite, with conifer forests draping a green blanket across large swaths of the park. This handful of tree species may be visually dominant, but there are about 1,200 species of native plants. Trying to categorize such a plethora of plants is a difficult—and incomplete—task, but ecologists begin by dividing the landscape into vegetation zones, defined by the tree or shrub community that is most common. Climatic influences of greatest importance in delineating vegetation zones are temperature and precipitation. Within Yosemite, broad-scale variations in temperature and precipitation are largely driven by changes in elevation. Temperature decreases with increasing elevation, and precipitation increases up to midelevations, beyond which it decreases slowly on the approach to the crest, then rapidly to the east of the Sierra Crest. The vegetation zones in—and around—Yosemite are as follows:

- **The foothill woodland and scrubland zone** occurs mostly below 4,000 feet.
- **The lower montane or mixed conifer forest zone** occurs between 2,000 and 7,400 feet, with the prevalence of white firs, a key

indicator species, peaking around 6,500 feet. Sugar pines, incense cedars, and ponderosa pines are also part of the mix.

- **The upper montane forest zone** is dominated by red firs and most widespread between 7,500 and 8,500 feet but continues to about 9,300 feet in moist locations, with occasional red fir stands existing above 10,000 feet. Western white pine, lodgepole pine, and, in dry locations, Jeffrey pine are also found in this zone.

- **The subalpine forest zone** has some patches occurring as low as 8,200 feet and extending up to the treeline; several different species can be dominant at these elevations, most commonly lodgepole pines, mountain hemlocks, and whitebark pines.

- **The alpine meadow and shrubland zone** occurs above treeline, which can be as low as 9,000 feet, but more commonly above 10,500 feet, and is defined as a region where full-size trees cannot establish. Whitebark pines are the stunted trees that grow right up to the alpine boundary.

- **The eastside forest and woodland zone** is found in the eastern Sierra, mostly between 5,200 feet and 7,200 feet.

Beyond elevation, water availability due to differences in topography plays the greatest role in the distribution of species. Because much of a winter's snow remains through late spring—and some remains throughout summer—most of Yosemite's vegetation has an adequate water supply during its peak flowering period; otherwise the flowers wouldn't be so spectacular! What changes is in which month the flowers are showiest, for snowmelt may be six weeks earlier or later at a location due to the winter's snowpack. Consider also just how much water supply varies with topographic position and how it affects the vegetation. Subalpine meadows exist in locations where conifers can't survive due to seasonally water-saturated soils. Elsewhere, especially in the vast granite slab country of northern Yosemite, shallow depressions in the granite create seasonal wetlands that erupt with colorful annuals following snowmelt but are soon parched due to their shallow soils. In contrast, on alpine rocky slopes, low-growing perennial species depend on snow cover for both insulation from extreme temperatures and desiccating winds and for moisture. In higher snowfall years when their soils retain moisture into midsummer, the flowers bloom robustly, while in drought years there are few flowers, the soils having dried before the temperatures were warm enough for flowering to begin. In contrast, streamside species often continue to flower colorfully for many months, irrigated from below, and can be showiest in years with early snowmelt when they experience a longer growing season. As an interesting side note, there were a lot of thick soils before glaciers removed them, and this altered the distribution of at least one notable species, the giant sequoia, which before glaciation was associated with red firs.

Fire is a second variable that creates a mosaic of habitats throughout the park. Historically, ground fires were common throughout Yosemite's montane forests and very important. In the process of clearing the ground and understory of thick brush, they significantly altered the populations of ground-dwelling plants and animals and everything associated with them. These fires would rarely have killed most of the canopy trees, allowing the landscape to rapidly recover from the fire. Then, from the late 1800s until 1971, fire suppression was a general Yosemite policy, and it led to the accumulation of thick litter, dense brush, and overmature trees— all prime fuel for a hot, destructive

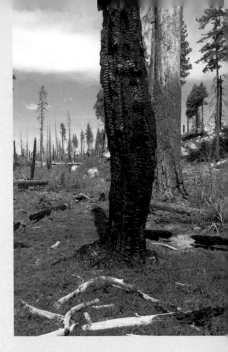

Burnt tree trunks *and orange moss are evidence of past wildfires along the trail to Kibbie Lake (see Trail 23, page 228).*

blaze when a fire inevitably sparked to life. Foresters now know that natural fires should not be prevented but only regulated. In recent decades, a combination of controlled burns (mostly alongside road corridors) and large wildfires (started by a combination of lightning strikes, careless campers, and arson) have cleared large swaths of forest of this brush. Unfortunately, years of fuel accumulation mean the large wildland fires also decimate the entire forest, often killing the vast majority of trees, a very different process to what ecologists project occurred previously.

Walking through the lower to midelevation reaches of Yosemite, you are immediately struck by just how much of the park has been scoured by fire in the past 25 years. North of Tioga Road, almost all the landscape below 7,500 feet has been burned—often multiple times—and the stands of rejuvenating conifers are mostly quite young. While the southwest of the park, from the south rim of Yosemite Valley to Wawona, mostly has intact, mature forest, areas farther east, including Little Yosemite Valley, Sunrise Creek, and Illilouette Creek, have also been charred. Some of the notable fires are the 2017 South Fork Fire (South Fork Merced east of Wawona), the 2017 Empire Fire (Empire Meadow to Mono Meadow), the 2014 Meadow Fire (Little Yosemite Valley and Sunrise Creek), the 2013 Rim Fire (much of the northwest area between Cherry Lake, Hetch Hetchy, and White Wolf), the 2003 Kibbie

Complex (north from Cherry Lake along Kibbie Ridge), the 1996 Ackerson Fire (similar to Rim Fire in extent), the 1991 Illilouette Fire (Illilouette basin), and the 1990 A Rock Fire (far western Yosemite, south of Crane Flat to Foresta), though many other smaller ones burned vegetated gaps left untouched by these big fires. Many of these fires have occurred following drought periods, and concern for additional behemoths is particularly high right now (2018) because a combination of the 2012–2016 drought and a bark beetle infestation has left the park's lands strewn with dead trees waiting to become bonfires. Sadly, the intensity and frequency with which fires are striking has led to predictions that much of the lower-elevation landscapes of Yosemite will remain scrubland for at least a century to come. The land has been too decimated for a forest to return anytime soon; in particular the soils have lost their organic matter and the landscape has, in places, lost every mature seed-providing tree, preventing rapid reestablishment.

Regarding the mosaic left by the fires, I strongly recommend visiting charred landscapes in spring and early summer, for vibrant blooms in the open areas partially compensate for the lack of shade. By midsummer the landscape simply feels dry and hot. Second, take a walk in an unburned dense fir forest, such as those you'll encounter walking to Dewey Point (Trail 36), before the clock marking ecological succession is reset in these lichen-draped forests. Third, if you walk a trail with regenerating trees that are starting to form cones (such as toward Ostrander Lake, Trail 42), smile at the dense thicket of young trees and be glad that the natural successional process is still working in some places. (In August 2017 the Empire Fire burned areas along parts of the Ostrander Lake Trail. Because this area has burned multiple times in the past decade, the fire is being described as a *good* one, leaving some stands intact and burning at low intensity.)

If you are interested in natural history, consult the list of books in Appendix C. In particular, my book *Wildflowers of the High Sierra and John Muir Trail* covers the flora you will see above 8,000 feet.

Fauna

Yosemite National Park has a diverse range of animal species whose presence throughout the park will most certainly enhance your visit. Fingers crossed, we are past the point where the commotion of bears in campgrounds is your most memorable Yosemite wildlife experience, and you will instead be treated to encounters with a collection of commonly seen—and maybe even not-so-commonly seen—animals as you embark on your hikes.

Of the park's vertebrate animals (that is, ignoring insects, spiders, and so on), birds are the most common, with about 250 species, of which 150 are relatively common. Which species garner your attention is quite dependent on elevation, with the black-crested blue Steller's jay among the most common from Yosemite Valley to around 7,000 feet in elevation. These birds are hopeless beggars and thieves—keep your food closely guarded as you picnic at the top of Vernal Fall. In the lodgepole pine forest encircling Tuolumne Meadows, it is the small gray, black, and white dark-eyed junco, a type of sparrow, that is near-ubiquitous. American robins, hopping along the ground in search of worms, are also a common sight in any forested or meadow landscape. At the highest elevations, ravens, Clark's nutcrackers, and maybe even a golden eagle vie for your attention. As your ears try and filter through the background chirps, a few calls may pique your interest. Most startling to the uninitiated are the bellowing "whomps" of the male blue (or dusky) grouse in search of mates. Common in late spring and early summer throughout conifer forests, I have on many an occasion jumped as one erupted from a tree quite close to me. The pecking of woodpeckers and sapsuckers always causes me to turn my head, as does the shriek of the goshawk and the shrill call of the belted kingfisher. The former is the only forest-dwelling hawk in Yosemite, and I encounter one most years while tromping through dense forest: a distinct hawk call often followed by the sight of a large bird deftly swerving among the trees as it flies to a new perch. Belted kingfishers inhabit open streamside locations—I have most frequently seen them in Lyell Canyon, diving from an unseen perch to snatch their prey from the water. Pick up a field guide, such as *Sibley Birds West* or *The Laws Field Guide to the Sierra Nevada,* and a pair of binoculars if you want to identify additional species.

Around 80 species of mammals inhabit Yosemite. As most of these mammals do a good job of staying hidden, you will likely see only the small number of species that are both diurnal, active during the daylight hours, and not terribly shy. Most common are the rodents, a group of species that includes mice and squirrels. One of the most frequently seen rodents is the yellow-bellied marmot, resembling an overgrown groundhog. It is most often seen at higher elevations, sunning itself atop a warm, flat boulder, although it also lives below treeline. The only common tree squirrel at high elevations is the chickaree (or Douglas squirrel), a small, dark-colored, and very loud squirrel that is quite skittish. Meanwhile, the western gray squirrel makes its home in Yosemite Valley and is most often seen in campgrounds or on the trail to the Vernal Fall bridge (Trail 32). Three common species of ground squirrels make their homes in Yosemite. Golden-mantled ground squirrels, which are found from 6,000 feet to above timberline, have a red-brown head and black-and-white stripes down their backs; they resemble overgrown chipmunks but lack the chipmunk's diagnostic face stripes. California (or Beechey) ground squirrels, regularly occurring up to 8,000 feet and on occasion up to above 10,000 feet, are grayish-brown, with a light gray patch on the backs of their necks and a long, furry tail. These are the cheeky squirrels very common from the Yosemite Valley floor up to the rim. Third are Belding's ground squirrels, which occupy dry flats and meadows from 6,000 to 11,500 feet, standing like sentries at their burrow entrances. They are a lighter, brown-beige color and have a short, nearly furless tail. Several species of chipmunks occur here, including the lodgepole chipmunk, which is widespread above 6,000 feet, and the largish shadow chipmunk. The chipmunks are quite difficult to visually distinguish among, especially because they are tiny and rarely stand still. All chipmunks have stripes on their faces and down their backs. Less commonly seen rodents include porcupines, beavers, montane voles (which leave the long soil runways across grassy meadows), and several types of mice.

There are also two species in the rabbit family that you might encounter. The white-tailed jackrabbit is large and inhabits subalpine and alpine environments—a species you might meet somewhere like Gaylor Lakes (Trail 7). This species molts from a pale brown in summer to white in winter to match the surroundings. Second are pikas, little round critters with Mickey Mouse ears that live in high-elevation talus piles or rock glaciers and emit an easy-to-identify "cheep-cheep" when disturbed. These are generally shy little critters, but you may see one along the trail from Virginia Lakes Basin to Green Creek (Trail 4) or on Mount Dana (Trail 6). They are also industrious, for, unlike most of the rodents, they do not hibernate. To feed themselves in winter, they spend summer harvesting and drying plants and stash their hay piles under rocks for the winter.

As for hoofed mammals, the mule deer is common throughout Yosemite, except on the highest peaks. So-called timberline bucks even venture well above treeline, while the does usually remain under forest cover. By midsummer many of the does have one or two delicately spotted fawns. While nearly every hiker will catch a glimpse of a mule deer, especially if you spend a few minutes in Yosemite Valley's meadows, only a few lucky hikers will get to see the Sierra Nevada bighorn sheep. These sheep require visually open, steep, rocky habitat that provides protection from predators. Amazingly, plants growing in this extreme environment provide sufficient nutrition. In Yosemite there are herds on the peaks around Mono Pass, at the head of Lundy Canyon (in the vicinity of Twenty Lakes Basin, Trail 5), and as of 2015, along the Lyell Fork of the Merced (the slopes around Mount Florence, east of Merced Lake). While few hikers are fortunate enough to see these sheep, it is wonderful to know their populations have been increasing in recent decades and they are inhabiting more of Yosemite than they have in at least 70 years.

The final group of mammals in the Sierra is the carnivores. Most discussed in Yosemite is the American black bear, which, despite its name, comes in a great variety of colors. They range throughout the Yosemite, even at quite high elevations. Luckily, you need only be concerned about your food, as this species is not aggressive toward humans. However, if you come across a mother with cubs, walk away from the bears. You may also be treated to seeing a coyote, for they are active at dawn, dusk, and occasionally even midday and range from sea level into the alpine—they are remarkably common in Yosemite Valley. Their loud choruses can be both eerie and engaging.

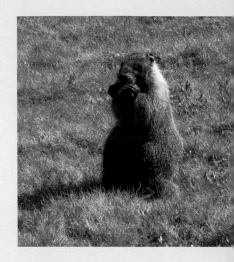

A marmot *near Tuolumne Pass (see Trail 12, page 131)*

Many other rarely seen carnivores inhabit Yosemite, including mountain lions, bobcats, short-tailed weasels, raccoons, and skunks. I have seen bobcats, raccoons, and mountain lions in Yosemite Valley, but never far from inhabited areas. I am sure the bobcats and lions have shared the forest with me on many other occasions, but the valley dwellers are probably more used to people and hence less skittish. Take note that whereas bears see you as bearers of food, mountain lions see you *as* food. Therefore, at elevations below 7,000 feet, in the evening it is best not to hike alone, and if you bring children, keep them close by, for their height is more similar to that of a deer. Should you be threatened, you may have to fight back. Running away invites attack because that is what prey does. All this said, no one has been attacked by a lion in Yosemite.

If you are lucky, you may spot a long-tailed weasel, a very skinny creature common across a wide range of elevations and habitats—I've mostly seen them in between 8,000 feet and treeline. Fishers, martens, and red foxes live in the park too but are very rarely seen—in hundreds of days hiking in the park, I have seen a single marten, on the trail from Ireland Lake to Lyell Canyon, and by amazing coincidence watched it chase a chickaree up and down a lodgepole tree, eventually watching it catch itself a meal.

Reptiles are represented by about two dozen species of lizards and snakes. Most notable are the western rattlesnakes because they are venomous. Rattlesnakes present a possible danger below 7,000 feet and are reasonably common in the Grand Canyon of the Tuolumne River area and along the Merced River Canyon but seemingly rare along trails elsewhere in Yosemite. The best advice here is that if you are in open, rocky canyon terrain, always look on the ground on the far side of a log before you cross it. The slopes rising above Yosemite Valley are prime habitat for them, but I suspect the density of people on the main trails encourages them to inhabit slightly quieter corridors. The most common snake at high elevations is the western terrestrial garter snake, which can occur in wet areas up to 12,000 feet. Long and skinny, with a bright yellow line running down the center of their black backs, they are most commonly seen in marshy grasslands, moving rapidly through the grasses or swimming elegantly in shallow water. Racers, with two stripes down their sides and which climb not only bushes but also steep cracks, are also regularly seen up to about 6,000 feet, while at higher elevations all the skinny, striped snakes are garter snakes. At the lower elevations, you will commonly see western fence lizards, with their blue bellies, sunning themselves on rocks. Also present are the larger northern alligator lizards, but they tend to hide under plants or rocks and are less commonly seen.

Worldwide, amphibian species are not faring well, and that is also true for Yosemite's species. A number of salamander species inhabit Yosemite, especially at lower elevations. Among these, it is the bright orange California newt you are most likely to see, for between November and May they are often out on wet days—I have seen them along the trails around Hetch Hetchy on many occasions in fall. Mount Lyell salamanders inhabit seeps up to at least 12,000 feet but are very rarely seen. Two species of frogs and a species of toad also live in Yosemite: the Pacific tree frog, the Yosemite toad, and the mountain yellow-legged frog. Of these, the Pacific tree frog is the most common. This species is just larger than your thumb and sports a characteristic black eye stripe. Its tadpoles are commonly seen in warm, shallow, temporary bodies of water, sometimes in large numbers. The quite rare Yosemite toad is wart covered and usually 2–3 inches in length. In the last decades, the mountain yellow-legged frog has garnered the greatest attention of Sierra Nevada amphibians. This large frog, with a mottled brown coloration pattern and light undersides, breeds mostly in high-elevation habitats. A combination of disease and nonnative trout in high-elevation lakes has now made them very rare, but dedicated conservation efforts are trying to ensure their numbers rebound in the Yosemite area. And please note that amphibians absorb chemicals through their skins, so if you see amphibians in a body of water, be extra careful not to contaminate it with sunscreen, insect repellent, or soap, and do not pick up the frogs.

Fish are native only to the lower elevations of Yosemite—the landscape below the first major waterfalls, for, quite understandably, the likes of Yosemite Falls, Vernal Fall, Chilnualna Falls near Wawona, and Wapama Falls at Hetch Hetchy create a natural barrier to upstream movement. The lower-elevation western Sierra, including Yosemite Valley, is the natural habitat of the rainbow trout. Why, then, will you see fish in just about every lake and stream in Yosemite? Fish stocking began in the 1870s to create a food source in the otherwise "barren" Sierra Nevada lakes and rapidly expanded the distribution of native and nonnative species alike. As a result, five species of trout are now common throughout Yosemite's waters: rainbow trout (native to lower-elevation western Sierra Nevada rivers), golden trout (native to the southern Sierra Nevada, including the Kern Plateau), Lahontan cutthroat trout (native to some eastern Sierra Nevada drainages and the Rocky Mountains), brown trout (native to Europe), and brook trout (native to the eastern United States). Though nonnative, these fish are tasty, and with a fishing rod, a fishing permit, and patience, you can supplement your daily dinners. Also note that stocking of fish ended in Yosemite three decades ago, and in light of the negative impact the nonnative fish have on native species, including the mountain yellow-legged frog, conservation efforts are now trying to restore some high-elevation lakes to their natural fish-free state.

When to Go: Weather and Seasons

If you are a typical hiker using this guidebook, you'll probably visit the park during the summer. Unlike most of America's mountain ranges, the Sierra Nevada is summer-dry, receiving only about 1.5 inches of precipitation during the summer months. The official summer period, June 22–September 21, matches well with the hiking season for most of Yosemite, though those exploring Yosemite Valley's trails will also find the second half of spring a spectacular time for a visit. For Yosemite, the last significant storm usually has just ended by the start of summer. In Yosemite Valley, in late June, the days will be in the 80s and the nights down to the 50s by the crack of dawn. Temperatures drop with elevation gain, and up at Tuolumne Meadows, which is about 4,500 feet higher than the valley, the summer temperatures are about 20°F cooler. This means that the early-summer temperatures at Tuolumne Meadows and other high-elevation areas are cool but acceptable. What limits hiker use is lingering snow. Unless the year has had far-above-average snowfall, by the start of summer all the park's major roads are open, with the spur roads to Tamarack Flat Campground, White Wolf, Yosemite Creek Campground, and the May Lake Trailhead sometimes not opening until early July. High trails, however, may be partly to mostly snowbound, so in June, unless you know it is a below-average snow year, it is best to confine your hiking to below about 8,000 feet elevation, such as along both rims of Yosemite Valley, up Little Yosemite Valley to Merced Lake, or up from Hetch Hetchy to Laurel Lake and Lake Vernon.

By the beginning of July the snow lines will have risen to at least 9,000 feet (in all but the heaviest snow years), and the afternoon temperatures are usually warm and the nights pleasant. However, July, like June, is a month of copious mosquitoes (and brilliant wildflowers), so if you backpack then, be sure to bring a tent. The dwindling snowpack also means that by mid- to late July, the volume of waterfalls is greatly diminished. Yosemite

Falls, in particular, is fed by a relatively low-elevation catchment and rapidly becomes less photogenic. Thunderstorms can occur anytime during the summer, but they become more common as monsoonal activity in the region around Arizona increases—usually sometime in July. The thunderstorms mostly occur from about midafternoon until sunset, and usually they are short-lived, drenching a local area for a few minutes before moving on. If ominous clouds are threatening you, be sure to take cover within a forest rather than staying in the open or under an isolated tree.

August is the most popular month for Yosemite hikers. The least snow is encountered and mosquito populations have dwindled to an acceptable level. Thunderstorms continue to be a possibility but are rarely more than a minor inconvenience. Also, lakes, which typically reach their maximum temperatures by late July (low to mid-70s for the lower lakes, mid- to high 60s for the higher lakes), are still nearly as warm and are fine for swimming. By the end of August or early September, the lakes definitely are cooling, and the Sierra may have had one or two weak frontal storms. After the Labor Day weekend, the park has fewer visitors. Should you backpack then, be sure to check the weather forecast for a possible storm, and certainly bring a tent if you will be out for more than one or two nights.

Autumn starts in late September, and now the days are considerably cooler. Yosemite Valley during the first half of autumn (through early November) is a favorite time for some. Whereas the nights may be crisp, the days are ideal, and the colors of turning foliage compensate for the valley's lesser waterfalls. These are also perfect months to complete the hikes starting at Hetch Hetchy Reservoir.

Backpackers at higher elevations need to be prepared for the season's first major storm, which may strike in early October or not until early November. Though most days are fair weather, I have a rule that, after October 15, I don't backpack more than a day's hike from the trailhead, making it unlikely that a storm will take me by surprise. If one does, I'll be close enough to plod through snow back to the trailhead. Tioga Road may close briefly in a minor snowstorm, but anytime after about late October that a major one hits, this road (along with U.S. Forest Service roads bordering the park) closes for the season.

November–mid-December is a time of solitude. The backcountry is virtually devoid of hikers, save for a few mountaineers. Likewise, the valley is empty, for the days are cool, the nights are nippy, and the ski season has not begun.

Winter starts in late December. This is the month with the least amount of daylight and the lowest noontime sun. Consequently, much of the valley's floor stays in the shadows, though much of the north wall may be sunlit. With little sunlight on the floor, its temperatures are downright cold. In some years, much of the valley's precipitation falls as snow and in other years rain dominates, but December and January tend to be mostly dreary months punctuated by days with blue skies. Snow can cover the valley's floor from about mid-December to mid-February, after which the cover will be at best patchy. Winter is ski season, and most folks driving up to the park head to Badger Pass for downhill skiing or cross-country skiing. Buses still bring in hordes of tourists to the valley, for indeed in the deep of winter, especially after a storm, the valley is a winter wonderland. Though the four months November–February produce the most precipitation, about 75% of it, most days are storm free, and when a storm does hit, it usually clears out in a day or two.

By March, the voracity of snowstorms tapers, though snow continues to accumulate at higher elevations through April. In March and April, temperatures usually get above freezing during part of the day but then drop below freezing during the night. Spring begins in late March, and March and April can have quite variable weather, pleasant in some years, wintry in others. You may experience balmy afternoons in the 70s or cold, blustery ones in the 40s or 50s, and the landscape in Yosemite Valley is still covered by dead yellow grass sheaths. By early May, daylight is about 13.5 hours long, and with the sun higher in the sky, the sun provides increasing radiation to bring spring to the valley floor. The deciduous trees produce leaves, and the meadows change from matted, brown, dead vegetation to a sea of green. The added radiation also increases snowmelt, sometimes augmented by the passage of a relatively warm rainstorm, and the valley's waterfalls reach their zenith from about early May through late June. The best time to visit these falls is around mid-May because most of the season's storms have abated but the summer tourist season is not yet in full swing.

Though all of the high country still lies under snow in May, some intermediate elevations are open to hikers. By May (or sometimes June), the rims of Yosemite Valley are largely snow-free, so you can hike up the Yosemite Falls Trail to the brink of Upper Yosemite Fall (Trail 30) or, in many years, even head to Merced Lake (Trail 35). Or you can start from Glacier Point and follow the Panorama Trail (Trail 41) to the floor. The Hetch Hetchy environs (Trails 23–25) are delightful early-spring destinations, often accessible as early as May. Finally, usually for Memorial Day, the National Park Service opens the cable route to the summit of Half Dome.

Trail Selection

Three criteria were used during the selection of trails for this guide. Only what I consider to be premier day hikes and overnight backpacking trips are included, based on beautiful scenery, ease of access, and diversity of experience. Because this area is Yosemite, most of the selected trails are very popular, and you can expect to see dozens to hundreds of other hikers along your route. Only on the longer or more remote routes, such as Trails 1, 27, and 44, might you meet few hikers.

The great majority of the trails included in this guide are out-and-back trips, requiring you to retrace your steps back to the trailhead—though the view is usually vastly different when facing the opposite direction. About a half dozen are loop or partial loop trips (some with options for straight out-and-back), and only five are point-to-point trails that are worthy of the required shuttle. However, for four of these, public transportation is available, so you don't need two vehicles.

Features and Facilities

Top Trails books contain information about features for each trail, such as lakes, great views, summits, waterfalls, and wildflowers. These are listed in the margin of each trail. Just beneath the list of features is a list of trailhead facilities, such as restrooms and water access.

Trail Safety

One danger is **getting lost**, though most of the trails in this book are very obvious routes. You can lose a trail where it crosses a lengthy stretch of bedrock that is not adequately marked by a line of rocks or by small piles of stones, called ducks or cairns. Also, in early season, patches of snow can obscure enough of your route that you lose it. In both situations it is important to look back before you cross the trailless stretch and note key features where you last see a distinct trail, so that if you fail to pick up the trail at the other end of the slab or snow patch, you then can recognize your way back toward the trailhead. While almost all trails are marked, maintained routes, the walks to Mount Dana (Trail 6) and Pothole Dome and the Tuolumne River (Trail 9) follow well-used social trails; there are no signposts along these routes.

Most of the park's trails are safe, but some spots are potentially dangerous, and these are identified in the text. At high elevations, especially above treeline, thunderstorms can be dangerous because they generate **lightning**. If the weather looks threatening, don't venture above the forest cover, even if the lightning is several miles away. Should you find yourself above trees (don't try to hide beneath isolated ones!), get rid of all your metal gear and get in the lightning position, both to reduce the likelihood of a direct strike and to reduce the seriousness of injury you are likely to sustain. The National Outdoor Leadership School recommends squatting or sitting as low as possible and wrapping your arms around your legs. This position minimizes your body's surface area, so there's less of a chance for a ground current to flow through you. Close your eyes, and keep your feet together to prevent the current from flowing in one foot and out the other. These storms usually pass overhead in about 15 minutes.

Both thunderstorms and frontal storms can chill you sufficiently that you can start slipping into **hypothermia**, and then you begin to lose physical coordination and mental judgment. Therefore, be sure you bring sufficient clothing to protect yourself from rain, snow, and cold winds. Even if you are on just a day hike, consider what you would need to survive a night, should you, say, break a leg and not get rescued until the next day.

Above 8,000 feet, you are more likely to suffer from **altitude sickness**, though most cases of altitude sickness occur above 10,000 feet in elevation. For unknown reasons, some people are much more prone to altitude sickness than are others—if you hike often at higher elevations, you will know how susceptible you are and how hard you can plan to push yourself at altitude. Generally, going slowly, staying hydrated, and keeping yourself eating some food are the best way to reduce your chance of experiencing the headaches and sense of nausea that are the most common symptoms of acute mountain sickness (AMS), the least severe and by far most common type of altitude sickness at Yosemite elevations. You can also reduce your chance of getting sick by camping one night above 6,000 feet elevation and then hiking the next day; any of the Tioga Road campgrounds would be ideal.

Sunburns can be particularly bad at high elevations, where the ultraviolet radiation is greater. You can even get burned on cloudy days because the radiation penetrates clouds. Therefore, always wear a wide-brimmed hat and apply sunscreen to all exposed skin, even if you are just hiking for an afternoon down in Yosemite Valley.

Besides staying on route and addressing the weather (which more often than not is fine), you should be aware of certain animals. **Mosquitoes** top my list as the most annoying, but so long as you have repellent, they are manageable. They are most plentiful before mid-July, especially around moist vegetated places such as meadows, grassy lakeshores, and lodgepole pine forests; before August, you'll likely want to backpack with a tent so that you can sleep in peace.

The largest animals are **black bears**, which almost always leave you alone but do want your food. Day hikers don't have to worry about bears—just keep your food at arm's reach during any breaks. However, because backpackers stand a very good chance of being visited by a bear during the night, they are required to keep their food in a bear canister. Bear-proof metal food-storage boxes are located at the campsites in Little Yosemite Valley and at the High Sierra Camps, but it is still recommended to carry a bear canister to the High Sierra Camp campsites to give you flexibility in your camping destination. With cash or a credit card, you can rent a park canister for a few dollars (plus a refundable deposit equal to the cost of the canister) at all locations that issue wilderness permits. They can be returned to any of these locations, and drop bins are available for after-hour returns at the wilderness permit–issuing locations as well as at the Arch Rock park exit (CA 140). If you've charged your deposit on a credit card, the charge will be

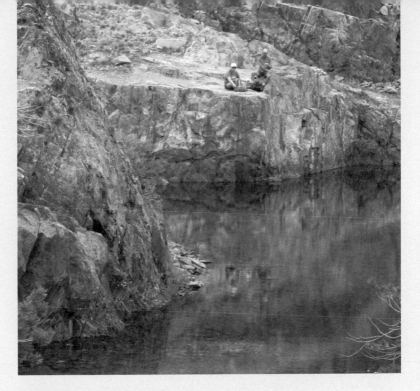

Nutter Lake *(see Trail 4, page 68)*

reversed. If you've used cash, then to get your money back, you will have to return the canister to one of the rental locations during business hours.

Rivers and waterfalls are the greatest danger to Yosemite's visitors, causing fatalities most years. Do not, do not, do not be tempted to swim in creeks at the tops of waterfalls. The rocks are as slick as glass from thousands of years of water pouring over them, and the current can be surprisingly strong. People have even slipped on the polished rock at the edge of the stream—that is, not in the water—into the stream and subsequently died. I look in horror at every picnicker sitting a few feet from the edge of Upper Yosemite Fall, hoping I never witness someone being unlucky. Stream crossings can also present a danger during periods of high snowmelt, in particular those along Trail 1 and Trail 44. Along Yosemite's popular trails, bridges or sturdy logs span most significant creeks, with notable exceptions detailed in the text. Nonetheless, winter storms and spring snowmelt often destroy some, so it is wise to check with rangers before setting out, especially in early summer. And note that, during peak snowmelt (usually in late June), river flows are much higher in the late afternoon than in the morning.

Fees

Not surprisingly, most trails start within Yosemite National Park, and to enter it you'll have to pay an entrance fee. The cost depends on which type of pass you purchase. The Standard Pass is $35/vehicle ($20 on motorcycle or on foot, bicycle, or bus), and it is good for seven days. The Annual Pass is $70/vehicle and is good for one full year from the date of purchase. Obviously, if you plan to visit the park more than twice within a 12-month period, the Annual Pass is the better deal. Should you plan to visit three or more national parks, purchase the $80 National Parks Pass. Finally, citizens or residents age 62 and older can get the $80 Golden Age Passport, which is good for a lifetime. US citizens or residents who are blind or permanently disabled get into all national entities for free and for life with the Golden Access Pass.

Camping and Lodging

Many hikers prefer to stay in campgrounds, and for the seven areas in this book, campgrounds near the trailheads are shown on the area maps. All campsites in and around Yosemite are also listed in Appendix A beginning on page 412. This section also includes basic information on the campsites. Here, additional information on the sites inside Yosemite is presented. In Yosemite Valley, reservations are required for sites at the North, Upper, and Lower Pines Campgrounds. The valley also offers Camp 4 (Sunnyside walk-in campground) on a first-come, first-served basis, but don't count on getting a site because climbers have a virtual monopoly on it. Other park campgrounds requiring reservations are Crane Flat, Wawona (reservations May–September), Hodgdon Meadow (reservations May–September), and half the sites in Tuolumne Meadows. The park's five other campgrounds, which are smaller and open only in the summer season, are on a first-come, first-served basis, and they fill up fast. These are Bridalveil Creek, along Glacier Point Road, and, from west to east on or near Tioga Road, Tamarack Flat, White Wolf, Yosemite Creek, and Porcupine Flat Campgrounds.

Visit nps.gov/yose/planyourvisit/camping.htm to learn more about the Yosemite campground reservation process and then make your reservation at recreation.gov. Briefly, reservations open in one-month blocks, and each time frame begins on the 15th of the month four months in advance. For example, if you wanted to camp between June 15 and July 14, you could reserve as soon as February 15. Note that as long as your reservation begins by July 14, you may book a stay that extends several days into the next reservation block. Because campsites in Yosemite's campgrounds fill incredibly quickly (within 10 seconds of becoming available for Yosemite Valley sites in summer), you should have backup campsites in mind when you get ready to make your reservations. And remember that if you are backpacking, you are eligible to spend the night before or after your trip in the backpackers' campsites in Yosemite Valley, in Tuolumne Meadows, and at Hetch Hetchy—no reservations required. If your plans for a Yosemite Valley campground fail, Appendixes A and B list all of the Yosemite region's campgrounds, public and private, as well as many resorts and lodges.

Aramark is the authorized concessionaire in Yosemite National Park and manages the park's hotels and lodges as well as the backcountry High Sierra Camps. The former include tent cabins and wood cabins in Half Dome Village (formerly Curry Village), Yosemite Valley Lodge, the Majestic Yosemite Hotel (formerly the Ahwahnee), Big Trees Lodge (that is, historical Wawona Hotel), Housekeeping Camp, and the tent cabins at White Wolf and Tuolumne Meadows. See travelyosemite.com/lodging for information about each of these. As for the High Sierra Camps, they are so popular that a lottery is held each December to determine the lucky relative few reservations for the following summer. To apply, visit travelyosemite.com/lodging /high-sierra-camps/high-sierra-camp-lottery. In a normal year, these facilities open around mid-July and close around mid-September. In years of heavy snowfall, the camps may not open at all! Backpackers may also seek to eat meals at the High Sierra Camps. Once, and only once, you have obtained a wilderness permit, you can request meals at the previously mentioned website—this is a way to greatly reduce your pack weight.

Permits

If you are going to spend one or more nights in the wilderness, be it in Yosemite National Park or in the wildernesses of adjoining U.S. Forest Service lands, you will need a wilderness permit. The notes for each hike that can be done as an overnight trip indicate the exact permit details you should request, including the issuing agency, the trailhead to request, and the location to pick up your permit.

Yosemite National Park's backcountry has quotas May–October, and 60% of each day's trailhead quota is available by reservation; the rest of the permits are given on a first-come, first-served basis beginning the day before the hike's start date. The rest of the year, virtually all of the high country will be under snow, and very few people will be backpacking, so you won't have to worry about any trailhead having its quota full. Though the flexibility of first-come, first-served permits is wonderful, most of Yosemite's trailheads are so popular that I strongly recommend you reserve your permit in advance. For popular trailheads, especially Happy Isles and those in the Tuolumne area, the reserved permit quota disappears quickly—that is, the same day it becomes available—and long lines can form well before dawn for the first-come, first-served permits. Starting on a Friday or Saturday, of course, only increases the permit competition. Detailed regulations are outlined at nps.gov/yose/plan yourvisit/wildpermits.htm. I strongly recommend that you check this website early in your planning process because Yosemite has changed various permit regulations and procedures several times in the last five years and is likely to continue fine-tuning their system.

Currently, you can get a permit from 24 weeks to 2 days in advance of your trip date. Though you can make a permit reservation by calling 209-372-0740, the reservation phone lines are often busy, and you may not get through. But the bigger problem is that permits faxed to the center over the previous 24 hours have priority to those made by phone. The reservation form to fill in is available on the website and can be faxed to 209-372-0739 up tp 24 hours in advance of the first date to make reservations; so that means you fax in your reservation request 24 weeks and 1 day before your hike starts. And yes, I know, no one has fax machines anymore—just fill out the sheet, sign it, scan it, or take a photo of it, and send it through one of the free online fax services, which convert your attached reservation form into a fax. The cost of confirmed permits is $5/ permit plus $5/person in the group.

Permits are also required to hike Half Dome as either a day hike or part of a backpacking trip. These were instated in 2011 to reduce overcrowding on the route, and now approximately 300 people per day are permitted on the cables, 225 day hikers and 75 backpackers. Most day hike permits are allocated by lottery, with applications accepted March 1–March 31, though 50 permits become available for a last-minute day-hike lottery two days in advance. Backpackers request their Half Dome permits together with their wilderness permit. Day hikers, see nps.gov/yose/planyourvisit/hdpermits .htm for details on permit applications; backpackers, see nps.gov/yose /planyourvisit/hdwildpermits.htm. The cost for all permits is $10/person.

There are five stations in Yosemite National Park that issue wilderness permits: the Yosemite Valley Wilderness Center, the Tuolumne Meadows Wilderness Center, the Big Oak Flat Information Station, the Wawona Visitor Center (at Hill's Studio), and the Hetch Hetchy Entrance Station. See nps.gov/yose/planyourvisit/permitstations.htm for maps of where each of these stations is located. It is requested that you pick up permits at the station closest to your trailhead, and if you are seeking a first-come, first-served permit, some level of preference is given to people at the "correct" (closest) station, but in the end, pick up your permit from the most convenient station to your trailhead.

Moving beyond Yosemite, if you are seeking a wilderness permit for the regions to the east of Yosemite (Trails 1–6), you need to obtain a wilderness permit from Humboldt-Toiyabe National Forest for the Hoover Wilderness trailheads, Virginia Lakes, Green Creek, and Robinson Creek, or from Inyo National Forest for permits for Twenty Lakes basin. The Hoover Wilderness trailheads all have quotas from the last Friday in June through September 15, with half the permits first come, first served and the others reservable for the summer beginning March 1. Though Robinson Creek quotas do fill in summer, obtaining these permits is much less competitive than are Yosemite permits. See www.fs.usda.gov/main/htnf/passes-permits for details. Permit reservations cost $3/person. These permits are picked up at the ranger station in far southern Bridgeport. The Saddlebag Lake Trailhead accessing Twenty Lakes basin does not have a quota, and permits can be obtained at the Mono Basin Scenic Area Visitor Center in northeastern Lee Vining or in Yosemite National Park at the Tuolumne Meadows Wilderness Center (but not other Yosemite permit-issuing centers).

Permits for Kibbie Lake (Trail 23) are obtained from Stanislaus National Forest. Though there is a quota for this trailhead (25 people per day), no advance reservations are possible. Instead, permits may only be obtained up to 24 hours in advance by contacting the Groveland Ranger District at 209-962-7825. It is located on the west side of Buck Meadow on CA 120—the street address is 24545 CA 120, Groveland, CA 95321. Yosemite permit centers can also issue permits for this trailhead (and other nearby trailheads entering Yosemite from Stanislaus National Forest), but it is not possible to make reservations.

Permits for the Isberg–Red Peak–Fernandez Passes Loop (Trail 44) and Vanderburgh Lake–Lillian Lakes Loop (Trail 45) are issued by Sierra National Forest. For this national forest, 60% of permits are first-come, first-served, and the remaining 40% are by reservation, year-round. Permits rarely fill for these trailheads, but given how far you have to drive to reach the trailhead, it is best to reserve a permit in advance to know one is waiting for you. Details on how to reserve permits are available at www.fs.usda.gov /detail/sierra/passes-permits. There is a $10/permit processing fee and $5/ person reservation fee. Monday–Friday permits can be picked up at the Bass Lake Ranger District at 57003 Forest Service Road 225, North Fork (559-877-2218), and seven days a week in summer at the Yosemite Sierra Visitors Bureau (559-658-7588), located in downtown Oakhurst (40343 CA 41, Oakhurst), or the Clover Meadow Ranger Station, located near the trailheads (559-877-2218, ext. 3136).

Topographic Maps

Topographic maps of various scales exist for all areas covered in this guidebook. The most detailed maps are those produced by the U.S. Geological Survey (USGS), generally referred to as the 7.5-minute (1:24,000 scale) topo series. These have become increasingly hard to purchase except directly from the USGS, but if you plan to explore off-trail, they are still the gold

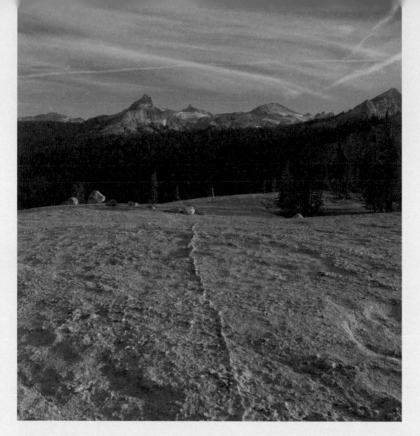

A dike rises above *the granite slabs on Pothole Dome (see Trail 9, page 110).*

standard. The data from these maps is available to the public, and you can download the maps to print yourself directly from the USGS. You can also view the content at a number of websites, such as Caltopo, and print your own maps covering the exact area you need for a walk.

A number of other cartography companies produce trail maps, topo maps annotated with trail distances. These vary in accuracy, but the two most commonly used are the Tom Harrison Maps and the National Geographic Trails Illustrated maps. The specific maps required for each hike are indicated in the introductory material for that hike.

Of course, for many of the walks in this book, the maps provided in the book should suffice and indeed are created to emphasize the information you should care most about. They are based on my own fieldwork, with all trails and campsite locations carefully logged on a GPS and then further edited and corrected. I estimate distances to be accurate within 2%.

On the Trail

Every outing should begin with proper preparation, which usually takes only a few minutes. Even the easiest trail can turn up unexpected surprises. People seldom think about getting lost or injured, but unexpected things can and do happen. Simple precautions can make the difference between a good story and a miserable outcome.

Use the Top Trails ratings and descriptions to determine if a particular trail is a good match with your fitness and energy level, given current conditions and time of year.

Have a Plan

Choose Wisely The first step to enjoying any trail, no matter the intended activity or the degree of difficulty, is to match the trail to your abilities. It's no use overestimating your fitness or experience—know your abilities and limitations, and use the Top Trails Difficulty Rating that accompanies each trail.

Leave Word About Your Plans The most basic of precautions is leaving word of your intentions with friends or family. Leave specific information such as your trailhead location and your daily itinerary. (I usually mark a copy of a map with my route.) Many people will hike the backcountry their entire lives without ever relying on this safety net, but every year you are likely to hear news reports about missing persons in the mountains. If you get caught in an unexpected storm, you can't be rescued if, first, no one knows that you are missing, and second, no one knows where you went hiking. In particular, if I am hiking solo, I make sure someone is expecting a brief message each time I return to the car.

> ### Prepare and Plan
>
> - Know your abilities and limitations.
> - Leave word about your plans.
> - Know your route and the area.

Review the Route Before embarking on any hike, read the entire description and study the map. It isn't necessary to memorize every detail, but it is worthwhile to have a clear mental picture of the route and general area. Because virtually all of the described trails are well used and easy to follow, you really don't need a topographic map for anything but the longest trails described.

Trail Essentials

- Dress to keep cool, but be ready for cold.
- Carry plenty of water.
- Have adequate food (plus a little extra).

Carry the Essentials

Proper preparation for any type of trail use includes gathering the essential items to carry. Your own checklist will vary tremendously by trail, conditions, and your personal preferences.

Clothing and Comfort In good summer weather, I prefer day hiking and backpacking in a short-sleeved shirt or long-sleeved sun shirt, shorts, and trail runners or lightweight hiking boots. That said, I am prepared for the worst, having a lightweight waterproof jacket as well as extra clothing should I be stuck overnight on a day hike gone astray.

Blisters can make your trip miserable, and you can avoid them two ways. First, wear broken-in, lightweight shoes or boots you know fit well. Second, wear wool socks, and have at least one spare pair should your feet get wet. Third, especially on a backpacking trip, bring along some blister bandages to cover a nasty blister; though expensive, they can turn a painful backpacking trip into one where your blisters are quickly forgotten. Leukotape is a wonderfully adhesive brand of tape to cover areas that you know are blister prone.

Backpackers definitely will want long pants and warm clothing, because in the high country, nights and mornings can be nippy even in the height of summer. Bundle up in the morning, then shed layers of clothing as you warm up. Pairs of lightweight thermal tops and bottoms together with a fleece or puffy jacket will be perfect. In the high country you'll also want a lightweight sleeping bag that keeps you warm down to about 20°F. Most people choose to carry a tent or tarp tent, especially during the mosquito season, but a ground tarp will certainly suffice for a short trip with a dry weather forecast.

Whether you day hike or backpack, bring sunscreen and, to be safe, mosquito repellent. Wear a wide-brimmed hat and bring dark glasses that you are certain offer UV protection (not just decorative darkening).

Water and Its Treatment On all walks longer than 15 minutes, you'll want to bring along one or more water bottles. My rule of thumb is that, on a hot day, I'll consume 1 quart for every 5 miles I walk—more if the hike is strenuous. If you backpack, you'll need to refill from creeks and/or lakes, which are usually safe for drinking, but on occasion may be contaminated with unseen giardia. Should you choose not to risk giardiasis, then use a water filter or chemical means of water purification.

Food Books give advice on the best food, but I say that, within reason, take what you like, especially on a day hike. Maintaining an appetite for the food you are carrying—and therefore eating it—is of the greatest importance. On a backpacking trip comes the added complication of needing to fit all your food into a bear canister, necessitating spatially dense food. If you are new to backpacking and struggling for suggestions, first visit some online forums to get ideas, and then repackage your food into lightweight zip-top bags. If you are going to be out longer than an overnight, bring extra food just in case you get lost or stuck in the wilderness. Especially in an unexpected snowstorm, you'll want to down a lot of calories.

Gear Depending on the remoteness and rigor of the trail, there are many additional useful items to consider. Even in my day pack I carry a headlamp, pocketknife, fire source (waterproof matches and/or lighter), and first-aid supplies. On backpacking trips, I may throw in duct tape and straps; you never know if you'll have to fix something, say, a broken pack or a broken bone. Every member of your party should carry basic survival items because groups sometimes get separated along the trail. I tuck an emergency blanket and whistle into each kid's pack, just to be sure.

For most folks, a topographic map and a compass are not necessary for these trails, but with them you can identify a lot of features not shown on this book's maps. Also, should you decide to leave your trail and go cross-country, say to a nearby lake, a topographic map is extremely valuable. Handheld GPS (global positioning system) receivers can be useful, but to me they supplement a map, not replace one; I have met a disturbingly large number of people with devices that were useless due to dead batteries or because they simply broke, leaving their owners with no alternative method of navigation. The same goes for cell phones: on the trail, the ability to communicate through them is essentially zero.

Solo hikers should be even more disciplined about preparation, should be more knowledgeable about potential hazards and their avoidance, and should carry more gear. Traveling solo is inherently more risky. With a group of three or more, should one be injured, another could stay behind with that person while another goes for help.

Weight Considerations Each person goes backpacking with a different amount of base weight, the weight of your gear before you add food or water. Among long-distance hikers, this weight differs from a staggering 8 to 30-plus pounds. Personally, I cannot imagine being comfortable at either end of this spectrum. I balance some combination of warm clothes, a warm sleeping bag, and comfortable backpack at one end and physical comfort at the other end. But I know people on both extremes who have thought through every item they are carrying and are very content with the decisions they've made. The important message is to think hard about every item you put in your pack and take out any you decide aren't essential. The less your pack weighs, the less you are carrying each step of the way, and having a lighter pack will most certainly enhance your trip.

I am likewise not inclined to tell people what shoes to wear—sometimes I'm in hiking boots and other times in lighter trail runners. Results from a large survey indicate that heavier footwear is associated with more blisters but fewer other foot problems, and people wearing boots suffer fewer falls. Make a considered choice, and then be comfortable with your decision.

Leave No Trace

The overriding rule on the trail is Leave No Trace. This is especially applicable to the more popular hiking destinations in and about Yosemite National Park, where during any summer hundreds of hikers will visit dozens of lakes.

Never Litter If you carried it in, pack it out. This includes any toilet paper you do not deposit in a pit toilet at one of the established backcountry campsites. It is not allowed—or acceptable—to attempt to bury toilet paper. Do not attempt to burn your litter—all you do is leave behind a plethora of half-burned foil linings for the next backpackers (and the rangers) to fume at. Try picking up any litter you encounter and packing it out—it's a rewarding feeling.

Trail Etiquette

- Leave no trace—never litter.
- Stay on the trail—never cut switchbacks.
- Share the trail—use courtesy and common sense.
- Leave it there—don't disturb plants or wildlife.

Don't Build Campsites Constructing fire rings or clearing the ground to place a tent or tarp transforms a pristine site into a human one—hardly a wilderness experience—not to mention it's illegal. Sure, you may move pinecones or small branches; just scatter them back over your tent site when you leave. Also, if you are going cross-country, don't mark your route. Let others do their own rewarding pathfinding just as you did.

Stay on the Trail Repeated shortcutting of switchbacks can lead to rapid erosion and time-consuming trail repair. Also, because shortcuts are steeper and have an uneven, sometimes bouldery tread, they can be dangerous, particularly for an exhausted backpacker in a hurry to get down. Don't risk broken bones or sprained ankles.

Share the Trail This book's trails attract many visitors, and you should be prepared to share the trail with others. Commonly accepted trail etiquette dictates that hikers yield to equestrians and their stock and that downhill hikers yield to uphill hikers. If a trail is wide enough to accommodate people passing, then ascending and descending hikers keep to their respective right side as they pass each other. Short tourist trails are severely impacted, hosting hundreds to thousands of visitors a day. You may meet an obnoxious person or two; don't become one and spoil someone else's day.

Leave It There Removal or destruction of plants, animals, and historical artifacts is both unethical and illegal.

Follow All Wilderness Regulations When you pick up your wilderness permit, you will be given a list of regulations to follow as a condition of obtaining the permit. While being handed the list and walked through it in terms of "do this, don't do this" can feel like a bit of a lecture, stop and consider each and every point and how they really do all make sense if we want to both use and preserve the Yosemite wilderness. For instance, the rule about no fires above 9,600 feet exists because, by that elevation, tree cover has thinned, and the small amount of deadwood on the ground is essential as homes for animals and, as it decomposes, as mulch for soil.

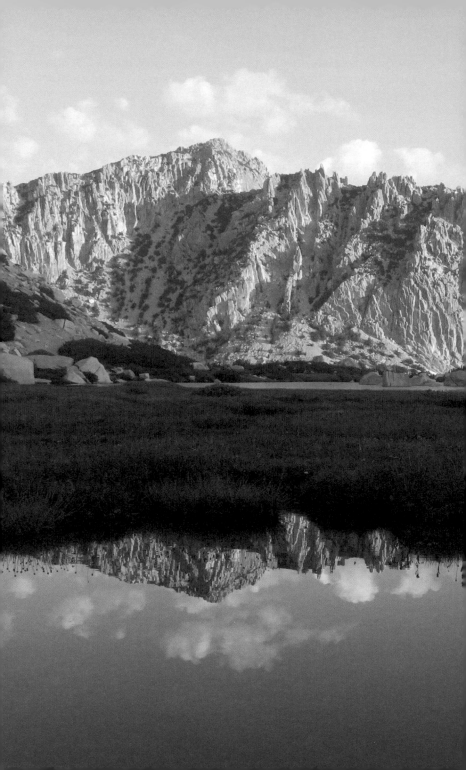

CHAPTER 1

Northeast Yosemite

As covered in this guidebook, the Northeast Yosemite country includes the lands extending from the park's northeast boundary southward along the Sierra Crest to Tioga Pass. The landscapes in this region are a mixture of granitic landscapes—John Muir's "Range of Light"—and metamorphic ones. Trails 1 and 2 traverse mostly granite, with its light gray shades, while the metamorphic rocks, with various earth tones of brown, brownish red, rust, and shades of ochre, make an appearance on the remaining trails. In addition to being more colorful, metamorphic rocks weather to produce more nutrients, so the lands with metamorphic soils support an abundance of subalpine and alpine wildflowers.

From US 395, roads climb west to trailheads north and east of Yosemite's Sierra Crest, and from these you can advance up canyons to the crest and then beyond into the lands of the northern third of the park. This area's landscape is characterized by many parallel or nearly parallel canyons, which, generally speaking, get progressively deeper toward the east. Many of the canyons are intersected by trails for just short stretches, increasing their remoteness. Indeed, only a single hike in this book, Trail 1, leads you through these north-country canyons, a 50-mile loop taking in trailed sections of several of the most famous canyons, including Piute Canyon near Benson Lake and Matterhorn Canyon. If the allure of northern Yosemite is strong, see *Yosemite National Park: A Complete Hiker's Guide* for descriptions of more trips in this region.

The remaining walks can all be completed as a day hike or overnight walk. Trails 2–5 start from eastern lands and visit lakes of the Hoover Wilderness that are east of the Sierra Crest. Trails 6 and 7 start from Tioga Pass, which, at about 9,940 feet, is the Sierra's highest pass and is traversed by CA 120 (also known as Tioga Road). Trail 6 ascends to the summit of Mount Dana, on the park boundary. Perhaps nowhere in the park or its vicinity can you obtain such expansive views of the Mono Basin than from this summit. And nowhere in the Sierra Nevada can you find a more easily

Opposite: *Tarn east of Mule Pass (see Trail 1, page 36)*

Northeast Yosemite

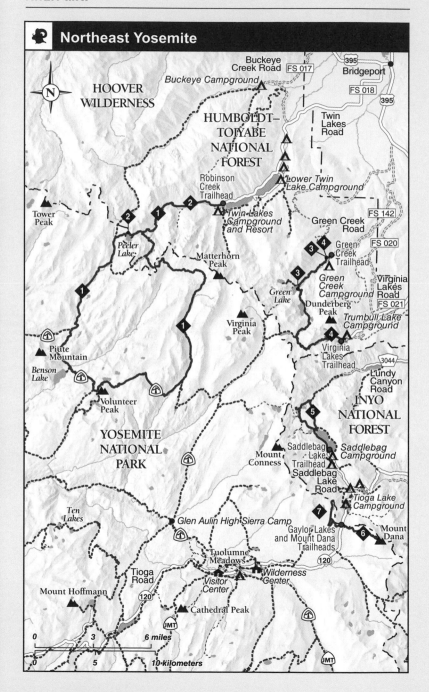

HOOVER
WILDERNESS

Buckeye
Creek Road FS 017

Buckeye Campground

395

Bridgeport

FS 018

395

HUMBOLDT–
TOIYABE
NATIONAL
FOREST

Twin
Lakes
Road

Robinson
Creek
Trailhead

*Lower Twin
Lake Campground*

Tower
Peak

*Peeler
Lake*

*Twin Lakes
Campground
and Resort*

Green Creek
Road

FS 142

Green
Creek
Trailhead

FS 020

*Matterhorn
Peak*

*Green
Creek
Campground*

*Green
Lake*

Virginia
Lakes
Road

FS 021

*Dunderberg
Peak*

*Trumbull Lake
Campground*

*Virginia
Peak*

Virginia
Lakes
Trailhead

3044

Piute
Mountain

*Benson
Lake*

Lundy
Canyon
Road

Volunteer
Peak

INYO
NATIONAL
FOREST

YOSEMITE
NATIONAL
PARK

Mount
Conness

Saddlebag
Lake

*Saddlebag
Campground*

Saddlebag
Trailhead
Saddlebag
Lake
Road

*Ten
Lakes*

*Tioga Lake
Campground*

Glen Aulin High Sierra Camp

Gaylor Lakes
and Mount Dana
Trailheads

Mount
Dana

Tuolumne
Meadows

Tioga
Road

120

Visitor
Center

*Wilderness
Center*

120

Mount Hoffmann

Cathedral Peak

JMT

0		3		6 miles

0		5		10 kilometers

JMT

Northeast Yosemite

Trail	Difficulty	Length	Type	USES & ACCESS	TERRAIN	NATURE	OTHER
1	5	50.3					
2	3–4	16.2					
3	2–3	6.3					
4	3	11.8					
5	2	7.5					
6	3	5.6					
7	2	4.0					

TYPE	USES & ACCESS	TERRAIN	NATURE	FEATURES
Point-to-Point	Day Hiking	Canyon	Autumn Colors	Great Views
Loop	Backpacking	Summit	Wildflowers	Camping
Out-and-Back	Horses	Lake	Giant Sequoias	Swimming
Balloon	Running	Stream		Secluded
	Wheelchair Access	Waterfall		Steep
DIFFICULTY	Stroller Access			Granite Slabs
− 1 2 3 4 5 +	Child-Friendly			Historical Interest
less more	Caution			Geological Interest

attained summit over 13,000 feet than Mount Dana. Finally, Trail 7 visits popular, easily accessed lakes west of and below the Sierra Crest, the subalpine Gaylor Lakes.

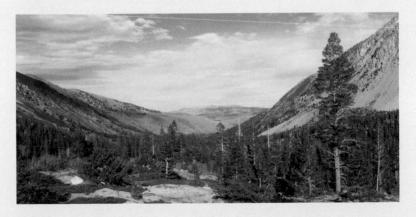

Green Creek drainage (*see Trail 3, page 63*)

Northeast Yosemite

Virginia Lakes Basin to Green Creek 68

The Virginia Lakes basin has much to offer. You can spend a relatively short time exploring the Virginia Lakes, or you can climb above them to the views at Burro Pass. Also, you can make either a long day hike or a moderate backpack beyond the pass down to the Green Creek Trailhead (described here). And you can either day hike to Summit Lake or backpack beyond it into upper Virginia Canyon, a classic glacier-smoothed subalpine valley.

Twenty Lakes Basin 77

This splendid balloon trip from Saddlebag Lake to Lake Helen and back passes more than one lake per mile, and in doing so offers you some of the Sierra's finest subalpine scenery along an easy grade. With the high and low elevations only about 400 feet apart, there are no significant ascents and descents. Still, at over 10,000 feet, you will notice the rarefied air if you try to hurry along. Though most people day hike this route, it also makes a superb, easy, family backpacking trip.

Mount Dana. 84

Dark glasses and good health are both necessary for this climb to the second-highest summit in Yosemite. Only Mount Lyell exceeds it—by about 60 feet—but the Lyell summit is distant. Because Dana is such an accessible big peak, it is very popular, and on weekends you may find dozens of people ascending it. Its summit views are among the Sierra's best.

Gaylor Lakes and Great Sierra Mine 90

Five subalpine lakes and sweeping panoramas await those who take this hike. Its endpoint provides a glimpse of the region's mining history. You also have the option of visiting the Granite Lakes by making a short cross-country hike. Camping is not allowed in the Gaylor Lakes area, including at the Granite Lakes.

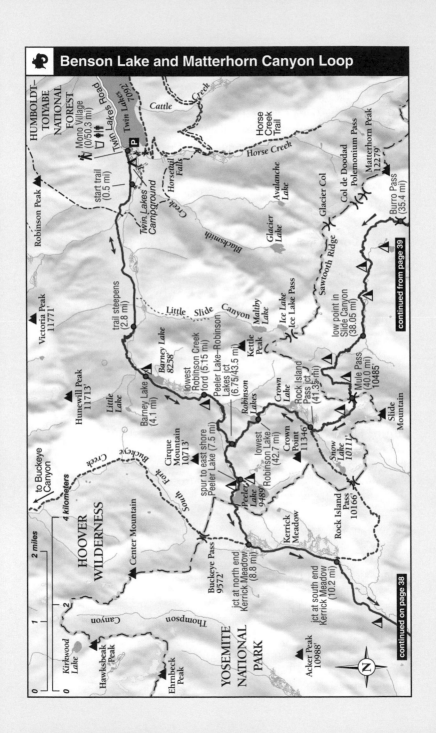

Benson Lake and Matterhorn Canyon Loop

HUMBOLDT-TOIYABE NATIONAL FOREST

Cattle Creek

Horse Creek Trail

Mono Village (0/50.3 mi)

Twin Lakes Road

Twin Lakes 7092'

P

Horse Creek

start trail (0.5 mi)

Horsetail Falls

Robinson Peak

Twin Lakes Campground

Creek

Avalanche Lake

Glacier Col

Col de Doodad

Polemonium Pass

Matterhorn Peak 12279'

Blacksmith

Glacier Lake

Victoria Peak 11171'

trail steepens (2.8 mi)

Little Slide Canyon

Maltby Lake

Ice Lake

Ice Lake Pass

Sawtooth Ridge

Burro Pass (35.4 mi)

continued from page 39

Barney Lake 8258'

lowest Robinson Creek ford (5.15 mi)

Peeler Lake–Robinson Lakes jct (6.75/43.5 mi)

Kettle Peak

low point in Slide Canyon (38.05 mi)

Hunewill Peak 11713'

Little Lake

Barney Lake (4.1 mi)

Robinson Lakes

Crown Lake

Rock Island Pass jct (41.35 mi)

Mule Pass (40.0 mi) 10485

Little Lake

Cirque Mountain 10713'

spur to east shore Peeler Lake (7.5 mi)

lowest Crown Robinson Lake (42.7 mi)

Crown Point 1134.6'

Snow Lake 10111'

Slide Mountain

to Buckeye Canyon

South Fork Buckeye Creek

Center Mountain

Peeler Lake 9489'

Kerrick Meadow

Rock Island Pass 10166

HOOVER WILDERNESS

Buckeye Pass 9572'

jct at north end Kerrick Meadow (8.8 mi)

Thompson Canyon

Kirkwood Lake

Hawksbeak Peak

YOSEMITE NATIONAL PARK

jct at south end Kerrick Meadow (10.2 mi)

continued on page 38

Acker Peak 10988'

Ehrnbeck Peak

4 kilometers

2 miles

0 1 2

0 1 2

N

Benson Lake and Matterhorn Canyon Loop

The vast lands of northern Yosemite cannot be reached on a weekend walk, because here the most sought-after destinations are all 15 miles or more from the trailhead. This loop takes you past many highlights of the area, introducing you to granite-ringed lakes; endless meadows; sharp-pointed ridges; and long, linear, U-shaped valleys scoured by glaciers. The well-traveled Pacific Crest Trail shares your route for a third of the distance, and indeed all the trails described receive reasonable traffic during the summer months, but you've nonetheless disappeared far into the wilderness.

Permits

Overnight visitors require a wilderness permit for the Robinson Creek Trailhead, issued by Humboldt–Toiyabe National Forest. Pick up your permit at the Bridgeport Ranger Station.

Maps

This trail is covered by the Tom Harrison *Hoover Wilderness Region* map (1:63,360 scale), the National Geographic Trails Illustrated *#308 Yosemite NE* map (1:40,000 scale), and the USGS 7.5-minute series *Buckeye Ridge, Matterhorn Peak,* and *Piute Mountain* maps (1:24,000 scale).

Best Time

Late July–mid-September is the best window for this walk. Northern Yosemite—with its abundant lakes, tarns, and meadows—is a mosquito haven, and the

TRAIL USE
Backpack, Horse

LENGTH
50.3 miles
(over 4–7 days)

VERTICAL FEET
±10,550'

DIFFICULTY
– 1 2 3 4 **5** +

TRAIL TYPE
Balloon

FEATURES
Canyon
Lake
Stream
Autumn Colors
Wildflowers
Great Views
Camping
Swimming
Secluded
Steep
Granite Slabs
Geological Interest

FACILITIES
Resort
Water
Campgrounds
Horse Staging

(continued on page 40)

37

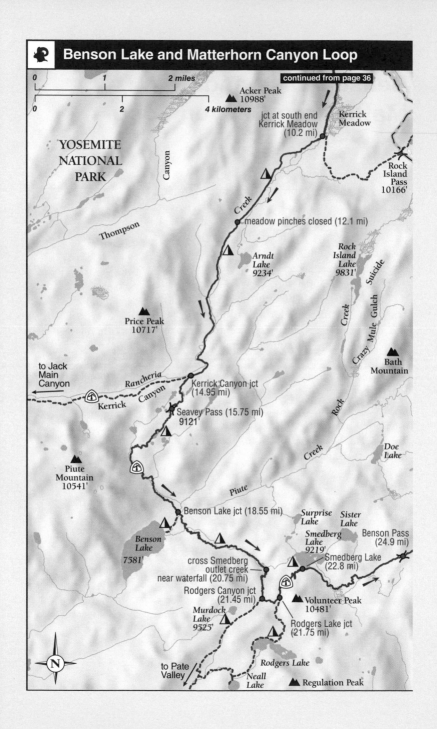

Benson Lake and Matterhorn Canyon Loop

0 — 1 — 2 miles

0 — 2 — 4 kilometers

continued from page 36

YOSEMITE
NATIONAL
PARK

Acker Peak
10988'

jct at south end
Kerrick Meadow
(10.2 mi)

Kerrick
Meadow

Rock
Island
Pass
10166'

Thompson Canyon

Creek

meadow pinches closed (12.1 mi)

Arndt
Lake
9234'

Rock
Island
Lake
9831'

Suicide

Price Peak
10717'

Crazy Mule Gulch

Creek

Bath
Mountain

to Jack
Main
Canyon

Rancheria

Kerrick Canyon jct
(14.95 mi)

Rock

Kerrick

Canyon

Seavey Pass (15.75 mi)
9121'

Creek

Doe
Lake

Piute
Mountain
10541'

Piute

Benson Lake jct (18.55 mi)

Surprise
Lake

Sister
Lake

Smedberg
Lake
9219'

Benson Pass
(24.9 mi)

Benson
Lake
7581'

cross Smedberg
outlet creek
near waterfall (20.75 mi)

Smedberg Lake
(22.8 mi)

Rodgers Canyon jct
(21.45 mi)

Volunteer Peak
10481'

Murdock
Lake
9525'

Rodgers Lake jct
(21.75 mi)

to Pate
Valley

Rodgers Lake

Neall
Lake

Regulation Peak

N

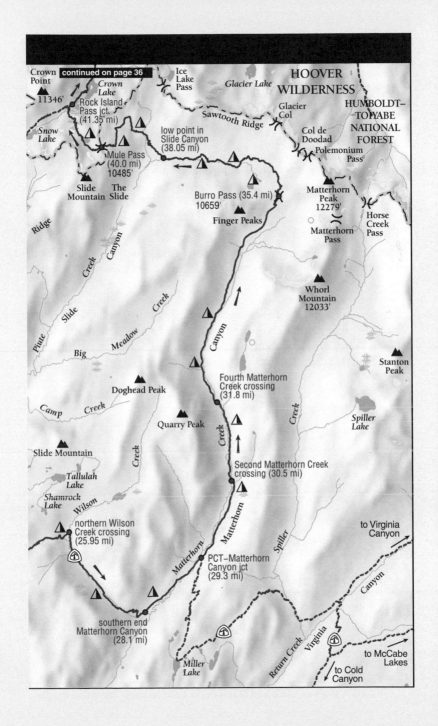

Crown
Point
11346'

continued on page 36

Crown
Lake

Ice
Lake
Pass

Glacier Lake

HOOVER
WILDERNESS

HUMBOLDT–
TOIYABE
NATIONAL
FOREST

Rock Island
Pass jct.
(41.35 mi)

Snow
Lake

Glacier
Col

Sawtooth Ridge

Col de
Doodad

low point in
Slide Canyon
(38.05 mi)

Polemonium
Pass

Mule Pass
(40.0 mi)
10485'

Slide
Mountain

The
Slide

Matterhorn
Peak
12279'

Burro Pass (35.4 mi)
10659'

Finger Peaks

Matterhorn
Pass

Horse
Creek
Pass

Ridge

Creek

Canyon

Slide

Creek

Piute

Meadow

Big

Whorl
Mountain
12033'

Canyon

Fourth Matterhorn
Creek crossing
(31.8 mi)

Doghead Peak

Camp   *Creek*

Quarry Peak

Creek

Creek

Stanton
Peak

Spiller
Lake

Second Matterhorn Creek
crossing (30.5 mi)

Slide Mountain

Tallulah
Lake

Shamrock
Lake

Wilson

Matterhorn

Matterhorn

Spiller

northern Wilson
Creek crossing
(25.95 mi)

PCT–Matterhorn
Canyon jct
(29.3 mi)

to Virginia
Canyon

Canyon

southern end
Matterhorn Canyon
(28.1 mi)

Matterhorn

Return Creek

Virginia

to McCabe
Lakes

Miller
Lake

to Cold
Canyon

(continued from page 37)

landscape cannot be fully appreciated if you feel unable to sit down and relax in your surroundings—especially on such a long trip. The mosquitoes start to wane in late July, and August is idyllic, with the large lakes warm enough for a swim.

By mid-September, temperatures drop and days are shorter. There are still a number of hikers completing long hikes, but it is wise to watch the weather forecast and ensure an early-fall snowstorm does not take you by surprise.

Finding the Trail

From US 395 near the northwest side of Bridgeport, take paved Twin Lakes Road southwest 13.6 miles to the entrance of Mono Village at the west end of upper Twin Lake.

The trailhead is at road's end in Mono Village, a private resort and campground. Overnight users must pay to park their cars here—drive about 0.1 mile past the day-use parking area where you first turn into the Mono Village complex to the overnight parking lot, located farther south along the lake's shore. Then visit the obvious campground entrance kiosk

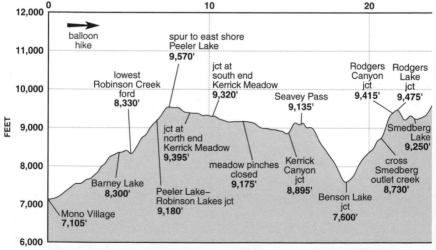

TRAIL 1 Benson Lake and Matterhorn Canyon Loop Elevation Profile

and pay $10 per trip, regardless if it is one night's parking or many. Water and toilets are present throughout the campground.

Trail Description

You begin in Mono Village, ►1 a private resort with cabins and a campground at the head of upper Twin Lake. Distances are measured from the campground's entrance booth, from which two main roads depart—either works, but the right (more northerly) option is slightly more direct, and after about 0.2 mile you reach the western end of the campground. The trail now skirts a meadow's edge as your route, a closed road, starts upcanyon. At the 0.5-mile mark ►2 the road veers left (south) across Robinson Creek on a bridge, and a sign marks the start of the Robinson Creek Trail; you follow the trail right. After walking west a couple of minutes, you pass low granitic outcrops, and just beyond them is a bulletin board with information on the area. The first part of your hike is open forest, dominated by Jeffrey pines on the dry slopes and aspens on wetter soils, particularly near unseen Robinson Creek. Less common trees include Fremont cottonwood and western juniper, both becoming more abundant upcanyon.

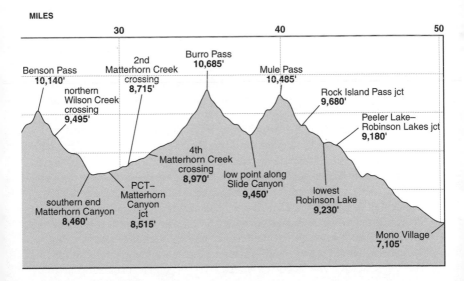

MILES

30   40   50

Benson Pass
10,140'

northern
Wilson Creek
crossing
9,495'

southern end
Matterhorn Canyon
8,460'

2nd
Matterhorn Creek
crossing
8,715'

PCT–
Matterhorn
Canyon
jct
8,515'

Burro Pass
10,685'

4th
Matterhorn Creek
crossing
8,970'

low point along
Slide Canyon
9,450'

Mule Pass
10,485'

Rock Island Pass jct
9,680'

Peeler Lake–
Robinson Lakes jct
9,180'

lowest
Robinson Lake
9,230'

Mono Village
7,105'

After crossing a stream chortling down from the basin between Victoria and Eagle Peaks, the trail winds gently up through more open terrain with sparse conifers, sagebrush, and bitterbrush, giving you your first unbroken views of the beautifully U-shaped glacial valley—the valley bottom is nearly flat, abruptly truncated to either side by steep valley walls, cascading watercourses, and sharp-tipped peaks. As your path continues on a westward course, the floor supports increasing numbers of mule ears and diminishing numbers of arrowleaf balsamroots, two large sunflowers whose names indicate the difference in their leaf shape. The pleasant amble leads to a welcome patch of shade beneath white fir cover (2.8 miles). ▶3 This is a good spot to stop for a drink and rest beside tumbling Robinson Creek before launching into the climb ahead.

The trail up the canyon headwall ascends a dozen well-graded but rocky switchbacks that lead north through head-high jungles of shrubs, staying always within earshot of unseen Robinson Creek. Above the switchbacks, the track is often wet, as water from springs dribbles along the trail, sustaining the abundant wildflowers that will distract you in summer. You continue up the gradual incline, often only a few steps from the bubbling creek's edge, and soon find yourself in a stunningly dense aspen forest. The ever-fluttering yellow and orange leaves will astound your senses in fall as you walk down the golden tunnel. Soon after stepping across a tributary draining Little Lake to the west, you reach the north end of a large flat that extends to the shore of Barney Lake (4.1 miles). ▶4 The lodgepole forest here is littered with campsites, with an additional selection of sites to the southeast of the creek (crossed on a large logjam just downstream of the lake's outlet) on a flat behind a granitic mass at the lake's northeast corner. Barney Lake's north shore has a sandy beach—growing gradually larger as water levels drop in late summer and into fall—a fine spot for a lunch break and perfect after a swim.

The western shoreline, which your trail follows, is a dry talus slope mixed with glacial debris. After rounding the base of a steep escarpment, a pair of switchbacks elevate the trail some 100 feet above Barney Lake's inlet. In sections the walking is fast, while elsewhere, protruding rocks break your stride. Once past Barney Lake, your gaze is drawn to the domain of industrious beavers, the marshy meadow upstream of the lake. This was once a lake itself and is slowly filling with sediment. Eventually you descend several short switchbacks; wind through broken rock, past avalanche-twisted aspens, and over two freshets draining Cirque Mountain; and slowly descend back to creek level. Beyond a small campsite to

the southwest of the path, the trail crosses Robinson Creek (5.15 miles),
▶5 a wet ford in early summer or a rock hop by midsummer.

From the far bank, you climb easily south above the riverbank through a mix of red fir and lodgepole pine. The trail soon leads back to the west bank of Robinson Creek, which you cross on rocks or (currently) a downed log; this crossing can be a wade and requires full attention at high flows—occasionally it can even be quite dangerous. Next the trail crosses the smaller cascading stream from Peeler Lake. Ahead lies a dry glacial till–covered slope, which you ascend via a long series of notably gentle switchbacks. Beyond you level off momentarily for a breather before darting north for a steeper ascent. The vistas east, to rough, ice-fractured outcrops of Kettle Peak, offer good excuses to stop frequently on this energetic climb. With increasing altitude, mountain hemlock, immediately identified by its drooping branch tips, now joins the mix of conifers on the cooler, more shaded aspects. Eventually you come to a small saddle at 9,185 feet and a trail junction (6.75 miles). ▶6 The left (southerly) fork is a trail bound for the Robinson Lakes, Rock Island Pass, and Slide Canyon and is the route on which you will return, while now you turn northwest (right) to Peeler Lake.

Walking moderately up in mixed open forest, cross the Peeler Lake outlet creek twice, and then switchback south up into a narrow gully. The wind can pick up as you ascend the gully, a sure sign that you're nearing the ridgetop. The final stretch is along a magical little shelf above the Peeler Lake outlet creek, replete with a collection of picturesque mountain hemlocks. Just as you sense the lakeshore is imminent, a spur trail leads left (south) to a collection of campsites on the lake's still unseen eastern shore (7.5 miles). ▶7 Continuing on the main trail, 9,489-foot Peeler Lake's often windswept waters suddenly come into view, back-dropped by rounded Acker and Wells Peaks in the west. A short descent leads you to—and then through—car-size granodiorite blocks that dam the lake's outlet and beyond to the dynamited trail tread on the north shore of Peeler Lake. The trail now undulates along the lakeshore, climbing and descending repeatedly to bypass small bluffs. The largest campsite is located in a forest pocket right along the north shore. At the lake's northwestern corner, you cross into Yosemite National Park and continue west toward Kerrick Meadow. Note that a number of areas are off-limits to camping along the lake's west shore.

The descent to Kerrick Meadow is pleasant, strolling in and out of lodgepole stands, across short stretches with slabs, and past fingers of meadow, all the while following alongside Peeler Lake's westerly outlet

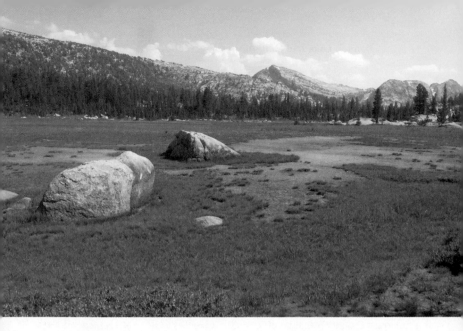

Kerrick Meadow

creek; yes, that's right, perched atop a ridge, water drains both east and west from Peeler Lake during high runoff. Your grade slowly lessens, and the line of lodgepole forest retreats to the north and the meadow pockets coalesce into a verdant cover of grass and dwarf bilberry as you slowly enter Kerrick Meadow. Though meadows dominate along the trail, heading north can yield some campsites on forested shelves and among small patches of slab—Kerrick Meadow is almost continually vegetated, making it off-limits to camping. Ahead you reach a junction where right (north) leads to Buckeye Pass, while you turn left (south) and cross Kerrick Meadow (8.8 miles). ►8

Though limited in camping opportunities to a few small sandy spots atop knobs, Kerrick Meadow is a stunning location, and following the trail through the middle of the meadow is especially picturesque in the early morning or late afternoon sun. Both tarns and small rocky outcrops add dimension to the meadow; the slightly elevated meadow patches turn yellow in late summer, while the depressions remain a bright green. As you stroll along, likely distracted by Belding's ground squirrels or marmots, dwarf bilberry, a heath species with small leathery leaves, continues to form a near-continuous mat at the meadow's edge. At the south end of the meadow you reach another junction, where left leads to Rock Island Pass, while you continue right in the direction of Benson Lake (10.2 miles). ►9

Beyond the junction the meadow narrows and the gradient steepens as you drop down through open lodgepole forest to reach a second, even longer meadow with Rancheria Creek meandering down its middle. The landscape here is drier than Kerrick Meadow, and as you walk along the sandy trail, you note that grass is less ubiquitous here, affording more opportunities to find campsites at the meadow's edge or atop shallow sandy knobs. Sandpipers, always seeming out of place in a subalpine setting, ply the sandbanks flanking the river for a meal. Your views now extend south to dark-colored Piute Mountain, around whose eastern base the trail will pass. After more than 30 minutes of walking, the meadow pinches to a close (12.1 miles). ►**10** If you were to cross the creek here—only a pleasant and safe endeavor after the main snowmelt flush has subsided—you would find a tributary creek that leads 0.6 mile south-southeast to Arndt Lake. Less visited than the trailside lakes, its slab-encrusted shores offer some good campsites.

Rancheria Creek now becomes a broken gorge, and we drop rockily down, walking on gravelly benches, only to strike another sandy meadow, this one with a flanking cluster of steep domes, some with black water stains and a striking red weathering patina. Walking through here the landscape feels not that different from the striking domes ringing Tenaya Lake, except that you are many miles from a road. As before, a little searching yields some camping choices. Dropping again you reach yet another expanse of meadow, in the middle of which you cross Rancheria Creek, a broad sandy wade in all but the driest conditions. Presently a master joint in the bedrock directs Rancheria Creek briefly east, and we follow its splashing course down over broken, porphyritic (large-crystaled) bedrock slabs, then back west on another master joint along shaded slopes to a junction with the Pacific Crest Trail (PCT) (14.95 miles). ►**11** Your route heads left, toward Seavey Pass and Benson Lake, while right leads down Kerrick Canyon toward Wilma Lake.

In comparison to the quick-paced meadow walking over the past 6 miles, the 8 miles along the PCT from now until Smedberg Lake are notoriously slow going—they have achieved an unfortunately negative reputation among PCT hikers, frustrated that they have to reduce their daily mileage through northern Yosemite. Instead, plan ahead, and accept that the continuous ups and downs for the coming miles will reduce your walking speed. Not only is the terrain never flat, but you are also winding between domes, descending gravelly slopes, and stepping over embedded rocks, and your stride is simply continually broken.

Such is the dome country of northern Yosemite, especially as the trail cuts across the landscape from one river drainage to another, from Rancheria Creek to Piute Creek (flowing into Benson Lake) to Matterhorn Creek. At higher elevations—that is, where you just were—are the long, linear valleys for which northern Yosemite is so celebrated; you will encounter these again as you ascend Matterhorn Canyon and descend Slide Canyon, but at the middle elevations, travel is more cumbersome.

Back to the route—heading uphill for the first time in many miles, you switchback up a steep slope bedecked with mountain hemlocks to a little passageway nestled between two domes. The trail bends slightly left to reach a cluster of small tarns, while straight ahead lies a lake with some camping options on its western side. Other camping options present themselves near the tarns, especially for hikers with small tents keen to spend the night in a patch of sand atop one of the view-rich domes. Winding along past small wildflower patches and between slabs, you cross Seavey Pass (15.75 miles) ▶12 and begin your descent. Gradual at first, you continue along a high shelf cradling additional lakes, all with slabs extending to their shores. No large campsites present themselves, but a small group will most certainly locate a flat, sandy patch to plop their tent—note that several of the lakes, including one below and west of the trail, have larger flat areas near their inlets. Scooting past the last in the series of lakes, the trail begins to descend more seriously on short switchbacks descending a steep, sheltered draw with lodgepoles and hemlocks.

The grade abruptly ends at a meadow at the imposing eastern base of Piute Mountain as the trail bends south (17.0 miles) to follow a tributary toward Piute Creek. Excepting brief forested glades, the trail diligently descends a dry slope of pine-mat manzanita and huckleberry oak, growing atop a mixture of light-colored granite and darker metamorphic rocks. Rounding a corner, you see Benson Lake ahead. Your trail eventually reaches the valley bottom, and after a short, flat stretch through lush forest, you reach a junction with a spur trail that leads to the lake's shore (18.55 miles). ▶13

Though not included in the mileage, a side trip to Benson Lake is hardly optional—this is one of the more remote lakes to which every Yosemite lover makes a pilgrimage. The 0.4-mile spur trail leads through nearly flat, lush forest of white fir, lodgepole pine, and the occasional aspen. To your side is Piute Creek, a gushing torrent in early summer, transforming to a lazy trickle with big sandbars by early fall. Just beyond, you reach the famous Benson Lake beach. The entire northeast shore is an open sandy bank, growing even wider as the lake's water level drops in late summer. Being relatively low-elevation, Benson Lake is remarkably warm for swimming, or you can simply bury your feet in the warm sand while staring across the expanse of water and the dark cliffs descending from Piute Mountain. You will find campsites at the back of the beach or in the forest at the far northeastern tip of the lake.

Back to the PCT, you quickly reach Piute Creek, just where two forks merge, both of which you cross independently on fallen logs. Should these logs be missing, this is a dangerous crossing in early summer, potentially requiring a retreat to quite deep but calmer waters near Benson Lake's shore. Now begins a long uphill along the banks of the Smedberg Lake outlet creek—more of a raging stream in early summer. Crossing over a rocky knob, with a possible campsite perched atop, you cross the creek on rocks and head up a dry slope, again a mixture of granite and metamorphic rocks. You note occasional junipers decorating exposed knobs and small clusters of lodgepoles or hemlock growing in flatter patches as you keep climbing slabs and through gravelly channels between outcrops. Crossing the creek again, you briefly enter a wet glade with possible campsites, and then revert back to dry, rocky terrain beside the cascading river. Passing a small tarn, you spy a headwall ahead, down which tumbles a small waterfall (20.75 miles). ▶14 Here you must again cross the creek, almost always a wade and a difficult one at high flow; head a little upstream of the trail for the best options.

The trail's gradient now increases, and you quite rapidly climb 700 feet via steep, tight switchbacks; thankfully the walking is on soft forest floor beneath cool hemlock cover. Soon after the ascent eases you reach your first trail junction in many miles, where right leads down Rodgers Canyon toward Pate Valley, while you turn left, toward Smedberg Lake (21.45 miles). ▶15 If it is nearing nightfall, one option for camping is to head an easy 0.5 mile south along the Rodgers Canyon trail toward Murdock Lake, where you will find quiet campsites to the south of the lake, with Volunteer Peak reflected in the shallows. Following our route along a lovely lodgepole pine and hemlock shelf, dwarf bilberry carpeting across the forest floor, the trail quite soon leads to another junction, where straight ahead leads to Smedberg Lake, while a right turn heads over a pass to Rodgers Lake, a longer detour to campsites (21.75 miles). ▶16

Continuing on toward Smedberg Lake, you wind along forested shelves and between narrow passageways in the pervading slabs and bluffs, all the while circumnavigating the base of near-vertical Volunteer Peak. Though vertical fractures adorn its face, the minimal talus at the peak's base attests to the rocks' integrity. Climbing again, admire the views west to massive Piute Mountain, Benson Lake visible at its foot. Stripes of trees across the landscape indicate where wide-scale fractures in the rock have allowed deeper soils to accumulate. Soon you crest a small pass and begin your final descent to Smedberg Lake. Small single-tent sites present themselves in sandy patches among the slabs as you descend, or as soon as you reach the lake, turn left to find abundant ▲ campsites along the lake's western edge (22.8 miles). ▶17 The campsites surrounding Smedberg Lake are well filled most midsummer nights and understandably so because this lake's location is strikingly beautiful; you may feel differently in early July, as I once did, when, having forgotten mosquito repellent, I walked past the lake without pause, desperate to part ways with the swarms of mosquitoes.

The landscape is now larger scale again, lacking the intricate slab passageways that defined the last many miles of trail, and the walking is correspondingly faster. Passing Smedberg Lake and some smaller campsites on slabs and in small lodgepole stands around its southern and southeast-▲ ern edges, you climb gradually alongside meadows and then more steeply as you trend toward Benson Pass. You mount a series of sand-and-slab benches. The rock here is predominately granite with large crystals—note the giant rectangular feldspar crystals in some outcrops—decomposing to a coarse-grained soil that creates a decidedly slippery walking surface atop underlying slabs. The gradient eases as you pass through a broad meadow, drying early and covered with lupines in late summer. It segues to a narrow, sandy gully that you ascend. Though unmarked on maps, this channel has water in it late into the summer. At its head the trail sidles south across a steep, gravelly slope, leading to the flat summit of Benson Pass (24.9 miles). ▶18

Continuing east, the trail descends through more slippery decomposing granite and then skirts north above a broad, often dry meadow landscape. A few camping options present themselves at the meadow's edge. The topography again steepens, and while the trail descends steep switchbacks, the creek pours down a narrow slot in rocks. Below you reach a small meadow opening ringed by lodgepole pines and then the shores of ▶ Wilson Creek, marking the halfway point in your loop (25.95 miles). ▶19 ▲ In the nearby lodgepole stands, you will find several campsites along the west side of the crossing.

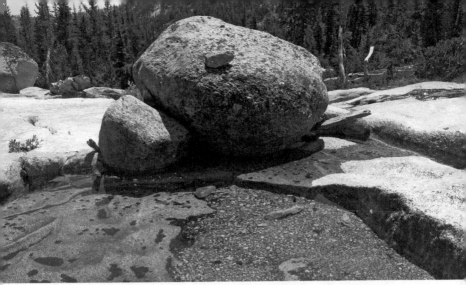

Granite slabs and pools *along Wilson Creek*

Crossing the creek atop logs or rocks, the trail now turns southeast to begin a 2-mile descent to Matterhorn Canyon. Each time I walk the length of this creek, my thoughts are immediately drawn to the massive scars down both canyon walls, a testament to the tremendous avalanches that tear down these slopes. The trees lay flattened, all pointing away from the flow of snow, meaning uphill directed trees were knocked down by slides that crossed the creek and flowed up the other side. Only beneath steep cliffs do mature forests persist because the cliffs slough snow continually, never letting it accumulate enough thickness for a more destructive slide. The beautiful slabs lining the creek also demand your attention, especially if your feet need a soak as you bask on the smooth, sunny rocks for lunch. Camping is limited on this descent to a few small forested shelves overlooking the stream. Toward the bottom of the straightaway, topography dictates that the trail twice crosses the creek, on rocks or downed logs, depending on water depth. Soon beyond the second crossing, the trail sidles away from Wilson Creek, leading you onto steep bluffs, where gnarled juniper trees clasp at small soil pockets, and your rocky route switchbacks steeply down among them. You are now staring at the lower reaches of Matterhorn Canyon, and quite soon your trail diverges for good from the banks of Wilson Creek, reaching the relative flat of the canyon floor (28.1 miles). ▶**20**

Now begins a long uphill as you walk the 7-mile length of Matterhorn Canyon to Burro Pass at its head. Excepting the final mile, the gradient is never steep. Surprising to me is how few campsites exist, especially during the upper miles: like many of northern Yosemite's canyons, the floor of Matterhorn Canyon is very wet, as endless seeps ooze water where the steep walls flatten. This means that for long stretches, you must search for small, flat, generally tree-covered knobs to make your home. But for this first stretch, campsites are everywhere. You are traipsing well west of Matterhorn Creek through flat lodgepole pine forests and will find an acceptable tent site just about anywhere you wish. Emerging into an open meadow, you reach a broad crossing of Matterhorn Creek, a wade in all but the lowest of flows and a wade over rounded boulders requiring caution at peak runoff, and just beyond reach a junction where you part ways with the PCT (29.3 miles). ▶21

Turning left and walking up along the stream's eastern bank, your route is mostly within lodgepole pine forest, occasionally trending into small meadow patches. The vegetation is mostly quite lush—grass grows beneath the lodgepole pine forests and the meadows are thick with color: a dense patch of tall purple delphinium in one place; corn lilies in marshier locales; Sierra tiger lilies along the banks of tributaries; and sagebrush on a dry, sandy knob. Crossing to the west bank of the creek, on rocks or wading at high flows (30.55 miles), ▶22 you traipse briefly along a narrower shelf above the creek and drop back to the creek to ford it again in the middle of a meadow. This time you cross on a series of rocks that only emerges at low water and otherwise have a long, broad wade. Back on the stream's eastern bank, the forest starts to thin as you approach the 9,000-foot mark. Your eyes are drawn upward to the steep eastern wall of Quarry Peak and the bright-white talus blocks that lie at its base. This stretch of Matterhorn Canyon is undeniably U-shaped, but while scoured clean and deepened by the glaciers, its orientation was achieved long before the ice fields covered the landscape. The sandy flats along this stretch of trail are the last guaranteed campsites for a large group as you head upward; from here until you cross Burro Pass, there are only a few sites with space for more than two tents. With the creek continuing to bubble by your side, you pass scattered stands of lodgepole pine and hemlock, cross sandy patches, and eventually cross Matterhorn Creek for the fourth time (31.8 miles). ▶23

About now you leave forest cover for good, marching upward along a meadow corridor. A small waterfall descends the slabs overhead. Evidence of endless avalanches partially explains the general lack of forest stands. The abundant moisture contributes as well—conifer species do not establish in locations where their roots are wet most of the summer growing season. This combination of factors gives the landscape a decidedly alpine feel, even though you are just above 9,000 feet, just barely higher than lodgepole-clad Tuolumne Meadows. Rounding one corner, the sharp-tipped Finger Peaks come into view, and then around the next bend, Sawtooth Ridge and Burro Pass are visible to the east. A drier patch of landscape affords some camping options in sandy patches, but it is soon marshy again from the endless springs at the cliff's base. With continued walking, the view becomes ever more dramatic. Whorl Peak, soon due east of the trail, demands ever more attention. Excepting a few particularly marshy areas, the walking is quite easy, with few rocks to break your stride. Belding's ground squirrels stand at attention throughout the meadows. I love watching the youngsters during the first weeks they are allowed to explore outside their burrows. Their juvenile curiosity almost gets the better of them as they stare at you approaching—then suddenly the instinct to escape overwhelms them and they race for their burrows, sometimes tripping themselves as they race forward and stare backward all at once.

Almost imperceptibly the slope increases, but at some point, around the 34-mile mark, it is noticeably steep, first continuing its due-north trajectory and then bending more eastward. Climbing through meadows and past little seeps, you soon begin an ascending traverse across the base of the Finger Peaks toward Burro Pass. The plants dwindle in height, while polished slabs and large boulders become more prominent—or maybe, you are just staring at the stunning granite summits that ring your location. Passing a few small sandy one-tent campsites that entice those wishing to spend their night with this vista, you soon find yourself climbing the first switchbacks since you entered Matterhorn Canyon. They lead purposefully to the summit of Burro Pass, where you will undoubtedly take a well-earned break (35.4 miles). ►**24** The view from here is stunning, especially north to Sawtooth Ridge. A few moments of staring at the odd-shaped protrusions and pinnacles on the skyline, and one immediately comprehends the inventive names assigned to these features: the Dragtooth, the Doodad, Three Teeth, and Cleaver Peak.

The north side of Burro Pass holds snow long into the summer season, so take care as you descend the uppermost switchbacks—my most recent crossing was in early August of a low snow year and there was still a patch of snow to navigate. Soon on flatter terrain, you begin your descent of upper Slide Canyon, walking through flower-filled wet meadow environments and across slabs, Sawtooth Ridge always looming over your right shoulder. White mountain heather with bell-shaped flowers, light purple alpine shooting stars, and orange-red-colored Peirson's paintbrush are

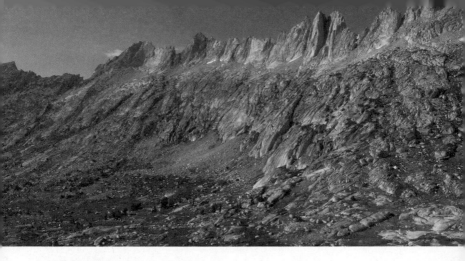

Sawtooth Ridge *from the summit of Burro Pass*

three of the most ubiquitous companions. Two small tarns lie on a shelf southwest of the trail, providing beautiful alpine campsites (albeit poor swimming choices), and are easily reached with a short detour off the trail. The trail is steep, rocky, and incised, dictating a slow pace as you pick your steps carefully. Continuing down, you pass occasional small campsites, eventually crossing the nascent Piute Creek. About here are your last uninterrupted views of the Sawtooth skyline, should that be a prerequisite for your campsite's location. You skirt a large, often marshy meadow and depart into the first continuous lodgepole pine forest you have encountered in many miles.

The going is pleasant as you continue downstream. Though still mostly a narrow trail, it is less eroded once under forest cover. Beautifully glacial-polished slabs glisten beside the trail, several with sandy flats at their centers that make enticing campsites. Piute Creek is a little to your south but easily within reach to fetch water. As you're walking down, look regularly ahead and to the left, where Slide Canyon bends southward—your route will diverge to the right by this point, but you should glean glimpses of a monumental rockslide that scarred the side of Slide Mountain, burying Slide Canyon under 2.5 million cubic yards of rocks. Some boulders rolled 200 feet *up* the east side of the canyon. This stretch of trail is also noteworthy for the tangles of downed logs, the aftermath of windstorms. A few last mediocre camping options present themselves to the south of the trail just before you reach the trail's low point in Slide Canyon (38.05 miles). ▶25

Climbing steadily through dry, open lodgepole pine forest, the trail first traverses up and left before completing six switchbacks. These lead toward a creek, which you follow upward through an increasingly open landscape, emerging into a finger of meadow before stepping across the creek. How quickly you find yourself back in an alpine environment always astonishes me—and in a lovely patch of meadow surrounded by flat slabs and sandy patches; camping options exist with a little snooping away from the trail and meadow corridor.

The trail meanwhile cuts west across a grassy shelf with scattered trees and then descends to enter a narrow slot positioned between two steep, polished granite slabs. Up through sandy, gravelly soil you walk, as this channel leads to a broad bench, in parts meadow covered and elsewhere with sandy flats. The east side of Mule Pass is a collection of steep granite bluffs and polished slabs, interrupted repeatedly by these flat benches, cre- ▲ ating a mysterious landscape—even staring at the map you keep wondering just where the trail will wind upward. Holding snow well into July—or beyond—the small streams bisecting the meadows flow through most of the summer, providing water should you wish to camp in one of the many ▲ sandy patches among slabs to the east of the trail. The view of the pinnacled Kettle Peak, Sawtooth Ridge, and Matterhorn Peak ringing the horizon, with the Finger Peaks in the foreground, is truly stunning in the evening light. Steep, rough switchbacks climb the final slope to the high point, as you turn back to savor the view east one final time. Facing forward, you are probably surprised to realize Mule Pass, the drainage divide, lies in the middle of the sandy flat to your west, so descending briefly you leave Yosemite National Park and reenter Hoover Wilderness (40.0 miles). ▶**26**

A brief set of switchbacks down a dry, sandy slope leads to a wet meadow, resplendent with diminutive meadow wildflowers, including ✳ yellow primrose monkeyflower, pink mountain laurel, and purple Lemmon's Indian paintbrush. At the northern end of the meadow lies a small whitebark pine–encircled lake. Following the labyrinth of sandy passageways between the stunted trees leads to some small campsites along ▲ the north and northeastern sides of the lake. Beyond, tight switchbacks descend to the east of a large rockslide, where massive, angular blocks fill the gully. Your sheltered passageway holds snow late into the year and can be icy early or late in the day—take care. The many points on Crown Point, straight ahead of you, exist due to joints in the rock, causing it to ✒ fracture along perfectly straight planes. Leveling out briefly, you descend again, this time on an old moraine deposit, before crossing the Snow Lake outlet creek and reaching the junction with the trail leading left to Snow Lake and Rock Island Pass, while you trend right toward the Robinson Lakes (41.35 miles). ▶**27**

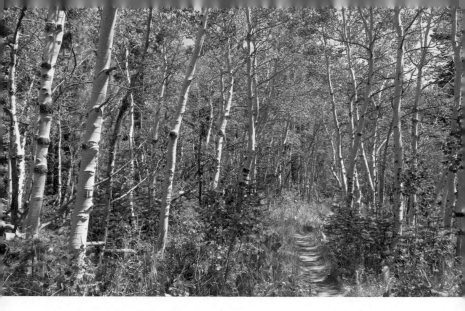

Aspen groves *below Barney Lake*

After briefly walking along a sandy slope above a series of tannin-rich tarns, you resume a switchbacking descent between fins of rock. The trail soon reaches the next flat, this one cradling Crown Lake. Camping is prohibited near the outlet of this well-used lake, but there are possible campsites if you head about 0.1 mile east of the outlet. Granite bluffs border the trail almost continually as you wind your way ever lower. Robinson Creek bubbles to the side, comical dippers bobbing endlessly on midstream boulders between brief forays into the water in search of insects; these dark-colored birds are also known as water ouzels. Dense glades of hemlock provide shade as you drop toward the largest—and lowest elevation—of the Robinson Lakes (42.7 miles). ▶28 Like Crown Lake, the cliff bands and boulder fields limit camping options around most of this lake; the best site is on a knob at the northwestern corner of the lake. Climbing gently, you promptly reach the next Robinson Lake, at which camping is prohibited. Skirting the edge of the lake leads to the final Robinson Lake, this one more a tarn, brilliant blue-green in color. Giant rock blocks, the aftermath of a long-ago rockfall, comprise part of its shoreline, with the clear water filling the gaps between the boulders. Passing a few places to camp on a pass beyond the lakes, the trail descends briefly through hemlock forest to reach a junction you will recognize from several days ago; you now turn right toward the trailhead, while left leads back to Peeler Lake (43.5 miles). ▶29 From here, retrace your steps to the Mono Village parking area (50.3 miles). ▶30

🚶 MILESTONES

▶1	0.0	Start at Mono Village parking area
▶2	0.5	Turn right from road onto Robinson Creek Trail
▶3	2.8	Trail steepens
▶4	4.1	Barney Lake
▶5	5.15	Lowest Robinson Creek crossing
▶6	6.75	Right at Peeler Lake–Robinson Lakes junction
▶7	7.5	Right at spur trail to Peeler Lake's east shore
▶8	8.8	Left at junction at north end of Kerrick Meadow
▶9	10.2	Right at junction at south end of Kerrick Meadow
▶10	12.1	Meadow pinches closed
▶11	14.95	Left at Kerrick Canyon junction
▶12	15.75	Seavey Pass
▶13	18.55	Straight ahead at Benson Lake spur junction
▶14	20.75	Cross Smedberg outlet creek near waterfall
▶15	21.45	Left at Rodgers Canyon junction
▶16	21.75	Left at Rodgers Lake junction
▶17	22.8	Smedberg Lake
▶18	24.9	Benson Pass
▶19	25.95	Northern Wilson Creek crossing
▶20	28.1	Southern end Matterhorn Canyon
▶21	29.3	Left at PCT–Matterhorn Canyon junction
▶22	30.5	Second Matterhorn Creek crossing
▶23	31.8	Fourth Matterhorn Creek crossing
▶24	35.4	Burro Pass
▶25	38.05	Low point along Slide Canyon
▶26	40.0	Mule Pass
▶27	41.35	Right at Rock Island Pass junction
▶28	42.7	Lowest Robinson Lake
▶29	43.5	Right at Peeler Lake–Robinson Lakes junction
▶30	50.3	Return to Mono Village parking area

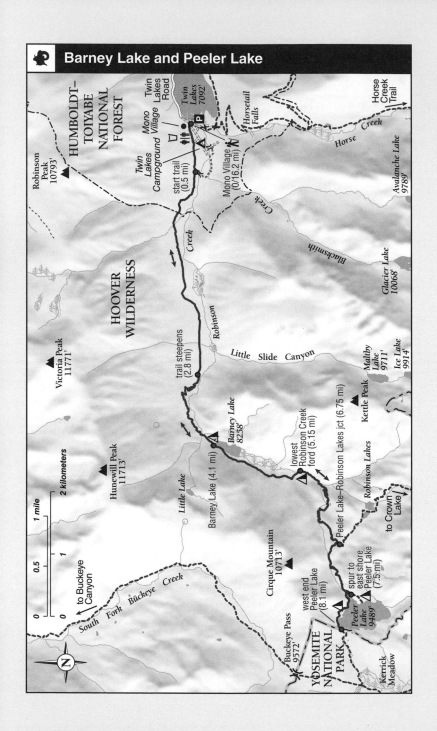

Barney Lake and Peeler Lake

HUMBOLDT–
TOIYABE
NATIONAL
FOREST

Twin
Lakes
Road

Twin
Lakes
7092'

Horsetail
Falls

Horse
Creek
Trail

Robinson
Peak
10793'

Mono
Village

Twin
Lakes
Campground Village

start trail
(0.5 mi)

Mono Village (0/16.2 mi)

Horse Creek

Avalanche Lake
9789'

HOOVER
WILDERNESS

Creek

Blacksmith

Glacier Lake
10068'

Victoria Peak
11771'

Robinson

Little Slide Canyon

trail steepens
(2.8 mi)

Maltby
Lake
9711'

Ice Lake
9914'

Kettle Peak

Barney Lake
8258'

lowest
Robinson Creek
ford (5.15 mi)

Peeler Lake–Robinson Lakes jct (6.75 mi)

Hunewill Peak
11713'

Barney Lake (4.1 mi)

Little Lake

Peeler Lake–Robinson Lakes jct

Robinson Lakes

to Crown
Lake

2 kilometers

1 mile

0.5

1

to Buckeye
Canyon

South Fork Buckeye Creek

Cirque Mountain
10713'

west end
Peeler Lake
(8.1 mi)

spur to
east shore
Peeler Lake
(7.5 mi)

Peeler
Lake
9489'

Buckeye Pass
9572'

YOSEMITE
NATIONAL
PARK

Kerrick
Meadow

N

Barney Lake and Peeler Lake

The Robinson Creek Trail is the most popular route through the Hoover Wilderness and into the Yosemite north country, and justifiably so. This relatively short, scenic trail leads quickly into breathtaking subalpine terrain. Glittering Peeler Lake, surrounded by frost-shattered and glaciated granite and windswept conifers, mirrors the region's grandeur. Intimate campsites beside its shore more than compensate for the day's tough climb. Alternatively climb only as far as Barney Lake, a popular and stunning day hike (or worthwhile overnight) destination. Finally, the 3-mile gentle ascent of the lower reaches of scenic Robinson Creek Trail to the start of its switchbacks is great for joggers.

Permits

Overnight visitors require a wilderness permit for the Robinson Creek Trailhead, issued by Humboldt–Toiyabe National Forest. Pick up your permit at the Bridgeport Ranger Station.

Maps

This trail is covered by the Tom Harrison *Hoover Wilderness* map (1:63,360 scale), the National Geographic Trails Illustrated *#308 Yosemite NE* map (1:40,000 scale), and the USGS 7.5-minute series *Buckeye Ridge* and *Matterhorn Peak* maps (1:24,000 scale).

Best Time

The first 3 miles up Robinson Creek canyon usually are snow-free by late May. Barney Lake is a desirable goal by mid-June, while Peeler Lake is best left for

TRAIL USE
Day Hike, Backpack, Horse, Run

LENGTH
16.2 miles, 6–10 hours (over 1–3 days)

VERTICAL FEET
One-way: +2,850', –385'
Round-trip: ±3,235'

DIFFICULTY
– 1 2 **3 4** 5 +

TRAIL TYPE
Out-and-Back

FEATURES
Canyon
Lake
Stream
Autumn Colors
Wildflowers
Great Views
Camping
Swimming
Secluded
Granite Slabs

FACILITIES
Campgrounds
Horse Staging
Resort
Water

early July—or later if you wish to avoid mosquitoes. Late September–mid-October, when abundant aspen trees turn a dazzling yellow, is a spectacular time to walk the Robinson Creek canyon and visit Barney Lake.

Finding the Trail

In September and October, you might spend a few minutes near the head of Twin Lakes to view the kokanee salmon run up Robinson Creek.

From US 395 near the west side of Bridgeport, take paved Twin Lakes Road southwest 13.6 miles to the entrance of Mono Village at the west end of upper Twin Lake.

The trailhead is at road's end in Mono Village, a private resort and campground. Day hikers will see a large parking area immediately to their left, alongside the lake; parking here is free. Overnight users must pay to park their cars—drive about 0.1 mile farther to the overnight parking lot, located farther south along the lake's shore. Then visit Mono Village's obvious campground entrance kiosk and pay $10 per trip, regardless if it is one night's parking or many. Water and toilets are present throughout the campground.

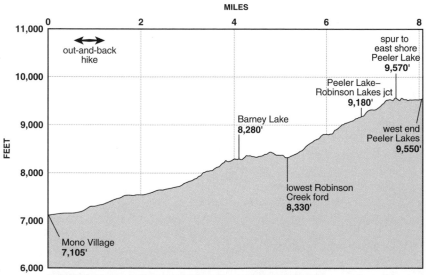

TRAIL 2 Barney Lake and Peeler Lake Elevation Profile

Trail Description

You begin in Mono Village, ▶1 a private resort with cabins and a camp-ground at the head of upper Twin Lake. Distances are measured from the campground's entrance booth, from which two main roads depart—either works, but the right (more northerly) option is slightly more direct, and after about 0.2 mile you reach the western end of the campground. The trail now skirts a meadow's edge, as your route, a closed road, starts upcanyon. At the 0.5-mile mark the road veers left (south) across Robin-son Creek on a bridge, and a sign marks the start of the Robinson Creek Trail; you turn right to follow the trail. ▶2 After walking west a couple of minutes, you pass low granitic outcrops, and just beyond them is a bulletin board with information on the area. The first part of your hike is open forest, dominated by Jeffrey pines on the dry slopes and aspens on wetter soils, particularly near unseen Robinson Creek. Less common trees include Fremont cottonwood and western juniper, both becoming more abundant upcanyon.

At the 1.2-mile mark, a short distance beyond the wilderness bound-ary marker, you reach a persistent stream, chortling down from the basin between Victoria and Eagle Peaks. Though never deep or dangerous, it is a broad crossing without a collection of large rocks on which to balance—at high flows some nimble jumps are required to keep your feet dry. Afterward, the trail winds gently up through more open terrain with sparse conifers, sagebrush, and bitterbrush, giving you your first unbroken views of the beautifully U-shaped glacial valley—the valley bot-tom is nearly flat, abruptly truncated to either side by steep valley walls, cascading watercourses, and sharp-tipped peaks. As your path continues on a westward course, the floor supports increasing numbers of mule ears and diminishing numbers of arrowleaf balsamroots, two large sun-flowers whose names indicate the difference in their leaf shape. At 7,600 feet (2.15 miles), you pass through a grove of aspens, ablaze with yel-low leaves in September, then amble through more sagebrush, scattered junipers, and boulders. The pleasant amble leads to a welcome patch of shade beneath white fir cover (2.8 miles) ▶3. This is a good spot to stop for a drink and rest beside tumbling Robinson Creek before launching into the climb ahead.

The trail up the canyon headwall ascends a dozen well-graded but rocky switchbacks that lead north through head-high jungles of aspen, bitter cherry, serviceberry, snowberry, and tobacco brush, staying always within earshot of unseen Robinson Creek. This section is short but stifling

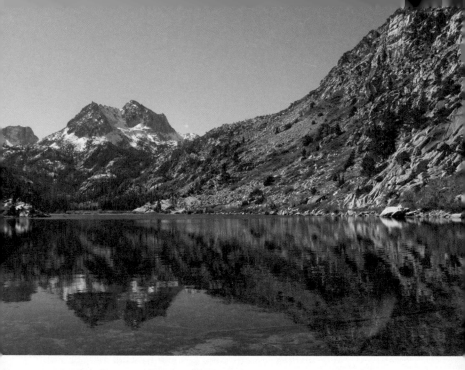

Barney Lake

on a hot summer's day because the tall brush blocks the mountain breezes. Soon after the switchbacks end, you step across a small rivulet merrily draining the slopes of Hunewill Peak (3.4 miles). The track through here is often wet, as water from springs dribbles along the trail, sustaining the abundant wildflowers that will distract you in summer. You continue up the gradual incline, often only a few steps from the bubbling creek's edge, and soon find yourself in a stunningly dense aspen forest. In the fall, the ever-fluttering yellow and orange leaves will astound your senses as you walk down the golden tunnel. Just below 8,300 feet you level out to step across a tributary draining Little Lake to the northwest.

Just ahead you reach the north end of a large flat that extends to the shore of Barney Lake (4.1 miles; 8,280'). ►4 The lodgepole forest here is littered with campsites, with an additional selection of sites to the southeast of the creek (crossed on a large logjam just downstream of the lake's outlet) on a flat behind a granitic mass at the lake's northeast corner. Barney Lake's north shore has a sandy beach—growing gradually larger as water levels drop in late summer and into fall—a fine spot for a lunch break and perfect after a swim. Admire the surroundings as you sit: 14-acre Barney Lake is nestled in a narrow, glaciated trough, rimmed on the east by the broken north spur of Kettle Peak.

The western shoreline, which your trail follows, is a dry talus slope mixed with glacial debris. After rounding the base of a steep escarpment, a pair of switchbacks elevates the trail some 100 feet above Barney Lake's inlet. In sections the walking is fast, while elsewhere, protruding rocks break your stride.

Once past Barney Lake, your gaze is drawn to the domain of industrious beavers, the marshy meadow upstream of the lake. This was once a lake itself and is slowly filling with sediment. Eventually you descend several short switchbacks; wind through broken rock, past avalanche-twisted aspens, and over two freshets draining Cirque Mountain; and slowly descend back to creek level. Beyond a small campsite to the southwest of the path, the trail fords Robinson Creek (5.15 miles). ►5 This crossing can be reasonably deep in spring and early summer, becoming a rock hop by midsummer. Rainbow and brook trout occur here, as in Barney Lake.

From the far bank, you climb easily south above the riverbank through a mix of red fir and lodgepole pine. The trail soon leads back to the west bank of Robinson Creek, which you cross on rocks or (currently) a downed log; this crossing can be a wade and requires full attention at high flows—occasionally it can even be quite dangerous. Next the trail crosses the much smaller cascading stream from Peeler Lake. Ahead lies a dry glacial till–covered slope, which you ascend via a long series of notably gentle switchbacks; only near the bottom of the ascent do you climb steeply, and there are a few times you find yourself stepping downhill while on your way *up*. Beyond you level off momentarily for a breather before darting north for a steeper ascent. The vistas east, to rough, ice-fractured outcrops of Kettle Peak, offer good excuses to stop frequently on this energetic climb. Adjacent to the trail are impressive rock fins, some nearly overhung, reflecting the jointed rock that is pervasive throughout this region.

With increasing altitude, mountain hemlock, immediately identified by its drooping branch tips, now joins the mix of conifers on the cooler, more shaded aspects. Eventually you come to a small saddle at 9,185 feet and a trail junction (6.75 miles). ►6 The left (southerly) fork is a trail bound for the Robinson Lakes, Rock Island Pass, and Slide Canyon, while those heading to Peeler Lake now turn northwest (right). You walk moderately up in mixed open forest to a small, shaded glade beside the Peeler Lake outlet creek and step across this stream twice before switchbacking south up into a narrow gully. The wind can pick up as you ascend the gully, a sure sign that you're nearing the ridgetop. The final stretch to Peeler Lake is along a magical little shelf above the Peeler Lake outlet creek, replete with a collection of picturesque mountain hemlocks. Just as you sense the lakeshore is imminent, a spur trail leads left (south) to a collection of campsites on the lake's still unseen eastern shore (7.5 miles). ►7 Continuing on the main trail, the often windswept waters of 9,489-foot Peeler Lake suddenly come into view, its waters backdropped by rounded Acker and Wells Peaks in the west. A short descent leads you to—and then through—car-size granodiorite blocks that dam the lake's outlet and beyond to the dynamited trail tread on the north shore of Peeler Lake. The trail now undulates along the lakeshore, climbing and descending repeatedly to bypass small bluffs. The largest campsite is located in a forest pocket right along the north shore.

Continue to the Yosemite National Park boundary at the lake's northwestern corner (8.1 miles) ►8. Areas near the trail are closed to camping, but exploring south along the lake's western shore will undoubtedly yield some private campsites among the extensive slabs. The lake margin, mostly rock, does have a few stretches of meadowy beach, where you can fly-cast for rainbows and brookies. When you are ready, backtrack to the trailhead (16.2 miles). ►9

🚶	**MILESTONES**	
►1	0.0	Start at Mono Village parking area
►2	0.5	Turn right from road onto Robinson Creek Trail
►3	2.8	Trail steepens
►4	4.1	Barney Lake
►5	5.15	Lowest Robinson Creek crossing
►6	6.75	Right at Peeler Lake–Robinson Lakes junction
►7	7.5	Right at junction with spur to Peeler Lake's east shore
►8	8.1	West end Peeler Lake
►9	16.2	Return to Mono Village parking area

Green Creek Basin

Large, attractive Green Lake is one of the most easily reached backpacker lakes in the northern Yosemite area, and the hike up to it is enjoyable because of the diverse vegetation and the impressive views down-canyon from the multistep climb. You can continue on to camp at East Lake, set before a dramatic back-drop of Page and Epidote Peaks. Or, from Green Lake you can make a day hike up to alpine West Lake and even explore cross-country the isolated lakes beyond. For those staying in the Bridgeport or Lee Vining areas, the relatively short trail up to Green Lake (and even to East Lake) is a great day hike.

Permits

Overnight visitors require a wilderness permit for the Green Creek Trailhead, issued by Humboldt–Toiyabe National Forest. Pick up your permit at the Bridgeport Ranger Station.

Maps

This trail is covered by the Tom Harrison *Hoover Wilderness* map (1:63,360 scale), the National Geographic Trails Illustrated #308 *Yosemite NE* map (1:40,000 scale), and the USGS 7.5-minute series *Dunderberg Peak* map (1:24,000 scale).

Best Time

The trail up Green Creek canyon usually is snow-free by mid-June, but snow can linger in shady patches at higher elevations into July, when the canyon's wildflower gardens lower down are already peaking. By late July, mosquitoes are abating and Green Lake is warm enough for swimming,

TRAIL USE
Day Hike, Backpack,
Child-Friendly

LENGTH
6.3 miles, 2.5–4 hours
(over 1–2 days)

VERTICAL FEET
One-way: +1,040', –90'
Round-trip: ±1,130'

DIFFICULTY
– 1 **2** 3 4 5 +

TRAIL TYPE
Out-and-Back

FEATURES
Lake
Stream
Autumn Colors
Wildflowers
Great Views
Camping
Swimming
Secluded

FACILITIES
Bear Boxes
Campground
Restrooms
Water

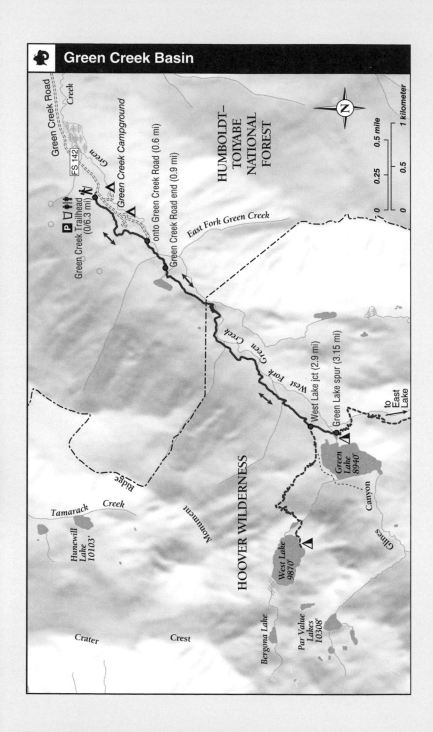

Green Creek Basin

Green Creek Road

Creek

Green Creek Campground

onto Green Creek Road (0.6 mi)

FS 142

Green Creek Trailhead
(0/6.3 mi)

Green Creek Road end (0.9 mi)

Green

East Fork Green Creek

HUMBOLDT–
TOIYABE
NATIONAL
FOREST

1 kilometer

0.5 mile

0.25   0.5

0

West Fork Green Creek

West Lake jct (2.9 mi)

Green Lake spur (3.15 mi)

to
East
Lake

Ridge

Green
Lake
8940'

Canyon

Tamarack   Creek

Monument

Hunewill
Lake
10103'

HOOVER WILDERNESS

Gillies

West
Lake
9870'

Crater   Crest

Bergona Lake

Par Value
Lakes
10308'

cooling a bit by mid-August. September and early October are also good months for Green Creek canyon, when the aspen trees and other deciduous vegetation put on a display of color and most of the hikers have gone.

Near the start is a 15-foot-high cliff, a basalt remnant that predates the recent glacial periods.

Finding the Trail

From Bridgeport, drive south on US 395 through the town to the Bridgeport Ranger Station, near its south edge. Continue 3.8 miles south on US 395 to a junction with Green Creek Road, Forest Service Road 142. If you're traveling north on US 395, you'll meet this junction about 8.1 miles north of US 395's Conway Summit. Take FS 142 about 3.5 miles to a T. To reach the Green Creek Trailhead, at the T you branch right, still on FS 142, and go 5.1 miles to an obvious trailhead parking area, with an outhouse and water spigot, on the right. (Just 300 feet past this is the Green Creek Campground. You first pass the group sites, on the left, and 0.25 mile farther you enter the campground proper.)

Trail Description

Behind the information signs in the trailhead parking area, ►1 the trail diverges north from the road to encircle a moist aspen glade—a dense stand of trees with a lush understory. The trail winds and undulates upcanyon before reintersecting the dirt Green Creek Road—indeed,

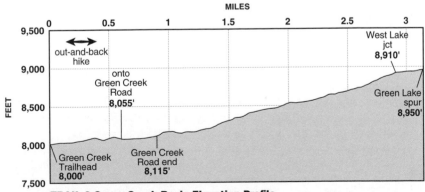

TRAIL 3 Green Creek Basin Elevation Profile

OPTION: **East Lake**

This is another popular and scenic lake, and from the Green Lake environs, ▶5 the 1.3-mile-long trail up to it is a moderate ascent through a relatively dense conifer forest. Partway up you'll cross the lake's outlet creek, which in early summer can be swift—take care not to slip into its cascading course. Above, you recross it, and after about a 500-foot elevation gain you make a leisurely ascent to a third crossing of the creek, just below 9,460-foot-high East Lake. This is a large subalpine lake, fully 0.75 mile long, and the trail parallels its east side for most of its length. From the outlet south to the southeast shore, there are scattered, usually small campsites on granite benches shaded mostly by whitebark pines.

following the road from the parking area is flatter and slightly shorter, but notably less scenic (0.6 mile). ▶2 The trail now temporarily ends and you must continue up the road 0.3 mile to its end at a small cabin and a trickle you step across (0.9 mile); note there is no parking here. ▶3 The proper trail now begins its multistep ascent. With a few steep switchbacks you quickly surmount a dry, juniper-dotted rocky knob and continue through open forest above the creek. Whereas you started in a forest dominated by Jeffrey pines, you now ascend through a moister forest of lodgepole pines and aspens. At 1.3 miles you cross into Hoover Wilderness and climb a dozen short, rocky switchbacks up to another step and rest as you catch your breath at these subalpine elevations.

Above the switchbacks, you pass beside a marshy flat, the confluence of Green Creek's two forks, and above encounter a stretch of lushly vegetated trail, irrigated by both a small tributary descending the steep slope to the right and Green Creek itself. Just muddy enough to be a possible nuisance for some early- and midsummer hikers, the trail cuts through a swath of luxuriant wildflowers that dazzle the eyes with myriad colors: the orange alpine lilies, lilac fireweed, and purple monkshood and larkspur. In fall this stretch of trail is especially colorful; the aspens are not much taller than a person, so you are literally in the middle of their bright yellow and orange canopies.

For a stretch the trail's meanders match those of the unseen creek, but then you diverge from the creek (2.3 miles) and complete a couple of switchbacks to a dry ridge above. For the first time you now have unbroken views of the surrounding mountains and back down Green Creek. You (usually) leave the bugs behind and can relax on a beautiful granite outcrop surrounded by juniper trees, a restful view spot. Just ahead you'll arrive at a trail junction (2.9 miles). ▶4 To the right is a trail that provides access to the northwest shore of Green Lake and to West Lake and its

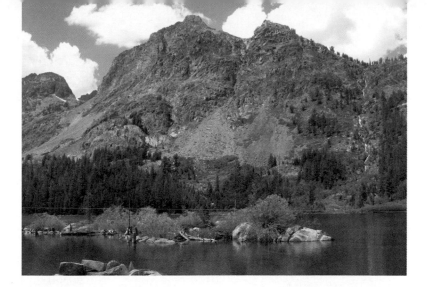

Green Lake

western outliers. For most folks, the steep 1.6-mile-long trail up to this 9,870-foot-high lake ringed by stark slopes is not on the agenda. Camping opportunities at West Lake are few, but the promise of unfettered views of colorful rocks may entice you higher.

Instead, from the trail junction, virtually all users turn left and make a brief jaunt 0.2 mile to a crossing of Green Lake's outlet creek. In spring and early summer this creek can be raging, and you'll need to find a log or two to cross it. Just after this creek, you can head west to the nearby lake to find some good campsites. At an elevation of 8,940 feet, Green Lake (3.15 miles) ►5 can be on the nippy side for swimming, but there are slabs for drying out and sunbathing. The relatively large volume and chilly temperatures are ideal for a good-size trout population. From here you can continue to East Lake or else backtrack to the trailhead (6.3 miles). ►6

MILESTONES		
►1	0.0	Start at Green Creek Trailhead
►2	0.6	Turn right onto Green Creek Road
►3	0.9	Green Creek Road end
►4	2.9	Left at West Lake junction, toward East Lake
►5	3.15	Green Lake spur
►6	6.3	Return to Green Creek Trailhead

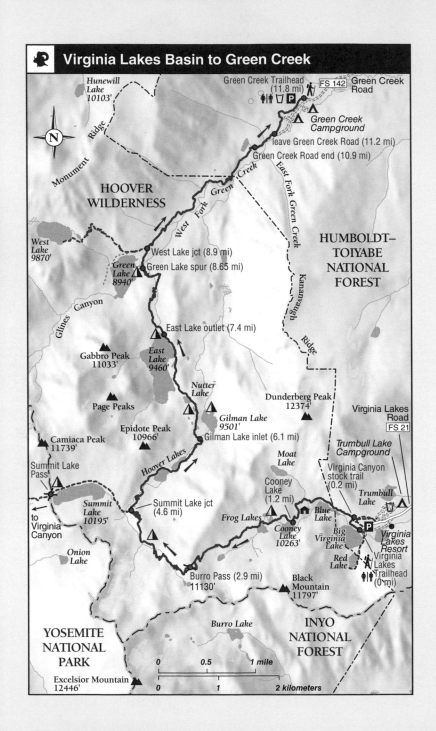

Virginia Lakes Basin to Green Creek

Hunewill
Lake
10103'

Green Creek Trailhead
(11.8 mi)

FS 142 Green Creek
Road

Green Creek
Campground

leave Green Creek Road (11.2 mi)

Green Creek Road end (10.9 mi)

Monument   Ridge

West Fork Green Creek

East Fork Green Creek

HOOVER
WILDERNESS

HUMBOLDT–
TOIYABE
NATIONAL
FOREST

West
Lake
9870'

West Lake jct (8.9 mi)

Green Lake spur (8.65 mi)

Green
Lake
8940'

Glines   Canyon

Kananaugh   Ridge

East Lake outlet (7.4 mi)

Gabbro Peak
11033'

East
Lake
9460'

Nutter
Lake

Dunderberg Peak
12374'

Virginia Lakes
Road

FS 21

Page Peaks

Gilman Lake
9501'

Epidote Peak
10966'

Gilman Lake inlet (6.1 mi)

Trumbull Lake
Campground

Camiaca Peak
11739'

Hoover Lakes

Moat
Lake

Virginia Canyon
stock trail
(0.2 mi)

Summit Lake
Pass

Cooney
Lake
(1.2 mi)

Trumbull
Lake

Summit Lake jct
(4.6 mi)

Frog Lakes

Blue
Lake

to
Virginia
Canyon

Summit
Lake
10195'

Cooney
Lake
10263'

Big
Virginia
Lake

P

Virginia
Lakes
Resort

Onion
Lake

Red
Lake

Virginia
Lakes
Trailhead
(0 mi)

Burro Pass (2.9 mi)
11130'

Black
Mountain
11797'

YOSEMITE
NATIONAL
PARK

Burro Lake

INYO
NATIONAL
FOREST

| 0 | 0.5 | 1 mile |

| 0 | 1 | 2 kilometers |

Excelsior Mountain
12446'

Virginia Lakes Basin to Green Creek

Virginia Lakes attracts a lot of outdoor enthusiasts (hikers, equestrians, anglers) because there is much to offer—and a paved road makes the drive there easy on the passengers. For the hiker there are several general possibilities. First, you can spend a relatively short time exploring one or more of the Virginia Lakes. Second, you can climb above them in rarefied air to Burro Pass to enjoy the views. Third, you can either make a long day hike or a moderate backpack beyond the pass down to the Green Creek Trailhead, passing 10 lakes and several ponds along a mostly descending route. And fourth, you can either day hike to Summit Lake or backpack beyond it down into upper Virginia Canyon, which is the easiest-to-reach classic glacier-smoothed subalpine gorge of the Yosemite north country. This route is popular with equestrians entering Yosemite.

Permits

Overnight visitors require a wilderness permit for the Virginia Lakes Trailhead (as described) or Green Creek Trailhead (hike in reverse), issued by Humboldt–Toiyabe National Forest. Pick up your permit at the Bridgeport Ranger Station.

Maps

This trail is covered by the Tom Harrison *Hoover Wilderness* map (1:63,360 scale), the National Geographic Trails Illustrated *#308 Yosemite NE* map (1:40,000 scale), and the USGS 7.5-minute series *Dunderberg Peak* map (1:24,000 scale).

TRAIL USE
Day Hike, Backpack, Horse

LENGTH
11.8 miles, 4–8 hours (over 1–2 days)

VERTICAL FEET
One-way:
+1,520', –3,370'

DIFFICULTY
– 1 2 **3** 4 5 +

TRAIL TYPE
Point-to-Point

FEATURES
Lake
Stream
Autumn Colors
Wildflowers
Great Views
Camping
Swimming
Secluded
Historical Interest

FACILITIES
Bear Boxes
Campground
Horse Staging
Resort
Restrooms
Water

Best Time

With a trailhead approaching 10,000 feet, small snow patches just below the pass can linger well into July. However, by early July the route to the pass is generally well traveled and easily passable—and the alpine wildflowers are at their height. To avoid crowds, hike in September, when fall colors abound.

Dunderberg Peak's periodic rockfalls create talus that is home for yellow-bellied marmots and pikas.

Finding the Trail

From Bridgeport, drive south on US 395 through the town to the Bridgeport Ranger Station, near its south edge. Continue 12.1 miles south on US 395 to Conway Summit and the Virginia Lakes Road (Forest Service Road 21) junction. If you're traveling from the south, Conway Summit lies 12.8 miles north of the CA 120 junction in Lee Vining.

Turning west onto Virginia Lakes Road, this broad, paved road climbs 4.5 miles to an easily missed junction with broad, well-graded Dunderberg Meadow Road (FS 20). This dirt road winds 9 miles north to a junction with Green Creek Road (FS 142) and is one

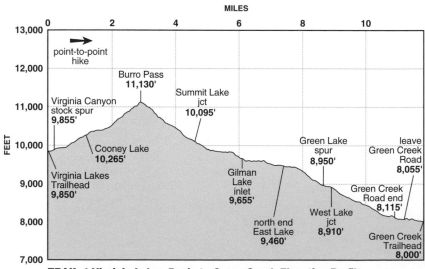

TRAIL 4 Virginia Lakes Basin to Green Creek Elevation Profile

route to the previous trip's trailhead and the shortest route to shuttle a second car to the ending point for this point-to-point walk. Once at the Green Creek Road junction, turn left (west) and follow FS 142 for 5.1 miles to an obvious trailhead parking area, with an outhouse and water spigot, on the right. You can also detour down to US 395 and drive up Green Creek Road from its junction with US 395 if you wish to minimize dirt road driving, but Dunderberg Meadow Road is in good condition and considerably faster.

As your hike starts from the Virginia Lakes Trailhead, for now continue straight an additional 1.6 miles along the paved Virginia Lakes Road up to a moderate-size trailhead at road's end, passing along the way first the Virginia Lakes Pack Station on the right, a tract of vacation homes, the Virginia Lakes Resort (with café) on the left, and finally the Trumbull Lake Campground on the right. Just past the campground, the road reverts to gravel. Trumbull Lake Campground has a water faucet.

Trail Description

At an elevation of 9,850 feet, the trail departs from the west side of the parking area, near the toilets and information signs. ▶1 Numerous use trails around Big Virginia Lake can make it difficult to discern the correct route—turn right (northwest) at the lake's edge and continue until the shoreline bends west. The trail now briefly jogs north, entering a stand of aspens, curving left again where you reach a junction with a horse trail merging from the right (0.2 mile). ▶2

Under sparse subalpine shade, your trail quickly passes a tarn and then reaches the Hoover Wilderness boundary. A fisherman's trail branches to the left, dropping slightly to 9,886-foot-high Blue Lake. Staying on the main route, Blue Lake comes into view a moment later, cupped in steep slopes of ruddy-brown hornfels—a metamorphic rock that doesn't have layers. Early summer colorful wildflowers emerge from the scant soil covering the rock. As you climb gently to moderately above the north shore of Blue Lake, you cross talus derived from rusty-weathered Dunderberg Peak high to your north.

At Blue Lake's western headwall, your way climbs steeply, the ascent pausing briefly as the trail rounds an immense talus fan to the verdant banks of Moat Lake's merrily descending outlet stream. Soon after you step across the creek, a steeply clambering use trail ascends to the unseen lake. Now your trail switchbacks more gradually up a forested hillside to reach a small miner's cabin in a clearing. After another short climb

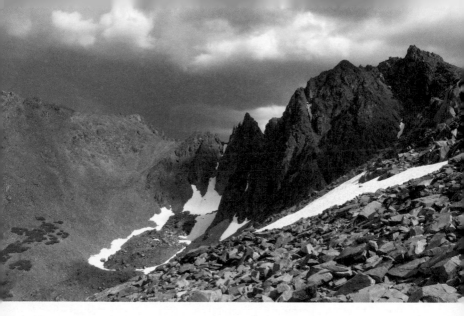

View south *from Burro Pass*

on steep bluffs, you arrive at the outlet of Cooney Lake (1.2 miles), ▶3 which occupies a low bench in this austere timberline upland. A few small camps are found south of the inlet in wind-tortured knots of whitebark pines, reached by a footpath across the low bench. As you leave the lake, views open to your trip's barren high point, Burro Pass (a local name; the pass is unnamed on maps). The pass saddles the western horizon; its metamorphosed tuffs look cream-colored against the surrounding, darker, metamorphosed lavas, such as Black Mountain, to your south.

Beyond Cooney Lake you ascend gently west into a rocky-meadowed draw. Just before you step across infant Virginia Creek, a short path leads north to several better camps. The creek is crossed via rocks and logs, requiring a keen sense of balance (or wet feet) during high flows but becoming a series of simple steps by midsummer. Across the creek you find a second rolling bench, which harbors a clutch of small lakelets—the Frog Lakes—named for once-numerous mountain yellow-legged frogs that have disappeared due to disease and nonnative, but tasty, trout. Now you swing south of the meadowy, lowest Frog Lake—often an early-summer mosquito haven—then ascend above some lush alpine turf, step across the river again, and reach the highest lake, where good camps are found among scattered whitebark pines.

You now leave the meadows and lakes behind and climb steadily through a rocky landscape dotted by whitebark pines. Finally, the trail resolves into switchbacks, then leaves the last whitebark pines behind for a true alpine ascent along the west wall of a cirque. The relatively warm, mineral-rich, easily weathered, water-holding metavolcanic soil here supports an abundance of alpine wildflowers rarely seen elsewhere along a trail. Views across the Virginia Lakes basin continue to improve, then after a burst of short switchbacks—often snow covered through much of July—you gain broad 11,130-foot-high Burro Pass (2.9 miles). ►4 By walking north just a minute from the trail's high point, you can also view the Hoover Lakes, at the base of Epidote Peak, and, in the northwest, Summit Lake, at the base of Camiaca Peak. Continuing off-trail a little higher along this ridge affords views to pointy-tipped Matterhorn Peak, another valley to the northwest.

From the barren, windswept crest, you make an initial descent south, then momentarily switchback northwest. Colorful wildflowers continue to emerge beneath the boulders, especially where you cross a small trickle. Your trail switchbacks northwest down through a small, stark side canyon to a sloping subalpine bench, with small campsites tucked north of the trail. After a third set of switchbacks, you arrive at a junction on a small bench (4.6 miles), ►5 just above East Fork Green Creek. Here you have a choice: Head over to Summit Lake (see the Option on page 75), or descend a popular route past a half dozen lakes and several ponds en route to the Green Creek Trailhead, the primary route described here.

From the junction, your Green Creek Trail descends northeast past a tarn to an excellent overlook downcanyon to the windswept, largely desolate Hoover Lakes. Beyond, light-colored granitic Kavanaugh Ridge peeks over the massive red shoulder of Dunderberg Peak. Heading north, you descend the bench you've been following to the drainage and step across East Fork Green Creek, then traverse across talus above the west shore of upper Hoover Lake before traversing its north shore. At the northeast corner of upper Hoover Lake, you cross its wide, rocky outlet stream (5.45 miles), and in this vicinity you could hike south briefly upslope to exposed camps on small flats above the lake's east shore. For those seeking more sheltered or larger sites, continue ahead to East Lake and Green Lake.

Below Hoover Lake, you drop easily over willowed benches, then circle above less-visited Gilman Lake to cross the East Fork Green Creek again, this time in a stand of hemlocks and whitebark pines (6.1 miles). ►6 Soon afterward, the gradient lessens, and your route rises gently to cross an expanse of bare rocks, still mostly red metamorphic rock. But you also pass outcrops of conglomerate rocks, easily recognized as a collection of pebbles, cobbles, and boulders cemented together. Once past Gilman Lake, you encounter a spur trail used to access campsites on the knob at the lake's north end, and then follow a shallow trench that leads shortly to small, green Nutter Lake (6.55 miles). Camps lie below your trail in subalpine conifers at Nutter Lake's west end. A short northwest climb from Nutter Lake on a pine-mat manzanita–patched slope next presents East Lake, the largest of the Green Creek lakes, spread 100 feet below you under the iron-stained talus skirts of crumbly Epidote Peak, Page Peaks, and Gabbro Peak. The trail parallels the east side of East Lake for most of its 0.75-mile length, passing scattered, usually small campsites on granite benches shaded mostly by whitebark pines. You then reach an extensive camping complex at East Lake's outlet (7.4 miles). ▶7 Fishing is good here for rainbow trout.

Your trail makes the first of three outlet creek crossings just past the lake, then makes an easy 0.3-mile descent to where it begins a moderate 500-foot drop in a relatively dense conifer forest, soon reaching a second crossing. In early summer the creek can be swift, and a slip here will send you down its cascading course—take care. Beyond a third crossing, also requiring care, the trail completes another set of tight switchbacks and then levels off, at which point you can branch left, west, toward Green Lake (8.65 miles) ▶8 and its excellent campsites. At an elevation of 8,940 feet, the lake can be on the nippy side; after a refreshing swim, you'll likely find yourself basking on nearby slabs. However, the lake's relatively large volume and chilly temperatures make it ideal for a good-size trout population.

From the lake you have to cross Green Lake's outlet creek, and in early summer it can be raging, so you'll need to find a log or two to cross it. You'll then make a brief jaunt to a junction (8.9 miles) ▶9 with a trail climbing steeply 1.6 miles up to West Lake, situated in a basin of barren rock—the shores have few trees and above lies a ring of rocky peaks.

From the junction, the Green Creek Trail, the right-hand option, starts a descent, and a rocky knob soon provides a great view down the Green Creek canyon, the best of several to come. Next, the trail descends through a swath of luxuriant wildflowers that dazzle the eyes with myriad colors. By early August, the display is diminished, but so is the water flowing down the trail. In fall this stretch of trail is equally showy, as the leaves on the scrubby aspen trees turn a brilliant yellow. Beyond, you

OPTION: Summit Lake

From the junction ▶5 you turn southwest and drop into a seasonally verdant—indeed downright marshy—meadow and cross three broad, shallow, cobble-paved freshets. Just beyond the meadow you step across the faster flowing outlet stream from Summit Lake and begin a short but steep and cobbly ascent, paralleling the outlet stream. Soon the climb moderates, and you traverse dry sedge flats and benches past some good—but small—hemlock-bower campsites. A tent is advisable because the scattered trees offer little wind protection. Nearing the outlet of usually windswept Summit Lake, you level off (0.4 mile from main route). Angling for small brookies is fair. Now begins a long traverse curving west along the north shore to Summit Lake Pass. In midsummer the moist flats you pass through are an astonishing burst of color, with dense fields of arnicas and lupines providing foreground for your photos. At the west end of the lake, you reach the Yosemite National Park boundary, barely rising above the 10,195-foot-high lake (1.05 miles from main route). Standing at the pass, you are gazing down into remote, lush Virginia Canyon. Staring at the skyline, you can readily identify Virginia Peak, a pointed metamorphic summit that rises above and north of the summits of Stanton Peak and Gray Butte. A few more exposed campsites can be found among clusters of whitebark pines near the pass. Sunset views can be quite spectacular from here.

reenter a taller forest dominated by lodgepole pines and aspens, and you soon descend a dozen short, rocky switchbacks. You soon cross out of Hoover Wilderness and traverse along a rocky bench. Below you, tall, stately Jeffrey pines dominate the forest, and you complete your descent with a brief drop to a step-across creek crossing and reach the dirt Green Creek Road (10.9 miles). ▶10 You follow the road for about 5 minutes before taking a trail branching left (11.2 miles), ▶11 which winds and undulates downcanyon, passing above the campground and reaching the parking area of the Green Creek Trailhead (11.8 miles). ▶12 (Note that you could follow the road all the way to the trailhead, and indeed this is the slightly quicker route, but the trail is a much more scenic way to end your excursion.)

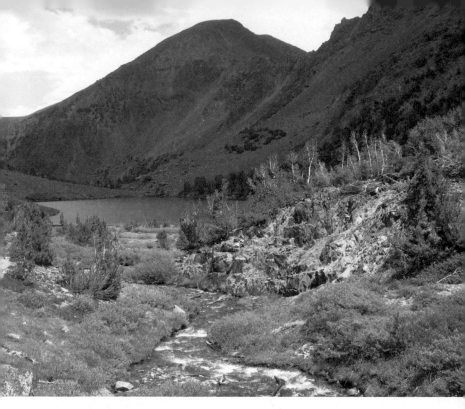

Looking north *to the Hoover Lakes*

Twenty Lakes Basin

This splendid balloon trip from Saddlebag Lake to Lake Helen and back passes more than one lake per mile, plus a number of ponds, and in doing so offers you some of the Sierra's finest subalpine scenery along an easy grade. With the high and low elevations only about 400 feet apart, there are no significant ascents and descents. Still, at over 10,000 feet, you will notice the rarefied air if you try to hurry along. Note that you can cut 3.1 miles off this loop by taking the ferry across Saddlebag Lake—just show up early to get your reservation on busy summer days.

Permits

Overnight visitors require a wilderness permit for the Saddlebag Lake Trailhead, issued by Inyo National Forest. Pick up your permit at the Mono Lake Scenic Area Visitor Center in Lee Vining or at the Tuolumne Meadows Wilderness Center (but not other Yosemite permit-issuing centers).

Maps

This trail is covered by the Tom Harrison *Yosemite High Country* map (1:63,360 scale), the National Geographic Trails Illustrated *#308 Yosemite NE* map (1:40,000 scale), and the USGS 7.5-minute series *Tioga Pass* map (1:24,000 scale).

Best Time

Because the loop trail through this basin is over 10,000 feet, snow can be long-lasting. You may not want to hike before mid-July nor after August, when wildflowers have set seed and temperatures

TRAIL USE
Day Hike, Backpack, Child-Friendly

LENGTH
7.5 miles, 3–6 hours
(over 1–2 days)

VERTICAL FEET
Round-trip: ±950'

DIFFICULTY
– 1 **2** 3 4 5 +

TRAIL TYPE
Balloon

FEATURES
Lake
Wildflowers
Great Views
Camping
Geological Interest

FACILITIES
Bear Boxes
Café
Campground
Restrooms
Water

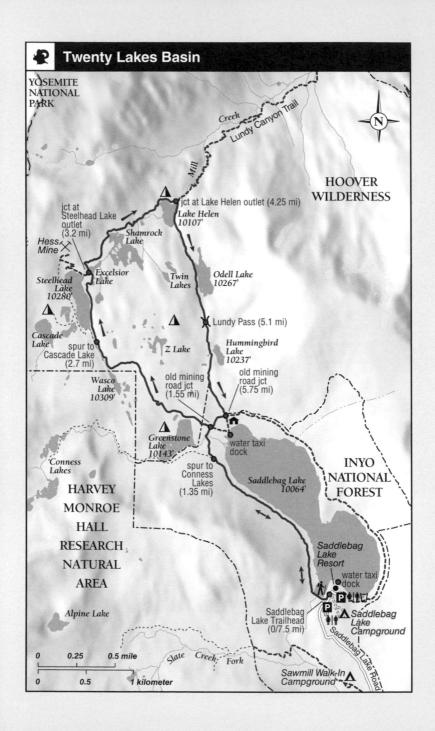

YOSEMITE
NATIONAL
PARK

Creek

Lundy Canyon Trail

Mill

HOOVER
WILDERNESS

jct at Lake Helen outlet (4.25 mi)

jct at
Steelhead Lake
outlet
(3.2 mi)

*Lake Helen
10107'*

*Shamrock
Lake*

*Hess
Mine*

*Excelsior
Lake*

*Steelhead
Lake
10280'*

*Twin
Lakes*

*Odell Lake
10267'*

*Cascade
Lake*

Lundy Pass (5.1 mi)

spur to
Cascade Lake
(2.7 mi)

Z Lake

*Hummingbird
Lake
10237'*

*Wasco
Lake
10309'*

old mining
road jct
(1.55 mi)

old mining
road jct
(5.75 mi)

water taxi
dock

*Greenstone
Lake
10143'*

'Conness
Lakes

spur to
Conness
Lakes
(1.35 mi)

*Saddlebag Lake
10064'*

INYO
NATIONAL
FOREST

HARVEY
MONROE
HALL
RESEARCH
NATURAL
AREA

*Saddlebag
Lake
Resort*

water taxi
dock

Alpine Lake

Saddlebag
Lake Trailhead
(0/7.5 mi)

*Saddlebag
Lake
Campground*

0   0.25   0.5 mile

0   0.5   1 kilometer

Slate   Creek   Fork

*Sawmill Walk-In
Campground*

Saddlebag Lake Road

start to drop. If you dress properly, the often chilly September days can be rewarding because the summer crowds are gone, and the blues of the lakes and sky seem to intensify.

Finding the Trail

From Tioga Pass drive 2.1 miles east on CA 120 (Tioga Road) down to the Saddlebag Lake junction, located a short distance beyond Tioga Pass Resort. Or, from US 395 just south of Lee Vining, drive 9.8 miles west on Tioga Road up to the junction. From the junction, drive 2.4 miles northwest up to Saddlebag Lake on a well-maintained but partially gravel road. Those on a day hike may park in the lot above the store (and restaurant), but backpackers need to use the lot adjacent to the group campground, reached by making a sharp right just as you pass the dam. There are toilets and water faucets near the backpacker parking area and at the parking lot closer to the ferry wharf.

> **The Twenty Lakes Basin is one of the most accessible Sierran locales for viewing alpine wildflowers, thanks to its nutrient-rich metamorphic rocks.**

Trail Description

The road ends in a fairly large trailhead parking area adjacent to the Saddlebag Lake Campground and the Saddlebag Lake Resort, which sells fishing licenses if you don't have one. ▶1 The resort's store also sells

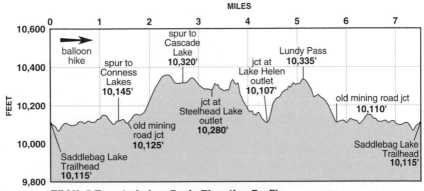

TRAIL 5 Twenty Lakes Basin Elevation Profile

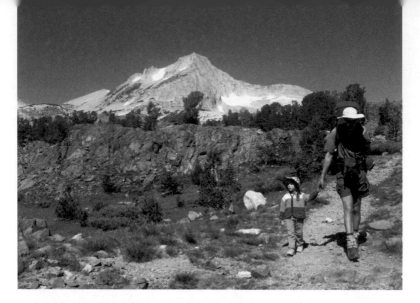

A perfect place *for a family backpacking trip*

fishing supplies and a few groceries, and its café serves breakfast and
lunch but not dinner. Saddlebag Lake often has quite a population of
 anglers in hot pursuit of brook, rainbow, and Kamloops trout. The resort
also offers water taxi service to the lake's far end, running nonstop all day;
if you wish to use this on the return, book a ticket for a prearranged time
before you leave.

To get to the 10,064-foot-high lake's far end, you could hike along a
closed former mining road that parallels the east shore, but a shorter alternative is to hike on a trail that parallels the west shore. From the trailhead
parking entrance, descend to the east end of the dam and cross on the dam
wall. Head across to the trail—a blocky tread cutting across open, equally
blocky talus slopes. This metamorphic rock talus may be uncomfortable to
walk on, but it creates soils superior to those derived from granitic talus,
and hence there is a more luxuriant growth of alpine plants.

About 0.5 mile north of the dam, your trail bends northwest, and
Mount Dana, in the southeast, disappears from view. Shepherd Crest,
straight ahead across Saddlebag Lake, now captivates your attention. Continuing on and on along the red talus slopes, you reach flatter terrain once
you round the end of the ridge. Among willows and a seasonally fiery field
 of Pierson's paintbrush, you pass an unsigned spur trail that leads to the
nearby south shore of 10,143-foot-high Greenstone Lake and beyond to
 Conness Lakes (1.35 miles). ▶2 Soon you reach the north end of Saddlebag
Lake and quickly meet the closed mining road on which water taxi riders

will be hiking, and above this shore your narrow road enters the Hoover Wilderness (1.55 miles). ▶3 Following the old road, you climb gently, staring southwest across Greenstone Lake to the granite wall sweeping up to a crest at Mount Conness, in whose shade lies the Conness Glacier, and due west to sharp-tipped North Peak. The northwest shore of Greenstone Lake sports many camping options, but note that camping is prohibited on the lake's southern shore as well as upstream toward the Conness Lakes. Your tread climbs northwest, and then beyond Z Lake it bends west, crosses the drainage divide, and slightly descends to relatively warm Wasco Lake and a string of tarns often filled with western tree frog tadpoles. You are now in the drainage of northeast-flowing Mill Creek—that was probably the easiest pass you have ever ascended. Just past the second tarn a use trail crosses the small drainage and climbs to Cascade Lake, the west shore of Steelhead Lake, and other hidden lakes, on a bench with the basin's choice campsites (2.7 miles). ▶4

Along the main loop, you quickly arrive at the south tip of 10,280-foot-high Steelhead Lake and follow the former jeep road north alongside the deep lake to its outlet. Diverse and colorful flowers—several species of penstemon, straggly yellow arnicas, and burgundy-colored roseroot— decorate the sandy slopes on either side of the trail. Just before reaching the outlet stream, the old road turns sharply left, crossing the creek west of your route and then continuing northwest above the lake's north shore to the Hess Mine. The main mine is blocked with boulders, but higher up the road is an unblocked mine that goes 150 feet into the mountainside. But even just a short detour up this road quickly gives you an aerial outlook and commanding view of Twenty Lakes Basin. The large, white, horizontal dikes on North Peak stand out well, and pointed Mount Dana pokes its summit just into view on the southeast skyline. You immediately see the distinction in landscape between the granitic peaks to the west and the metamorphic summits to the east; the nearby mines lie near the contact between the two rocks where ore is most likely to be found.

As you cross Steelhead Lake's outlet ▶5 (3.2 miles)—Mill Creek—you are leaving the old road behind and now embark on a route that follows a narrow use trail—generally very obvious, but there are a few places where it becomes faint. You head downstream, scramble over a low knoll, and quickly descend to the west shore of tiny Excelsior Lake, unnamed on most maps. At the north end of Excelsior Lake, you go through a notch just west of a low metamorphic rock knoll that is strewn with granitic glacial erratics. A long, narrow pond quickly comes into view. Your trail

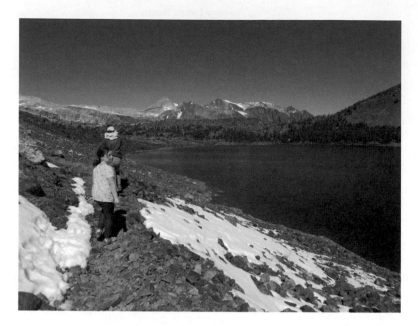

Walking around *Saddlebag Lake*

skirts its west shore, then swings east to the west shore of adjacent, many-armed Shamrock Lake.

Your ducked (marked with stones) route—more cross-country than trail along this section—crosses a talus fan along Shamrock Lake's northern shore, continues northeast over a low ridge, and descends steep slabs and bluffs to reunite with Mill Creek on flatter terrain. You traipse past two ponds and reach the west shore of Lake Helen, sporting some small campsites beneath whitebark pines. Encircling the lake's north shore on a good trail through dark talus, the trail loops down to the narrow channel through which Mill Creek exits Lake Helen, and crosses the creek on a log or rocks. A step beyond the crossing is a junction: your route is to the right (south) toward Lundy Pass and Odell Lake, while the left branch is a rough trail descending to Lundy Canyon (4.25 miles). ▶6

Heading south, the trail is better again, as you skirt the eastern shore of Lake Helen on red scree and then follow an inlet stream upward through a straight, narrow gully that transforms into a wildflower garden as soon as the late-lasting snow melts; the columbines are particularly showy here. The trail continues alongside the remarkably straight creek channel until you climb above the creek's western bank and shortly approach Odell Lake. Climbing gently above the lake's shore, you parallel the west shore southward while observing the lobes of slowly seasonally flowing talus just east of the lake. The most gradual of climbs continues to Lundy Pass (5.1 miles), ►7 another astoundingly shallow pass that drops you back into the Lee Vining Creek drainage. Turning west from this gap will take you to some small campsites near Z Lake, while the trail continues south toward Hummingbird Lake, boasting terrific lakeshore for an afternoon break. Beyond, the trail parallels the east side of the sea- sonal outlet creek to reach a four-way junction where you again intersect the old mining road (5.75 miles). ►8 The main route around the lake is right (west), a 0.5-mile-longer route around the lake is left (east; along the old mining road, passing some spectacular wet gullies of flowers), and straight ahead (south) takes you to the water taxi dock on Saddlebag Lake. If you decide to retrace your steps from this morning, turn right and you will soon reach a junction where you turn left (south); this was the junction you passed as you began the loop. Now retrace your steps to the trailhead (7.5 miles). ►9

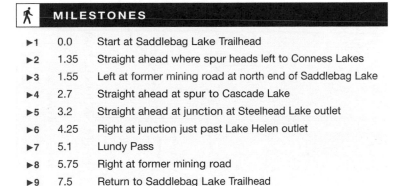

👣	**MILESTONES**	
►1	0.0	Start at Saddlebag Lake Trailhead
►2	1.35	Straight ahead where spur heads left to Conness Lakes
►3	1.55	Left at former mining road at north end of Saddlebag Lake
►4	2.7	Straight ahead at spur to Cascade Lake
►5	3.2	Straight ahead at junction at Steelhead Lake outlet
►6	4.25	Right at junction just past Lake Helen outlet
►7	5.1	Lundy Pass
►8	5.75	Right at former mining road
►9	7.5	Return to Saddlebag Lake Trailhead

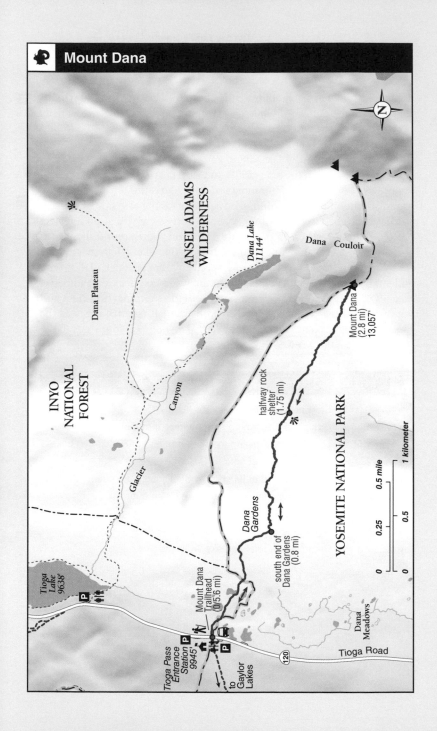

Mount Dana

ANSEL ADAMS WILDERNESS

INYO NATIONAL FOREST

Dana Plateau

Dana Lake 11144'

Canyon

Dana Couloir

Glacier

Mount Dana (2.8 mi) 13,057'

halfway rock shelter (1.75 mi)

Dana Gardens

south end of Dana Gardens (0.8 mi)

YOSEMITE NATIONAL PARK

Tioga Lake 9638'

Mount Dana Trailhead (0/5.6 mi)

Dana Meadows

Tioga Pass Entrance Station 9945'

to Gaylor Lakes

Tioga Road

120

0   0.25   0.5   0.5 mile

0   0.5   1 kilometer

Mount Dana

Dark glasses and good health are both necessary for this climb to the second-highest summit in Yosemite. Only Mount Lyell exceeds it—by about 60 feet—but the Lyell summit is distant, and it requires mountaineering skills. Because Dana is such an accessible big peak, it is very popular, and on weekends you may find dozens of people ascending it. Its summit views are among the Sierra's best, but turn back if the weather looks threatening.

Maps

This trail is covered by the Tom Harrison *Yosemite High Country* and *Mammoth High Country* maps (1:63,360 scale), the National Geographic Trails Illustrated *#308 Yosemite NE* map (1:40,000 scale), and the USGS 7.5-minute series *Tioga Pass* and *Mount Dana* maps (1:24,000 scale).

Best Time

Because this route is between just under 10,000 feet and just over 13,000 feet, snow can linger and obscure parts of the trail, particularly on the middle section, until early July. Higher up, on the windswept slopes, snow often is blown away during winter storms and is snow-free earlier. Both July and August are good months for the ascent, with warm temperatures, but be sure to check the weather forecast; this is not a hike to embark on if thunderstorms threaten. September is fine too, cooler, but with a lower chance of thunderstorms terminating your summit bid. If you dress properly, the usually chilly early- and mid-October days can

TRAIL USE
Day Hike
LENGTH
5.6 miles, 4–6 hours as a day hike
VERTICAL FEET
One-way: +3,140', –20'
Round-trip: ±3,160'
DIFFICULTY
– 1 2 **3** 4 5 +
TRAIL TYPE
Out-and-Back

FEATURES
Summit
Wildflowers
Great Views
Steep
Geological Interest

FACILITIES
Bear Boxes
Campgrounds
Entrance Station
Restrooms
Shuttle Stop

Probably in the 1930s, Yosemite's eminent botanist, Carl Sharsmith, established this route to minimize impact to the fragile alpine environment. In 2013 Yosemite National Park restored many of the parallel trails created by hikers and formalized a single main route, again to protect the surrounding vegetation. Please keep to the trails in a location where vegetation grows by the inch and dies by the foot.

be rewarding because the crowds are gone and the sky is a brilliant blue.

Finding the Trail

The trail begins on Tioga Road (CA 120) at Tioga Pass, the park's eastern entrance. The entrance station is 7 miles east of the Tuolumne Meadows Campground and 12 miles west of the US 395–CA 120 junction in Lee Vining. If you are coming from Lee Vining (from the east), consider parking in the large pullout just before you reach the entrance station because parking is quite limited once in the park. For those coming from the Tuolumne Meadows direction, the Gaylor Lakes Trailhead or a parking lot across the street from it are the best choices.

There are three shuttle buses a day from the Tuolumne Meadows Lodge; if you are staying at the Tuolumne Meadows Campground and wish to use this service, the times are detailed in the newsletter you received when you entered the park. There are toilets across the street at the Gaylor

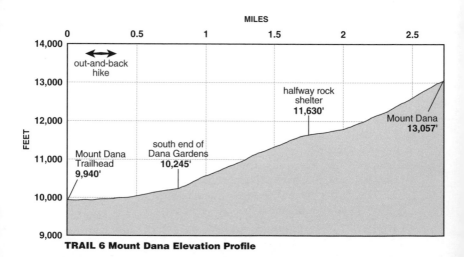

TRAIL 6 Mount Dana Elevation Profile

Lakes Trailhead, but the closest water is at Tuolumne Meadows or one of the campgrounds east of Tioga Pass.

Trail Description

From Tioga Pass, ►1 the footpath starts due east, then meanders southeast between two ponds that are among two dozen that developed when the last major glacier retreated. After 0.4 mile your path starts a moderate ascent, but shortly flattens again and turns south for a delightful traverse through the aptly named Dana Gardens. A mixture of the nutrient-rich metamorphic soils and moisture seeping down the slope makes this one of the most colorful wildflower patches in Yosemite—and that is saying a lot. Indeed all elevations on Mount Dana boast an astounding diversity of species. All too soon the flattish botanical interlude abruptly ends and a steep climb ensues (0.8 mile), ►2 though endless flowers continue to decorate the rocky soils: larkspur, monkshood, spotted fritillary, phlox, western flax, and, soon after the snow melts, the delicate little rock star flowers. The steep, vaguely switchbacking trail continues relentlessly upward, bidding the last trees goodbye, passing a jumble of boulders that marmots and pikas call home, and slowly leaving behind the vegetated lower slopes. Continuing on talus and passing some long-lasting snow slopes, the slope rolls over to an alp. Having completed half the climb, a rest is due in this miniature alpine pasture, and a handy wind shelter is the perfect place to lean back and relax as you stare at the expanding vista (1.75 miles). ►3

The landscape is briefly flatter as you traverse a flower-dotted plain—alpine tundra—toward the rocky slopes above. Several use paths, one more prominent than the others, head up the rubbly slopes of ancient rock to the windblown summit. Up here, it's necessary to wear a hat and dark glasses and cover your skin with sunscreen to protect yourself from the strong rays. Continuing in a southeasterly direction you follow the steep trail straight up the slope ahead. The path is bouldery and you are constantly high-stepping to surmount the next rock. Tall cairns—rock towers—indicate the direction the trail takes, first leading you straight up and then slowly trending south (right). As you climb, the panorama continually expands with elevation, saturating the optic nerves with overpowering vistas. What you don't see until you are just feet from the top is the summit itself—you just sense that the trail is becoming steeper and the ridges to your left and right are converging. Take the ascent slowly because the atmosphere is thin and in your euphoria you can easily

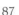

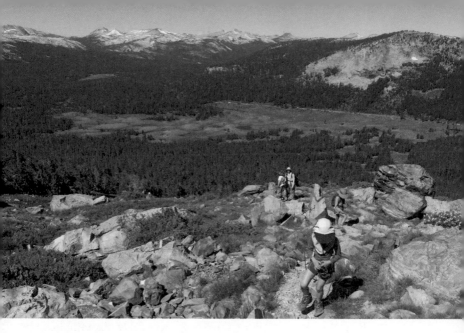

View back to Tuolumne Meadows *on the hike up Mount Dana*

overexert yourself. Being above the 12,000-foot elevation, July hikers may see the sky pilot blooming, with its dense head of blue flowers.

At Mount Dana's summit (2.8 miles), ▶4 at about 13,057 feet, your exhausting efforts are rewarded by a stupendous 360-degree panorama. The Sierra's eastern escarpment can be viewed as far as the Wheeler Crest, about 40 miles to the southeast. East of it extends a long north-south mountain chain, the White Mountains. At the north end of the White Mountains stand the pale, isolated twin summits of Montgomery and Boundary Peaks, both over 13,000 feet high. Below these twin summits rises Crater Mountain, the highest of Mono Domes' (formerly Mono Craters) many volcanic summits and, like most of them, fewer than 10,000 years old. The youthfulness of Mono Domes strongly contrasts with the age of the ancient giant, orbicular Mono Lake, directly north of them, which may be over 1 million years old. During glacial times, Mono Lake was much larger than today. At its maximum size, Lake Russell—glacial Mono Lake—was about 345 square miles in area and up to 950 feet deep, versus about 86 square miles and 186 feet deep in historic time before Los Angeles started diverting water away from it.

Continuing your counterclockwise scan west, you see deep-blue Saddlebag Lake and, above it, the serrated Shepherd Crest. Next comes pointed North Peak, then a true "Matterhorn," Mount Conness. Beyond a sea of dark-green lodgepoles lies Tuolumne Meadows and its sentinel,

Lembert Dome, whose bald summit appears nearly flat from this altitude. On the skyline above them stand Tuolumne Peak and Mount Hoffmann, while south of these stand the craggy summits of the Cathedral Range. Examining the range counterclockwise, you can identify blocky Cathedral Peak, north-pointing Unicorn Peak, clustered Echo Peaks, and the adjacent Cockscomb plus the finlike Matthes Crest extending south from it. A bit farther are sedate Johnson Peak, more profound Rafferty Peak, and broad Tuolumne Pass, through which former Tuolumne glaciers overflowed into the Merced drainage.

To the south-southwest stands the park's highest peak, Mount Lyell (13,114'), flanked by Mount Maclure to the west and pointed Rodgers Peak to the southeast. Mount Ritter and Banner Peak barely poke their triangular summits above Kuna and Koip Peaks, while more rounded Parker Peak and Mount Wood stand above closer Mount Gibbs, and Mount Lewis, of intermediate distance, projects just east of them.

On your descent to your trailhead, try to retrace the way you ascended, resisting the temptation to attempt a different route down (5.6 miles). ►5 While your path was straightforward, albeit exhausting, all other routes ascending Mount Dana are trickier, and most use trails peter out before the bottom.

🚶	**MILESTONES**	
►1	0.0	Start at Mount Dana Trailhead at Tioga Pass
►2	0.8	South end of Dana Gardens
►3	1.75	Halfway rock shelter
►4	2.8	Mount Dana's summit
►5	5.6	Return to Mount Dana Trailhead

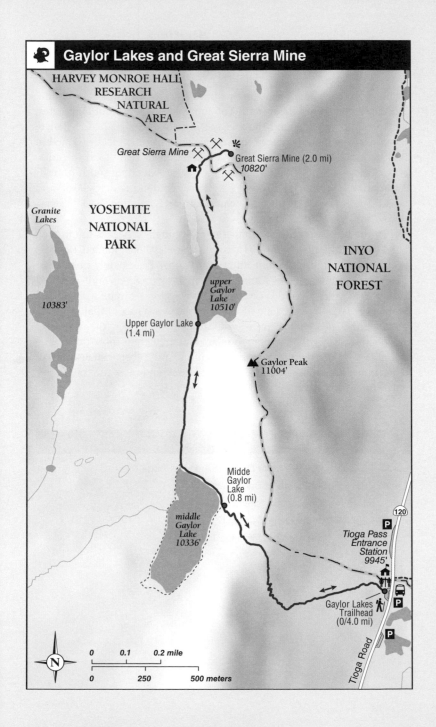

Gaylor Lakes and Great Sierra Mine

HARVEY MONROE HALL
RESEARCH
NATURAL
AREA

Great Sierra Mine

Great Sierra Mine (2.0 mi)
10820'

*Granite
Lakes*

YOSEMITE
NATIONAL
PARK

INYO
NATIONAL
FOREST

*upper
Gaylor
Lake
10510'*

10383'

Upper Gaylor Lake
(1.4 mi)

▲ Gaylor Peak
11004'

Midde
Gaylor
Lake
(0.8 mi)

Tioga Pass
Entrance
Station
9945'

*middle
Gaylor
Lake
10336'*

120

Gaylor Lakes
Trailhead
(0/4.0 mi)

P

P

P

0   0.1   0.2 mile

N

0   250   500 meters

Tioga Road

Gaylor Lakes and Great Sierra Mine

Five subalpine lakes and sweeping panoramas await those who take this hike and its optional side trip, though most visitors visit only middle and upper Gaylor Lakes and perhaps the mining cabins above them. To reach the Granite Lakes, you have a cross-country hike. Camping is not allowed in the Gaylor Lakes area, including the Granite Lakes.

Maps

This trail is covered by the Tom Harrison *Yosemite High Country* map (1:63,360 scale), the National Geographic Trails Illustrated *#308 Yosemite NE* map (1:40,000 scale), and the USGS 7.5-minute series *Tioga Pass* map (1:24,000 scale).

Best Time

Because this route is between about 9,940 and 10,800 feet, snow can be long-lasting. You can usually hike the trail by early July but may encounter patches of snow at the higher elevations, and the stretch of trail beyond middle Gaylor Lake is often soggy. So while late July–early August may be the best time for a good trail tread, late June–July provides the maximum display of wildflowers. By late August the ground cover will begin to adopt fall-colored yellow and red hues, providing a subtler collection of colors that last through much of September. When weather permits, days of mid-September–mid-October offer brisk hikes with bright blue skies and relative solitude.

TRAIL USE
Day Hike,
Child-Friendly

LENGTH
4.0 miles, 2–4 hours

VERTICAL FEET
One-way: +1,110', –240'
Round-trip: ±1,350'

DIFFICULTY
– 1 **2** 3 4 5 +

TRAIL TYPE
Out-and-Back

FEATURES
Lake
Wildflowers
Great Views
Geological Interest
Historical Interest

FACILITIES
Bear Boxes
Campgrounds
Entrance Station
Restrooms
Shuttle Stop

Finding the Trail

The trail begins on Tioga Road (CA 120) at Tioga Pass, the park's eastern entrance. The entrance station is 7 miles east of the Tuolumne Meadows Campground and 12 miles west of the US 395–CA 120 junction in Lee Vining. If you are coming from Lee Vining (from the east), consider parking in the large pullout just before you reach the entrance station because parking is quite limited once in the park. For those coming from the Tuolumne Meadows direction, the best choices are the Gaylor Lakes Trailhead or a parking lot across the street and a bit to the south from it.

In these meadowy uplands are many marmots and Belding's ground squirrels, plus spotted sandpipers, shorebirds identified by their bobbing walk.

Three shuttle buses a day leave from the Tuolumne Meadows Lodge; if you are staying at the Tuolumne Meadows Campground and wish to use the shuttle service, look at the newsletter that you received when you entered the park; it details the times the shuttle runs.

There are toilets at the trailhead, but the closest water is at Tuolumne Meadows or one of the campgrounds east of Tioga Pass.

Trail Description

From the small parking area southwest of the Tioga Pass Entrance Station, ▶1 your rocky trail ascends steeply through lodgepole forest, and

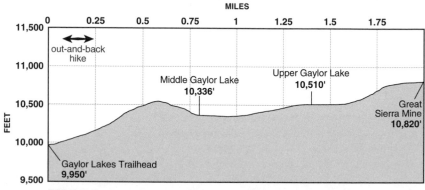

TRAIL 7 Gaylor Lakes and Great Sierra Mine Elevation Profile

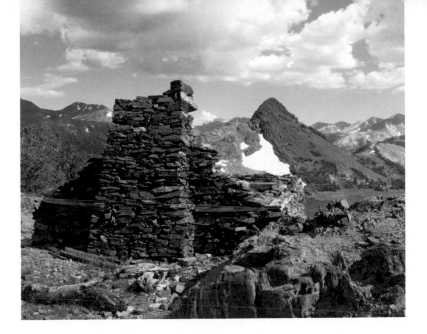

Ruins of *one of the Great Sierra Mine cabins*

in season you pass a profusion of wildflowers. You may also see whitebark pines, and while its bark resembles that of lodgepoles, lodgepole
pines have two needles per bunch while whitebarks have five. Your
steep trail, rutted, incised, and lacking the well-graded switchbacks
of Yosemite's stock trails, begins to level off near the top of the ridge,
and once atop it you have a well-earned view that includes, clockwise
from the north, Gaylor Peak, Tioga Peak, Mount Dana, Mount Gibbs,
the canyon of the Dana Fork Tuolumne, Kuna Peak, Mammoth Peak,
Lyell Canyon, and the peaks of the Cathedral Range. From the vantage
point you can see where red metamorphic rocks to the northeast are in
contact with gray granites to the southwest.

As you move west on the ridgetop, the rocks underfoot become
quite purplish, a hue shared by the flowers of penstemon and lupine,
which obtain their mineral requirements from these rocks. Now the
trail descends steeply past clumps of whitebark pine to middle Gaylor
Lake (0.8 mile) ▶2 and skirts the lake's north shore. On the other side,
the peaks of the Cathedral Range seem to be sinking into the lake, their
summits barely poking above the water. For those wishing to explore
this lake's environs instead of pushing higher, a use trail encircles middle
Gaylor Lake, letting you admire the shimmering waters from all aspects.

The main trail leads up the inlet stream, making a short, gradual
ascent to upper Gaylor Lake (1.4 miles). ▶3 The meadows through here

are strikingly lush in comparison to most Sierran landscapes because the soils derived from the metamorphic rocks provide the plants with a greater supply of nutrients and minerals, allowing a dense carpet of plants to establish. Large boulders dot the landscape—favorite perches of marmots.

Wandering along the shore of the upper lake, you cross the inlet stream, resume a steeper climb, and soon you can see a rock cabin, a century-old relic, built by a mining company that sought to tap the silver veins that run somewhere under Tioga Hill, directly north of the lake. Should you go to the cabin, you can admire the skill of the dry-rock mason who built this long-lasting house near the Sierra Crest. Farther up the hill are other works—including one dangerous hole—left by the miners, in various states of return to nature. Several other cabins are in this area, and they are all that are left of the envisioned "city" of Dana, the site of the (not so) Great Sierra Mine.

Atop Tioga Hill (2.0 miles) ►4, which is just beyond the cabins, you have all the earlier views plus a view down into Lee Vining Canyon. A scant mile northeast of and below Tioga Hill is another "city," Bennettville, which in the 1880s sprang up near the mouth of a tunnel being dug to exploit the silver lodes. Its founder mistakenly projected that its population would rise to 50,000, but at its heyday it did feature several dozen buildings, including a post office. From this vicinity, most folks return to the trailhead (4.0 miles), ►5 but with map in hand, from upper Gaylor Lake, you could navigate 0.4 mile southwest to relatively close alpine lower Granite Lake, following the lake to its southern edge and then returning southeast to middle Gaylor Lake.

🚶	**MILESTONES**	
►1	0.0	Start at Gaylor Lakes Trailhead
►2	0.8	Middle Gaylor Lake
►3	1.4	Upper Gaylor Lake
►4	2.0	Great Sierra Mine
►5	4.0	Return to Gaylor Lakes Trailhead

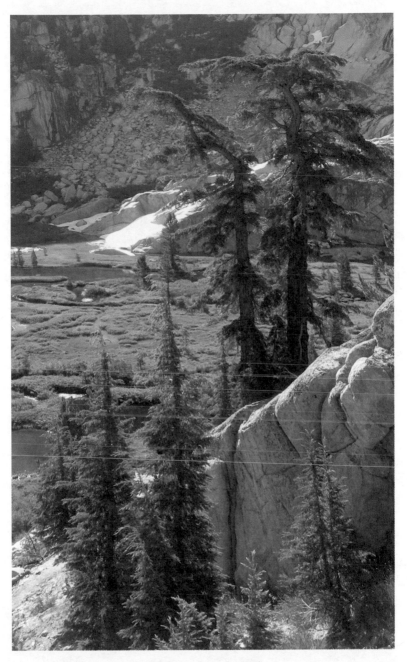

Hemlocks just above Crown Lake *(see Trail 1, page 36)*

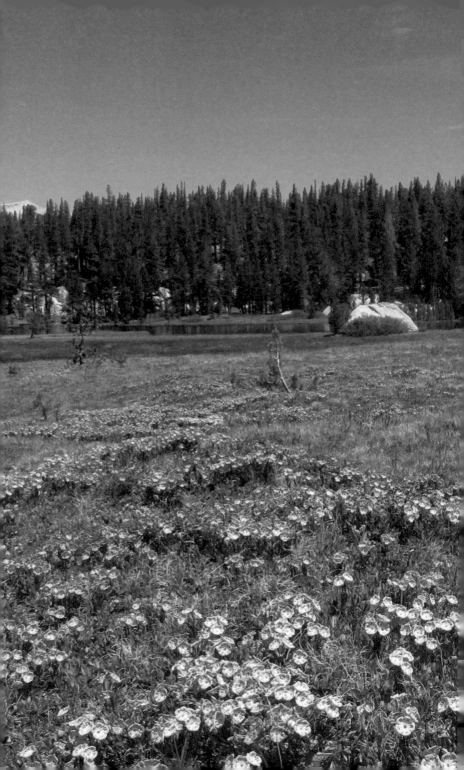

CHAPTER 2

Tuolumne Meadows

The Tuolumne Meadows area receives intensive backpacker use. Consequently, you should reserve a wilderness permit for your overnight hike as early as possible—currently 24 weeks in advance to be precise. The extreme popularity of this area is due in part to its supreme scenery, which is dominated by the Cathedral Range and the Sierra Crest. Its accessibility, thanks to Tioga Road (also known as CA 120), which traverses east-west along the meadows, is the second contributor. From the meadows' trailheads, you can hike in just a few hours' time to crest passes and subalpine lakes. How can one forget the alpenglow on the metamorphic Sierra Crest? The form of twin-towered Cathedral Peak? The beauty of an alpine wildflower garden? The dashing waterfalls and cascades above and below Glen Aulin? These and many other sights continue to lure backpackers and day hikers to this area year after year.

The top trails I've selected for Tuolumne Meadows are mostly relatively easy and short, ranging from an hour or two to three days in length. The only exception is Trail 16, which is the longer part of the High Sierra Camps Loop, which lies south and east of Tioga Road, and is usually hiked in four days.

Trails 15 and 16, when combined, comprise the entire 46.9-mile High Sierra Camps Loop. Along this loop are five High Sierra Camps, each spaced a convenient day's hike from the next. Hikers can either stay at the concessionaire-run camps or camp in nearby campgrounds, most with potable water and toilets. Other visitors make this loop on horseback. Those staying at the camps must carry little more than a day pack because the camps provide meals and bedding. Unfortunately the camps are so popular that a lottery is held each December to determine the lucky relative few who are allowed reservations for the following summer. For a lottery application, visit travelyosemite.com/lodging/high-sierra-camps and submit your application between September 1 and October 31. A few people are also able to obtain

(continued on page 100)

Opposite: *Fields of bog kalmia near the middle Young Lake (see Trail 10, page 115)*

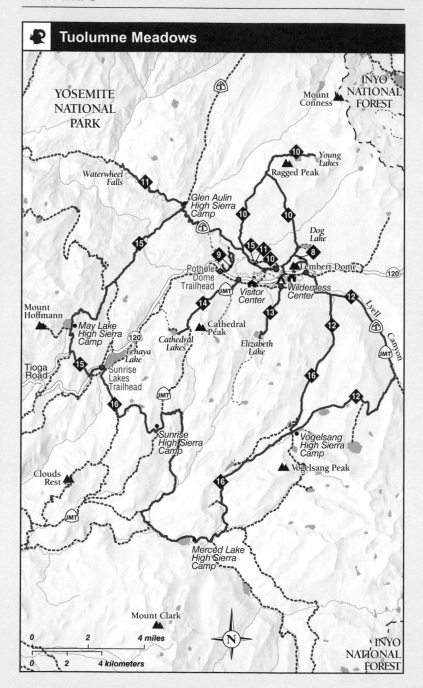

Tuolumne Meadows

YOSEMITE
NATIONAL
PARK

INYO
NATIONAL
FOREST

Mount
Conness

Young
Lakes

Ragged Peak

Waterwheel
Falls

Glen Aulin
High Sierra
Camp

Dog
Lake

Pothole
Dome
Trailhead

Lembert Dome

120

Visitor
Center

Wilderness
Center

Mount
Hoffmann

May Lake
High Sierra
Camp

Cathedral
Peak

Elizabeth
Lake

Lyell
Canyon

Cathedral
Lakes

Tenaya
Lake

Tioga
Road

Sunrise
Lakes
Trailhead

JMT

JMT

Sunrise
High Sierra
Camp

Vogelsang
High Sierra
Camp

Clouds
Rest

Vogelsang Peak

JMT

Merced Lake
High Sierra
Camp

Mount Clark

0   2   4 miles

0   2   4 kilometers

N

INYO
NATIONAL
FOREST

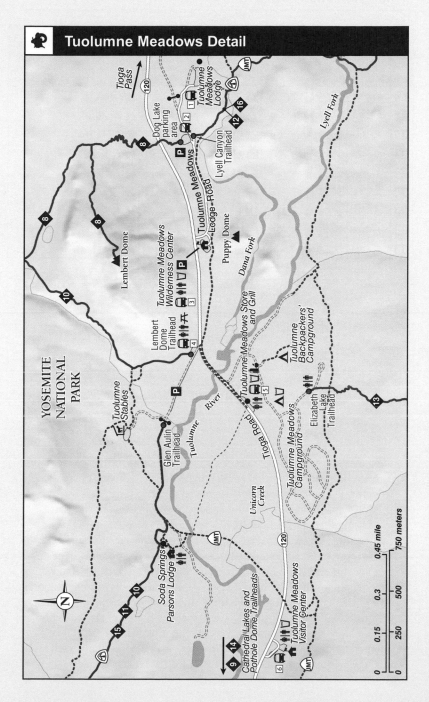

Tioga Pass

120

Tuolumne Meadows Lodge

JMT

Dog Lake parking area

Lyell Fork

1
2
16
12

8

Lyell Canyon Trailhead

P Tuolumne Meadows Lodge·Road

Lembert Dome

8

8

Tuolumne Meadows Wilderness Center

P

Puppy Dome

Dana Fork

10

3

Tuolumne Meadows Store and Grill

Lembert Dome Trailhead

4

Tuolumne Backpackers' Campground

YOSEMITE NATIONAL PARK

Tuolumne River

5

Elizabeth Lake Trailhead

13

P

Tuolumne Stables

Glen Aulin Trailhead

Tuolumne Meadows Campground

Tioga Road

Unicorn Creek

JMT

120

10

Soda Springs Parsons Lodge

11

15

N

Cathedral Lakes and Pothole Dome Trailheads

14

9

Tuolumne Meadows Visitor Center

6

JMT

0.15   0.3   0.45 mile
0 250 500 750 meters

Tuolumne Meadows

Trail	Difficulty	Length	Type	USES & ACCESS	TERRAIN	NATURE	OTHER
8	2	3.9	Out-and-Back	Day Hiking, Child-Friendly	Summit, Lake		Great Views, Swimming, Granite Slabs
9	2	3.0	Loop	Day Hiking, Child-Friendly	Summit, Stream		Great Views, Swimming, Granite Slabs, Geological Interest
10	3	14.1	Loop	Day Hiking, Backpacking, Horses, Running	Lake	Wildflowers	Great Views, Camping
11	4	17.6	Out-and-Back	Day Hiking, Backpacking, Horses, Running	Canyon, Stream, Waterfall		Great Views, Camping, Steep, Granite Slabs, Geological Interest
12	4	19.3	Loop	Day Hiking, Backpacking, Horses	Lake, Stream	Wildflowers	Great Views, Camping, Swimming, Granite Slabs
13	2	4.6	Out-and-Back	Day Hiking, Child-Friendly	Lake	Wildflowers	Great Views
14	2	7.2	Out-and-Back	Day Hiking, Backpacking, Running, Child-Friendly	Lake		Great Views, Camping, Swimming, Granite Slabs
15	4	16.8	Point-to-Point	Day Hiking, Backpacking, Horses, Running	Canyon, Lake, Stream, Waterfall	Wildflowers	Great Views, Camping
16	5	30.1	Point-to-Point	Backpacking, Horses	Canyon, Lake, Stream	Wildflowers	Great Views, Camping, Swimming, Steep, Granite Slabs

TYPE	USES & ACCESS	TERRAIN	NATURE	FEATURES
Point-to-Point	Day Hiking	Canyon	Autumn Colors	Great Views
Loop	Backpacking	Summit	Wildflowers	Camping
Out-and-Back	Horses	Lake	Giant Sequoias	Swimming
Balloon	Running	Stream		Secluded
	Wheelchair Access	Waterfall		Steep
DIFFICULTY	Stroller Access			Granite Slabs
– 1 2 3 4 5 +	Child-Friendly			Historical Interest
less more	Caution			Geological Interest

(continued from page 97)

their meals from the High Sierra Camps, but camp in the backpackers' campgrounds nearby. If this option appeals to you, you must first obtain a wilderness permit and then contact the High Sierra Camps (at the website previously mentioned) to see if meals are available for your trip dates.

I've omitted other long hikes, principally because most hikers do two- to three-day weekend hikes, not because walks deeper into the wilderness surrounding Tuolumne Meadows are less appealing. The most famous omissions are along the tristate Pacific Crest Trail (PCT) heading either south toward Mammoth Lakes (33 miles to Devils Postpile National Monument; concurrent with the John Muir Trail for most of this distance) or north to Sonora Pass some 77 miles away. There are also many other remote loops through northern Yosemite that branch off the PCT at various points north of Tuolumne Meadows. Trail 1 is the only such walk included in this book, following the PCT for 14.3 of its 50 miles; if longer, more remote walks sounds enticing, pick up a copy of the more comprehensive *Yosemite National Park: A Complete Hiker's Guide,* also published by Wilderness Press.

In terms of logistics, note that Tioga Road rarely opens before Memorial Day weekend (late May) and not until late June in high snowfall years. The road generally remains open into November, but overnight parking along the road is prohibited after October 14, effectively ending backpacking to Tuolumne Meadows destinations.

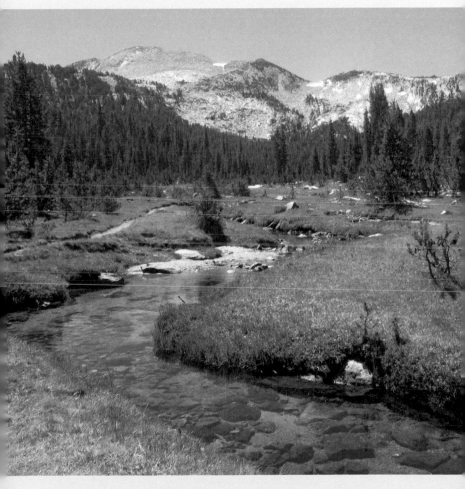

View south *from near Elizabeth Lake (see Trail 13, page 139)*

Tuolumne Meadows

Lembert Dome and Dog Lake 105

This is perhaps the finest short day hike in the Tuolumne Meadows area. If you have just an hour or two, then hike only to the top of Lembert Dome or visit Dog Lake, while a half day suffices to visit both locales. The view from the summit of Lembert Dome contends with the panoramas from much taller peaks. This entire route, being within 4 miles of Tuolumne Meadows, is off-limits to camping.

Pothole Dome and the Tuolumne River 110

Because Pothole Dome is Yosemite's most accessible dome, there are nearly always a few parties ascending its slabs. Its upper slopes and summit provide outstanding views of Tuolumne Meadows and the surrounding peaks and domes. Combining the summit with a visit to the nearby Tuolumne River is a perfect day's outing. There is no camping along these trails.

Young Lakes 115

The Young Lakes are the only reasonably accessible lakes north of Tuolumne Meadows at which camping is allowed, making this isolated cluster of lakes backdropped by the scenic Ragged Peak crest quite popular. Most visitors will backpack to the Young Lakes, but those in good shape can day hike to and from them. This is a relatively long day hike, but the ascent is gradual for most of the route, with a moderate 2,300-foot ascent and descent on the 12.4-mile round-trip hike to the lower lake. The climb to the upper lake is steeper, adding 1.7 miles and 300 feet of elevation gain and loss to your day.

Glen Aulin and Waterwheel Falls ... 122

The popular hike to Glen Aulin is noted for the scenic pools, rapids, cascades, and falls that it passes. Though particularly awe-inspiring with high, early-summer water flows, the polished rock and pools along the Tuolumne River are eye-catching through the summer hiking season. Because the hike descends from Tuolumne Meadows, it is ideal for hikers unaccustomed to high elevations and is also among the first Tuolumne area hikes to be snow-free.

TRAIL 11

Day Hike, Backpack, Horse, Run
17.6 miles,
Out-and-Back
Difficulty: 1 2 3 **4** 5

Vogelsang High Sierra Camp and Lyell Canyon. 131

At 10,130 feet, subalpine Vogelsang is by far the highest of the park's High Sierra Camps, surrounded by near-vertical granite walls, lovely flower-filled meadows, and austere lakes. An extra plus is that with the thin air, you are treated to very starry nights. At such a high elevation, nights and mornings can be brisk. While you can stay at the camp, most folks camp at one of the nearby lakes. Some hikers return directly to Tuolumne Meadows from Vogelsang, but if time permits, looping back over Evelyn Lake and Lyell Canyon showcases some more of Tuolumne Meadows' wonderful surroundings.

TRAIL 12

Day Hike, Backpack, Horse
19.3 miles, Balloon
Difficulty: 1 2 3 **4** 5

Elizabeth Lake. 139

Due to its accessibility, Elizabeth Lake ranks with Dog Lake in popularity. Though Dog Lake is considered the better swimming lake due to its notably warmer water, Elizabeth Lake is the winner for scenery. Sitting on the shore, you stare up to Unicorn Peak or take an after-lunch exploration through the nearby meadows. Camping is prohibited in this drainage.

TRAIL 13

Day Hike, Child-Friendly
4.6 miles,
Out-and-Back
Difficulty: 1 **2** 3 4 5

Lembert Dome and Dog Lake

I would consider this the most breathtaking short walk in the Tuolumne Meadows area and a must-do for all visitors who are comfortable scrambling up the slabs near the summit of Lembert Dome. If you have only an hour or two to spare, then hike only to the top of Lembert Dome. The distance to the summit is short, but remember you are at high elevation and the trail is steep; keep a slow, steady pace to avoid overexerting yourself. If you hike only to the top of Lembert Dome, the round-trip distance is 2.1 miles; if only to Dog Lake, then the round-trip distance is 2.9 miles. This entire route, being within 4 miles of Tuolumne Meadows, is off-limits to backcountry camping.

Maps

This trail is covered by the Tom Harrison *Tuolumne Meadows* map (1:42,240 scale), the National Geographic Trails Illustrated *#308 Yosemite NE* map (1:40,000 scale), and the USGS 7.5-minute series *Tioga Pass* map (1:24,000 scale).

Best Time

Though Tioga Road usually opens by late May, snow patches may persist through much of June. If there is still snow, the trail can be hard to follow, especially on the relatively flat lands between Lembert Dome and Dog Lake, where abundant snow can accumulate and, where under forest cover, it will persist the longest. Around the Dog Lake environs, mosquitoes can be abundant through July, diminishing by early August. Should you want to swim at the lake, early to mid-August is optimal; beyond

TRAIL USE
Day Hike,
Child-Friendly

LENGTH
3.9 miles, 2–4 hours

VERTICAL FEET
One-way: +890', −420'
Round-trip: ±1,010'

DIFFICULTY
− 1 **2** 3 4 5 +

TRAIL TYPE
Out-and-Back with
Spur

FEATURES
Summit
Lake
Great Views
Swimming
Granite Slabs

FACILITIES
Bear Boxes
Campground
Restrooms
Shuttle Stop
Store
Visitor Center
Water

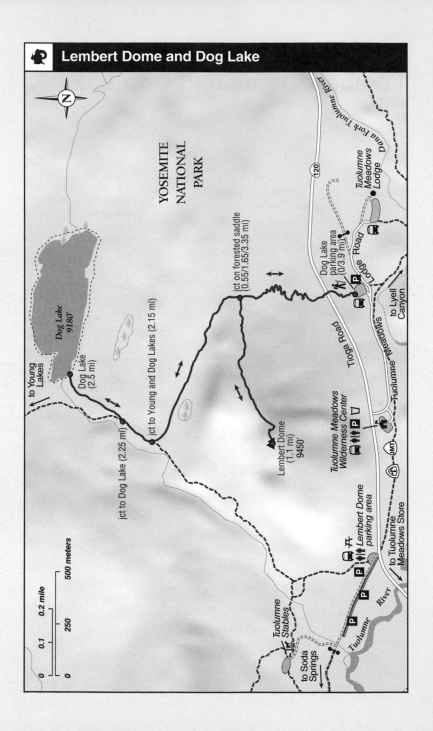

YOSEMITE NATIONAL PARK

Dog Lake 9180'

to Young Lakes

Dog Lake (2.5 mi)

jct to Dog Lake (2.25 mi)

jct to Young and Dog Lakes (2.15 mi)

jct on forested saddle (0.55/1.65/3.35 mi)

Lembert Dome (1.1 mi) 9450'

Tuolumne Meadows Lodge

Dog Lake parking area (0/3.9 mi)

Lodge Road

to Lyell Canyon

Tioga Road

Tuolumne Meadows

Tuolumne Meadows Wilderness Center

JMT

Lembert Dome parking area

Tuolumne Stables

to Tuolumne Meadows Store

Tuolumne River

to Soda Springs

120

Dana Fork Tuolumne River

500 meters

250

0.2 mile

0.1

0

that, this subalpine lake begins to cool considerably. Nonswimmers can appreciate the lake mosquito free in August and September. Beyond that, air temperatures cool notably, so dress warmly.

Finding the Trail

Start from the large parking lot for hikers and backpackers, on the left, 0.4 mile along Tuolumne Meadows Lodge Road. To reach this lot from Tuolumne Meadows Campground (the only campground in the area), drive 0.6 mile northeast on Tioga Road, turning right onto Tuolumne Meadows Lodge Road. If you are descending from Tioga Pass, drive 6.4 miles southwest to the only road that branches left before you reach Tuolumne Meadows; you pass it just beyond a pedestrian crossing and reduced speed limit signs. Along Tuolumne Meadows Lodge Road, pass the Tuolumne Meadows Wilderness Center parking area and a collection of employee houses before reaching the parking lot. The closest water and toilets are at the Tuolumne Meadows Wilderness Center or the Tuolumne Meadows Store.

> Like all glaciated domes, this one is more gently sloped on its upcanyon side and steeply sloped on the opposite side.

Trail Description

From the north end (back) of the parking lot, ▶1 you make a brief, moderate climb on an obvious trail to a crossing of Tioga Road. Onward, you switchback up at a generally moderate grade through dry lodgepole pine forest to a junction just a few steps shy of a broad, lodgepole-forested

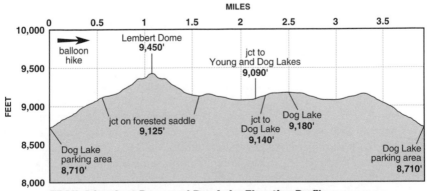

TRAIL 8 Lembert Dome and Dog Lake Elevation Profile

OPTION: Alternate Return

An alternate 0.9-mile-longer return route to your trailhead is, from ►4, to descend a steep trail southwest to a parking lot at the foot of Lembert Dome, then cross Tioga Road and follow the Pacific Crest Trail/John Muir Trail through a meadow back to your starting point. ►8 While this return adds diversity to your walk, I don't find the alternative striking enough to justify the extra distance.

saddle (0.55 mile). ►2 To climb Lembert Dome, branch left and ascend westward on a trail that at first stays just below the crest, winding through open forest to reach a minor gap at 0.95 mile; a subsidiary peak, Dog Dome, lies to the north.

To reach the summit of Lembert Dome, head west across the bedrock slopes. Nearly flat at first, the ridge soon rises steeply before you. At this point veer to the left, descend very slightly, and then arc right up the shallower (but still steep) slabs in front of you. A close examination of the rock will reveal undulations and cracks in the rock; walk along the flatter sections and climb back to the ridge where fractures break the slabs. The best route is identified by a line of hardy plants and whiter rock from the wear of thousands of previous hikers, and you soon reach the summit (1.1 miles). ►3 Even if you pick the perfect route, it can be intimidating, so if you feel unsure, don't do it! Enjoy a long rest on your aerie, admiring the massive red metamorphic summits to the east and the pinnacles of Cathedral Range to the southwest. After exploring the glaciated Lembert Dome summit, retrace your steps first to the minor gap and then to the junction just shy of the forested saddle (1.65 miles). ►4

Onward toward Dog Lake, you turn sharply left, opposite the way you came previously. Beyond the saddle you drop briefly west-northwest, then traverse in the same direction, having a view of the north cliffs of Dog Dome and skirting a pond that in midsummer has wild onions growing in wet ground near its shore. Just a few minutes beyond it you cross the outlet creek of an unseen sedge-filled pond, and soon thereafter reach a trail junction (2.15 miles). ►5

Turning right, head northwest up this trail toward Dog Lake, soon reaching a second junction (2.25 miles); ►6 the left (more westerly) branch is the trail to Young Lakes (Trail 10), while you veer right and make an easy ascent to the outlet at the western end of Dog Lake (2.5 miles). ►7 The official trail ends here, but you could go either right, along the lake's south shore, or left, along its north shore. Encircling the lake is difficult until late summer, due to boggy ground by its eastern end; if you head in this direction, be prepared to detour far from the lakeshore to

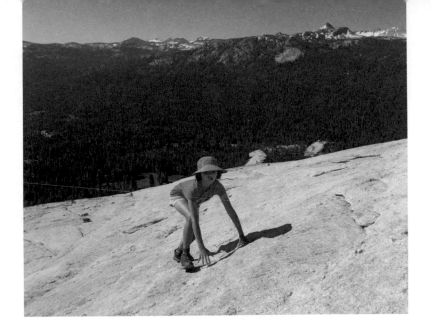

Climbing *Lembert Dome*

avoid disturbing the delicate wetland vegetation. No camping is allowed here because the lake is within 4 miles of Tuolumne Meadows.

From the lake's west shore just north of the outlet creek, you obtain views of Mount Dana, Mount Gibbs, and also Mount Lewis. A long peninsula extends east into the lake from your shoreline, and on it you can walk—usually in knee-deep water—well out into the middle of this large but shallow lake. Because it is shallow, it is one of the high country's warmest lakes, suitable for swimming and just plain relaxing. Leaving Dog Lake, retrace your steps back to the trailhead, but skip the detour up Lembert Dome (3.9 miles). ▶8

🚶	**MILESTONES**	
▶1	0.0	Start at Dog Lake parking area
▶2	0.55	Left at junction on forested saddle
▶3	1.1	Lembert Dome summit
▶4	1.65	Left at junction on forested saddle
▶5	2.15	Right at junction to Young Lakes and Dog Lake
▶6	2.25	Right at junction to Dog Lake
▶7	2.5	Dog Lake
▶8	3.9	Return to Dog Lake parking area

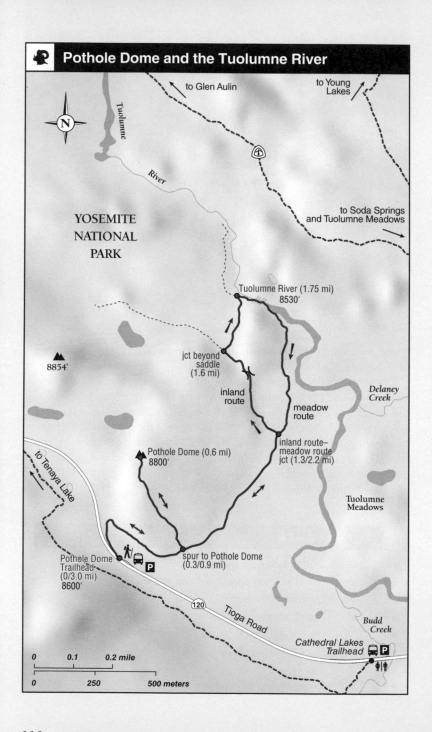

Pothole Dome and the Tuolumne River

to Glen Aulin

to Young
Lakes

YOSEMITE
NATIONAL
PARK

Tuolumne

River

to Soda Springs
and Tuolumne Meadows

Tuolumne River (1.75 mi)
8530'

8854'

jct beyond
saddle
(1.6 mi)

inland
route

meadow
route

Delaney
Creek

inland route–
meadow route
jct (1.3/2.2 mi)

Pothole Dome (0.6 mi)
8800'

Tuolumne
Meadows

to Tenaya Lake

spur to Pothole Dome
(0.3/0.9 mi)

Pothole Dome
Trailhead
(0/3.0 mi)
8600'

P

120

Tioga Road

Budd
Creek

Cathedral Lakes
Trailhead

P

0   0.1   0.2 mile

0   250   500 meters

Pothole Dome and the Tuolumne River

Because Pothole Dome is Yosemite's most accessible dome, there are nearly always people ascending its slopes, but the broad summit area means that you will find your own patch of slab for your break on top. Its upper slopes and summit provide outstanding views of Tuolumne Meadows and the surrounding peaks and domes. Not all visitors climb the dome; many instead take a nearly level use trail to granite slabs along a very scenic stretch of the Tuolumne River.

Maps

This trail is covered by the Tom Harrison *Tuolumne Meadows* map (1:42,240 scale), the National Geographic Trails Illustrated *#308 Yosemite NE* map (1:40,000 scale), and the USGS 7.5-minute series *Falls Ridge* map (1:24,000 scale).

Best Time

If you plan only to climb Pothole Dome, its approach is mostly snow-free by the time Tioga Road opens (late May–mid-June, most years), and once on its summit you'll be above the swarming mosquitoes. Mosquitoes can, however, be prevalent in marshy areas as you head toward the Tuolumne River, especially June–mid-July. Waiting until August is also sensible if you hope to swim in the Tuolumne River—in many years it can be a life-threatening torrent through mid-July, but it almost always will be safe for frolicking in its brisk water in August. If you just want a leisurely stroll, then September is fine, when the river's turbulent flow will be reduced to a

TRAIL USE
Day Hike,
Child-Friendly

LENGTH
3.0 miles, 2–4 hours

VERTICAL FEET
One-way: +260', –330'
Round-trip: ±400'

DIFFICULTY
– 1 **2** 3 4 5 +

TRAIL TYPE
Balloon

FEATURES
Summit
Stream
Great Views
Swimming
Granite Slabs
Geological Interest

FACILITIES
Shuttle Stop
Store
Visitor Center

near trickle and it will be the polished rocks in the riverbed that you will be enjoying.

Finding the Trail

Park in a roadside lot at the westernmost edge of Tuolumne Meadows, 1.25 miles west of the Tuolumne Meadows Visitor Center; Pothole Dome stands prominently across a meadow. The closest water and toilets are at the Tuolumne Meadows Visitor Center or the Tuolumne Meadows Store.

Trail Description

From the trailhead, ▶1 take a trail that starts northwest, looping left along the perimeter of the often-boggy meadow; first parallel CA 120 and then turn east along the base of the dome. Begin your ascent of the dome as soon as you feel safe; the initial slopes are steep but a fun challenge for those partial to a scramble. Continuing to the dome's eastern base reveals slopes with a mellower grade because, like other glaciated Yosemite domes, Pothole Dome has gentle upcanyon slopes and steep downcanyon slopes. If you were to detour north along the dome's western face or climb the steep slabs on the south side, you'll see one or more large potholes, hence the dome's name. These formed as high-velocity streams beneath former glaciers turbulently churned boulders that over time drilled progressively deeper into the bedrock.

The safest routes up to the low dome's summit begin where your trail curves from southeast to northeast (0.3 mile). ▶2 From this spot or

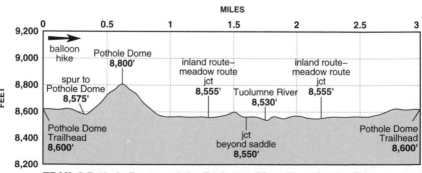

TRAIL 9 Pothole Dome and the Tuolumne River Elevation Profile

any spot north of it, an ascent of Pothole Dome is only a walk up, with an average gradient of about 20%. This is nonetheless steep to walk straight up, and because you are over 8,500 feet, the air is thin; switch-backing up the open bedrock reduces the effort. Already well below the summit you will have an unobstructed view across Tuolumne Meadows, as well as views north, east, and south toward the high peaks beyond the meadows, but continue to the actual summit for a 360-degree panorama that includes most of the park's north country (0.6 mile). ▶3 As you ascend—and descend—Pothole Dome, admire the vestiges of glacial activity. Shallow, parallel scratches indicate the direction in which ice and entrained sand scraped across the rock. Much of the rock is magnificently polished—smooth to the touch and indeed slippery underfoot. Scattered boulders are glacial erratics, rocks entrained in the glacier that were dropped atop the bedrock.

To reach the Tuolumne River, return to the trail at the eastern base of the dome (0.9 mile), ▶4 turn left, and continue, traversing along the dome's eastern base. The trail skirts between the base of the dome and the west edge of the meadow, traversing through meadow stretches and young forest as well as along the base of the dome. In 0.4 mile the trail forks (1.3 miles). ▶5 Both directions reach the Tuolumne River—and indeed combining them into a loop walk is the suggested route. If you are embarking on this walk before mid-July, it is recommended that you start by heading left on the fainter trail because the right fork requires you to walk on steep slabs just above the swiftly flowing river's edge; in times of high flow this is intimidating at a minimum and occasionally dangerous. This section is just before the walk's destination and you'd hate to have to turn back—you can make the decision on the return whether it is sensible to complete the loop or retrace your steps.

The northwest-trending use trail takes you away from the meadow, skirting the northeast base of Pothole Dome, and soon crosses a very minor divide. Ahead your use trail is more poorly defined; if you lose it, note that within minutes of descending from the saddle, the trail reaches a cryptic junction (1.6 miles) ▶6 where you head right, curving north in the direction of the often-audible river and soon reach its banks (1.75 miles). ▶7 This stretch has pools and rapids, and when the water is low, the pools may be safe for swimming, but not when the flow is swift. The water is never warm, but summer days often are and allow you to warm up on glacier-smoothed slabs after a brisk swim. On your return, if water levels make it safe, follow the river's edge on slabs up past a short stretch of cascades. It leads to the northwestern tip of Tuolumne

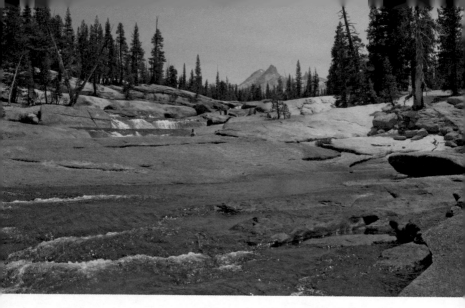

By midsummer *the Tuolumne River is perfect for swimming among slabs and pools.*

Meadows. Because these slopes are water polished in spots and therefore slippery, don't take this route in time of high water, when a slip into the raging river could be fatal; instead retrace your steps on the inland route. If you continue, you'll reach the flat expanse of Tuolumne Meadows as soon as you're above the slabs, pick up a more distinct use trail, and follow it back south, past Pothole Dome and to the trailhead (3.0 miles). ▶8

🚶	MILESTONES	
▶1	0.0	Start at Pothole Dome Trailhead
▶2	0.3	Left on spur trail to Pothole Dome
▶3	0.6	Pothole Dome summit
▶4	0.9	Left on main trail
▶5	1.3	Left at junction between inland and meadow routes
▶6	1.6	Right at cryptic junction beyond saddle
▶7	1.75	Tuolumne River
▶8	3.0	Return to Pothole Dome Trailhead

Young Lakes

The Young Lakes are the only reasonably accessible lakes north of Tuolumne Meadows at which camping is allowed, making this isolated cluster of lakes backdropped by the scenic Ragged Peak crest quite popular. Most visitors will backpack to the Young Lakes, but those in good shape can day hike to and from them. This is a relatively long day hike, but the ascent is gradual for most of the route, with a moderate 2,300-foot ascent and descent on the 12.4-mile round-trip hike to the lower lake. The climb to the upper lake is steeper, adding 1.7 miles and 300 feet of elevation gain and loss to your day.

Permits

Overnight visitors require a wilderness permit for the Young Lakes via Glen Aulin Trailhead (loop as described) or Young Lakes via Dog Lake (loop in reverse), issued by Yosemite National Park. Pick up your permit at the Tuolumne Meadows Wilderness Center, located in the parking lot a short way down Tuolumne Meadows Lodge Road.

Maps

This trail is covered by the Tom Harrison *Tuolumne Meadows* map (1:42,240 scale), the National Geographic Trails Illustrated *#308 Yosemite NE* map (1:40,000 scale), and the USGS 7.5-minute series *Tioga Pass* and *Falls Ridge* maps (1:24,000 scale).

Best Time

Though Tioga Road usually opens by late May (or late June in high snowfall years), this hike is likely to have snow patches well into June, especially in

---

TRAIL USE
Day Hike, Backpack, Horse, Run

LENGTH
14.1 miles, 7–12 hours (over 1–2 days)

VERTICAL FEET
One-way: +1,980', –340'
Round-trip: ±2,620'

DIFFICULTY
– 1 2 **3** 4 5 +

TRAIL TYPE
Balloon

FEATURES
Lake
Wildflowers
Great Views
Camping

FACILITIES
Bear Boxes
Campground
Horse Staging
Picnic Tables
Restrooms
Shuttle Stop
Store
Visitor Center

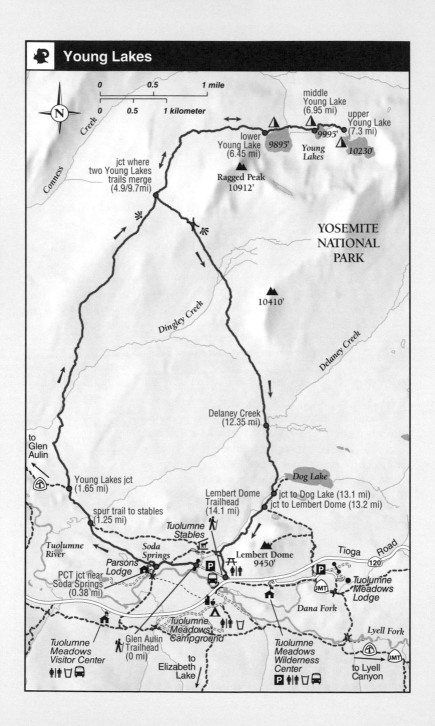

0   0.5   1 mile

0   0.5   1 kilometer

N

Conness   *Creek*

middle
Young Lake
(6.95 mi)

upper
Young Lake
(7.3 mi)

lower
Young Lake
(6.45 mi)

9995'

10230'

9895'

*Young
Lakes*

jct where
two Young Lakes
trails merge
(4.9/9.7mi)

Ragged Peak
10912'

YOSEMITE
NATIONAL
PARK

10410'

Dingley Creek

Delaney Creek

Delaney Creek
(12.35 mi)

to
Glen
Aulin

Dog Lake

Young Lakes jct
(1.65 mi)

jct to Dog Lake (13.1 mi)
jct to Lembert Dome (13.2 mi)

spur trail to stables
(1.25 mi)

Lembert Dome
Trailhead
(14.1 mi)

*Tuolumne
Stables*

*Tuolumne
River*

*Soda
Springs*

*Parsons
Lodge*

Lembert Dome
9450'

Tioga   Road

120

PCT jct near
Soda Springs
(0.38 mi)

P

P

*Tuolumne
Meadows
Lodge*

JMT

Dana Fork

Lyell Fork

*Tuolumne
Meadows
Campground*

Glen Aulin
Trailhead
(0 mi)

*Tuolumne
Meadows
Visitor Center*

to
Elizabeth
Lake

*Tuolumne
Meadows
Wilderness
Center*

to Lyell
Canyon

JMT

P

the shaded glades north of Ragged Peak. In the Young Lakes environs, mosquitoes can be abundant through July, diminishing by early August.

Should you want to swim at these rather cool lakes, late July–early August is optimal; beyond that, these subalpine lakes begin to cool considerably. The air temperatures begin to cool notably in September, though the walk is still pleasant for a day hike or an overnight walk for those with warm layers.

John Lembert sold the Soda Springs lands to the Sierra Club in 1912, and for 60 years club members then enjoyed their own private campground in Tuolumne Meadows.

Finding the Trail

Toward the east end of Tuolumne Meadows, immediately northeast of the Tuolumne River, turn left off Tioga Road onto a dirt road starting west from the base of Lembert Dome. This road passes the small Lembert Dome parking area (where this loop ends) and continues 0.3 mile to a locked gate; you can park anywhere along this stretch because you will have to walk the length of the road at either the start or end of your hike. Alternately, just before the locked gate, turn right (north) to the Tuolumne Stables, where there is a large parking area. You can retrace your steps to the official trailhead, or use the connecting trails fanning out from the stables parking area; both are a similar hiking distance. The mileage is measured from the locked gate (Glen Aulin Trailhead). The closest water and toilets are at the Tuolumne Wilderness Center or the Tuolumne Meadows Store.

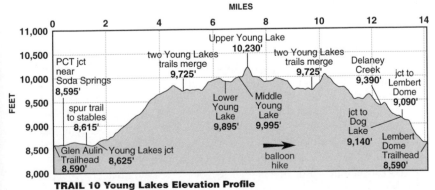

TRAIL 10 Young Lakes Elevation Profile

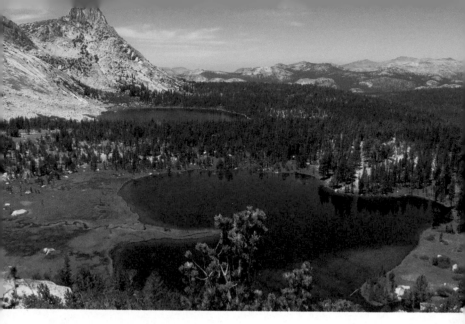

Looking down *on the two lower Young Lakes*

Trail Description

Leaving the spread-out parking area, you pass a locked gate ▶1 and continue west along an old road at the edge of Tuolumne Meadows. On it you are treated to fine views south toward Unicorn Peak, Cathedral Peak, and some of the knobby Echo Peaks. After about 0.25 mile you meet a trail heading northeast to the horse stables, and about 600 feet past this junction, you face a split (0.38 mile). ▶2 The more prominent left branch heads over to a bridge across the nearby Tuolumne River, but take the right path marked as the Pacific Crest Trail (PCT). It veers right, slightly uphill, and quickly encounters a spur trail that leads to the still-bubbling natural Soda Springs. It is worth a detour to look at the springs and historic Parsons Lodge before arcing right and continuing on your way along the trail signposted for the PCT and Glen Aulin.

Trending to the northwest, your trail undulates past a reed-filled tarn, across dry granite flats, and through a forest of sparse, small lodgepole pines to reach a spur trail coming from the stables (1.25 miles). ▶3 If you parked at the stables, this is most likely where you will join the described route. Just beyond, the trail descends to cross Delaney Creek, a possibly intimidating crossing. Currently there are no logs spanning the flow, and during the high water flows common on warm June days, you will want to cross early in the day; amazingly, by late summer you can boulder-hop the channel. Beyond a second smaller tributary, you reach the junction to Young Lakes (1.65 miles), ▶4 on which you branch right, north, while the PCT continues left along the Tuolumne River toward Glen Aulin.

Turning right, you ascend slightly and cross a broad expanse of boulder-strewn, grass-pocketed, glaciated sheet granite. An open spot affords a look south across broad Tuolumne Meadows to the line of peaks from Fairview Dome to the steeplelike spires of the Cathedral Range. Ascending the open, glacier-polished granite, you follow a line of boulders denoting the route, for a trail cannot be constructed on bedrock. Beyond, the trail tread resumes and climbs northward on a tree-clothed slope, the first 2 miles moderately, the next mile gently, to a ridge. The trail remains just south of the ridge, denying the hiker spectacular northward vistas. Detour just 100 feet north from the trail, and on the other side of the ridge, a new panoply of peaks appears in the north—majestic Tower Peak, Doghead and Quarry Peaks, the Finger Peaks, Matterhorn Peak, Sheep Peak, Mount Conness, and the Shepherd Crest. From this high viewpoint a moderate descent leads to a step-across crossing of a usually flowing tributary of Conness Creek and, just beyond, a junction with a southeast-climbing trail, the other Young Lakes Trail, your return route (4.9 miles). ▶5

Now you start a roller coaster traverse northeast through a cool forest of mountain hemlocks, lodgepoles, and western white pines. On a level stretch of trail, you cross a diminutive branch of Conness Creek and then switchback 0.25 mile up to a plateau from where the view is fine of the steep northwest face of Ragged Peak. After rounding the edge of a meadow, you descend to the lower Young Lake (6.45 miles), ▶6 whose north shore easily has the most campsites of the three lakes—and indeed most hikers camp here, though it is recommended that everyone visit the upper lakes as a side trip. Backpackers should bring a tent because there can be hordes of mosquitoes at any of the Young Lakes in the morning and evening (or all day) until late July or early August. Furthermore, afternoon to evening thunderstorms can occur anytime during the summer months. At about 9,900 feet, lower Young Lake lies in the subalpine realm, so it still has sufficient trees for shade and to diminish the sometimes strong late-afternoon winds.

From the lake's northeast corner you can hop its outlet creek—a possibly wet ford in early summer if logs aren't available—and take a trail east. Remaining on the north side of the inlet stream, the route parallels the creek east moderately up to the relatively small middle

Young Lake (6.95 miles). ►7 The most-used campsites are on a rocky ridge above the middle lake's northwest shore, but there are also options farther to the northeast, nestled in a grove of lodgepole pines.

To reach the uppermost lake, after encircling the middle lake's north shore, most people follow a use trail just north of the creek, but it is narrow, eroded, and often muddy. A better, if sometimes cryptic, use trail stays just slightly farther to the north, meandering eastward up to benchlands across which you make an easy, nearly level, open, scenic traverse southeast to the upper Young Lake (7.3 miles). ►8 At about 10,230 feet, it lies in the lower alpine realm, and small clusters of whitebark pines offer little protection from the elements. A few small campsites are along its north and west shores; for some the open views from their campsites are a sublime treat, while others prefer the greater protection afforded at the lower lakes. If you do camp here, remember that the alpine turf is fragile, and restrict your site selection to sandy, previously used locations.

After exploring the Young Lakes area, retrace your steps to the junction where the two Young Lakes trails merge (9.7 miles). ►9 Turning left, you will now take the route that passes close to Dog Lake. First make a steep ascent on a boulder-dotted slope under a forest cover of lodgepoles and hemlocks. As the trail ascends, the trees diminish in density and change in species to a predominance of whitebark pines. From the southwest shoulder of Ragged Peak, the trail quickly enters and then descends through a very large, gently sloping meadow. This broad, well-watered expanse is a wildflower garden in season, laced with meandering brooks. Numerous species of wildflowers in the foreground set off the marvelous views of the entire Cathedral Range, strung out on the southern horizon—indeed the reason for completing the loop in this direction is to imbibe this view as you descend. (If you were thinking of camping here, note that you are just under 4 trail miles from the trailhead, making it an illegal place to pitch your tent.)

Near the lower edge of the meadow, you hop across multiple small creeks as you cross the headwaters of Dingley Creek. Beyond you descend steeply at times, past exfoliating Peak 10,410, to reach a seasonal creek in a mixed forest of lodgepole and hemlock. Another seasonal creek is crossed, and then you make a short but noticeable climb to the crest of a large, bouldery ridge. Down its gravelly slopes (that is, slower walking), you descend to a very large, level meadow, above which the reddish peaks of Mounts Dana and Gibbs loom in the east. Here Delaney Creek forms a deep channel as it meanders lazily through the sedges and grasses (12.35

miles). ►**10** You cross on a collection of logs because the channel is too wide to leap across and would be a deep (but easy) wade.

After climbing briefly over the crest of a second bouldery ridge, your route drops once more toward Tuolumne Meadows. Lembert Dome can be glimpsed through the trees along this stretch of trail. After 0.4 mile of an easy descent east, your trail levels off in a small, linear meadow and turns south to parallel it. Should you wish to visit Dog Lake, which defi- nitely is worthwhile, the quickest way is to leave the trail just after you hop across its outlet stream and then continue east, reaching its shores in about 400 feet. By adhering to the trail, continue south to reach a junction with the ascending lateral to Dog Lake (Trail 7) (13.1 miles). ►**11**

Turning right, away from Dog Lake, after another 0.1 mile, you reach a junction with a trail that leads east along the north side of Dog and Lembert Domes (13.2 miles). ►**12** You keep southwest (right), parallel the outlet creek from Dog Lake, and switchback quite steeply down a rocky, dusty trail. As the gradient lessens, there are two spur trails west (right) to the stables, while you continue south (left) on beautiful white polished slabs to the west side of Lembert Dome. Passing through a few lodgepole pines, you reach the Lembert Dome parking area (14.1 miles). ►**13**

🚶 MILESTONES

►1	0.0	Start at Glen Aulin Trailhead
►2	0.38	Right on the PCT toward Soda Springs
►3	1.25	Left at junction with stables spur trail
►4	1.65	Right at junction to Young Lakes
►5	4.9	Left where two Young Lakes trails merge
►6	6.45	Lower Young Lake
►7	6.95	Middle Young Lake
►8	7.3	Upper Young Lake
►9	9.7	Left where two Young Lakes trails merge
►10	12.35	Delaney Creek
►11	13.1	Right at lateral to Dog Lake
►12	13.2	Right at Lembert Dome junction
►13	14.1	Finish at Lembert Dome Trailhead

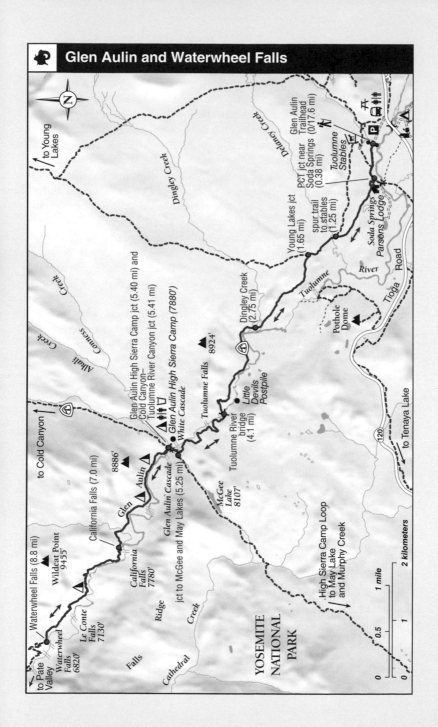

Glen Aulin Trailhead (0/17.6 mi)

PCT jct near Soda Springs (0.38 mi)

Tuolumne Stables

spur trail to stables (1.25 mi)

Young Lakes jct (1.65 mi)

Soda Springs Parsons Lodge

Tuolumne River

Tioga Road

to Young Lakes

Dingley Creek

Dingley Creek (2.75 mi)

Pothole Dome

120

to Tenaya Lake

Conness Creek

Alkali Creek

Glen Aulin High Sierra Camp jct (5.40 mi) and Cold Canyon–Tuolumne River Canyon jct (5.41 mi)

Glen Aulin High Sierra Camp (7880')

8924'

Tuolumne Falls

Little Devils Postpile

to Cold Canyon

White Cascade

8886'

Glen Aulin

Glen Aulin Cascade

California Falls (7.0 mi)

Tuolumne River bridge (4.1 mi)

McGee Lake 8107'

High Sierra Camp Loop to May Lake and Murphy Creek

jct to McGee and May Lakes (5.25 mi)

Waterwheel Falls (8.8 mi)

Wildcat Point 9455'

Le Conte Falls 7130'

California Falls 7780'

Falls Ridge

Creek

Cathedral

to Pate Valley

Waterwheel Falls 6820'

YOSEMITE NATIONAL PARK

1 mile

2 kilometers

0   0.5   1

0   1   2

N

Glen Aulin and Waterwheel Falls

Up to Glen Aulin, this trail coincides with the High Sierra Camps Loop (Trail 15), the Pacific Crest Trail, and the Tahoe–Yosemite Trail. Scenically, this popular hike to Glen Aulin is noted for the pools, rapids, cascades, and falls it passes. Because this hike takes you downhill first, it is ideal for hikers unaccustomed to high elevations. Spending a night at Glen Aulin or farther down along the Tuolumne River gets you partly acclimated, preparing you for the hike back up to your trailhead.

If you are hiking when the river is still swift, which it usually is before mid-July, then it is worth your while to descend an additional 3.4 miles to Waterwheel Falls, which are most dramatic during maximum runoff. However, from Glen Aulin to Waterwheel Falls, you descend (and later ascend) 1,420 feet, more than doubling the elevation gain and loss of your trip.

Permits

Overnight visitors require a wilderness permit for the Glen Aulin Trailhead (first night at Glen Aulin backpackers' camp) or Glen Aulin Pass Thru (first night beyond Glen Aulin backpackers' camp), issued by Yosemite National Park. Pick up your permit at the Tuolumne Meadows Wilderness Center, located in the parking lot a short way down Tuolumne Meadows Lodge Road.

Maps

This trail is covered by the Tom Harrison *Tuolumne Meadows* map (1:42,240 scale), the National Geographic Trails Illustrated *#308 Yosemite NE* map

TRAIL USE
Day Hike, Backpack, Horse, Run

LENGTH
17.6 miles, 7–12 hours (over 1–3 days)

VERTICAL FEET
One-way: +430', –2,200'
Round-trip: ±2,630'

DIFFICULTY
– 1 2 3 **4** 5 +

TRAIL TYPE
Out-and-Back

FEATURES
Canyon
Stream
Waterfall
Great Views
Camping
Steep
Granite Slabs
Geological Interest

FACILITIES
Bear Boxes
Campground
Horse Staging
Picnic Tables
Restrooms
Shuttle Stop
Store
Visitor Center

(1:40,000 scale), and the USGS 7.5-minute series *Falls Ridge and Tioga Pass* maps (1:24,000 scale).

Best Time

Though Tioga Road usually opens by late May (or late June in heavy snow years), shaded sections near the beginning of this walk may have patches of snow well into June, and Glen Aulin proper (the flat valley below the High Sierra Camp) is a near marsh. Through mid-July is also the season when mosquitoes can swarm in unbelievably high numbers around Glen Aulin. Because the falls and cascades above and below Glen Aulin are at their best from about mid-June into early July, those wanting to see Waterwheel Falls in all its glory will simply have to put up with these inconveniences. By August the volume of the Tuolumne River diminishes, changing your experience: now lower water makes for great, if brisk, swimming in its pools, and instead of watching water roar and dash down the granite slopes, you will admire the beautiful polished rock decorated with narrow tentacles of gliding water. For a quieter experience, take this walk in September, when Glen Aulin's High Sierra Camp shuts down, the summer crowds leave, and you pretty much have the backpackers' camp to yourself. With campsites below 8,000 feet, the fall temperatures will be a bit milder than at other Tuolumne-area locations.

Finding the Trail

Toward the east end of Tuolumne Meadows, immediately north of the Tuolumne River, turn off Tioga Road onto a dirt road starting west from

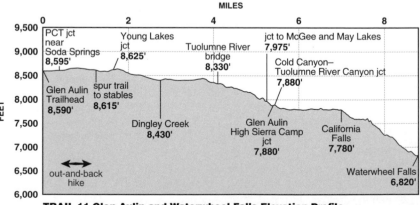

TRAIL 11 Glen Aulin and Waterwheel Falls Elevation Profile

the base of Lembert Dome. This road passes the small Lembert Dome parking area and continues 0.3 mile to a locked gate, the start of the walk; you can park anywhere along this stretch but closer to the gate shortens your walk. Alternately, just before the locked gate, turn right (north) to the Tuolumne Stables, where there is a large parking area. You can retrace your steps to the official trailhead, or use the connecting trails fanning out from the stables parking area; both are a similar hiking distance. The mileage is measured from the locked gate. The closest water and toilets are at the Tuolumne Wilderness Center or the Tuolumne Meadows Store.

Little Devils Postpile is an 8 million-year-old andesite outcrop that fractured to form "columns," much like the columnar basalt observed at its namesake near Mammoth. This rock, however, solidified underground— otherwise it would not have survived the erosive action of subsequent glaciers.

Trail Description

The first 4-plus miles are nearly level, which makes it ideal for joggers. Should you jog, get acclimatized first or else take it very easy when you start.

From the locked gate ▶1 you walk along a service road that skirts the northern edge of Tuolumne Meadows, traipsing through meadow interspersed with clusters of lodgepole pines. On it you are treated to fine views south toward Unicorn Peak, Cathedral Peak, and some of the knobby Echo Peaks. You may also see an occasional marmot foraging for food or Belding's ground squirrels standing upright by their rodent holes. After 0.25 mile you meet a smaller trail heading northeast to the horse stables, and soon thereafter the main trail splits (0.38 mile). ▶2 The left branch heads to a bridge across the nearby Tuolumne River. Your route—the alternative—veers right, slightly uphill, still on an old road, and quickly encounters a spur trail to the bubbling natural Soda Springs. You can follow the spur trail west across this vicinity or continue on the main trail, which arcs counterclockwise; the two reconnect just 0.1 mile to the north. The main trail passes alongside land that was the private holding of John Lembert, namesake of Lembert Dome, from 1895 to 1897 and the site of the old Sierra Club–owned Soda Springs Campground from 1912 to 1976.

From the effervescent Soda Springs, your westbound trail traverses past a shallow tarn and then open sandy flats interspersed with lodgepole

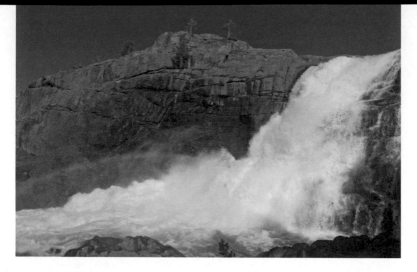

Tuolumne Falls

pine groves where large-scale rock fractures allow deeper soils to accumulate. Another spur trail from the stables soon merges from the southwest (right) (1.25 miles), ▶3 and just beyond you descend to cross Delaney Creek. With significant flow during June and early July, you will want to search for a log to balance across; later on, boulder-hopping will do. High spring runoff in 2017 dislodged the previously used logs, making this crossing dangerous in the afternoons of the highest flow periods—usually in mid-June. Crossing a second smaller tributary, you soon reach the junction to Young Lakes (1.65 miles), ▶4 on which those taking Trail 10 will branch right, north.

You instead veer left (northwest), winding through scattered lodgepoles then descending some bare granite slabs and entering a flat-floored forest. You are now northwest of Tuolumne Meadows, and the unseen Tuolumne River is cascading down slabs just 0.2 mile to your south. A glimpse at a satellite photo would show that your route is carefully chosen: your rambling traverse across the granite slabs picks a route that follows a series of shallow, forested depressions, making for easier walking. A mile's pleasant walking brings you to the west end of a huge meadow near the bank of the Tuolumne River and then to three branches of Dingley Creek (2.75 miles). ▶5 The channels are broad with cobble underfoot; without conveniently located logs they are a wade, albeit never a deep one, during high flows, so make sure to stay in your water shoes (or barefoot) until you've passed all three. From here, the nearly level trail often runs along the river, and in these stretches by the stream, there are numerous glacier-smoothed granite slabs on which to take a break—or dip, if the river's current is slow.

After a mile-long winding traverse, the trail leaves the last slabs to climb briefly on a granite outcrop to get around the river's gorge. You can leave the trail and walk toward a brink, from where you'll see, on the south side of the gorge below you, Little Devils Postpile, which is an 8 million-year-old lava remnant. Back on the trail you wind down to reach a sturdy Tuolumne River bridge (4.1 miles). ▶6 Immediately beyond the bridge you can look north up long Cold Canyon to Matterhorn Peak and Whorl Mountain and, to their right, Mount Conness. The river now flows rapidly down a series of sparkling rapids separated by large pools and wide sheets of water spread out across more slightly inclined granite slabs. The trail alongside this beautiful stretch of river also descends more steeply; you will find the walking rockier, slower, and most certainly harder on the knees. As you descend, give yourself time to gaze at Tuolumne Falls in particular.

The trail twice trends into moist glens west of the river corridor; in the second you pass a junction with the trail to McGee Lake and May Lake (5.25 miles) ▶7 (Trail 15). Just beyond is White Cascade, best viewed before you cross another bridge high above the churning Tuolumne River. During high runoff, you may have to wade just to reach this bridge—note the expanse of rounded river cobble and boulders strewn across the trail. From here it is only a few minutes' walk to the junction (5.4 miles) ▶8 to Glen Aulin High Sierra Camp, which is reached on a spur trail by crossing a bridge over Conness Creek. From the camp a short spur trail leads north past the High Sierra Camp's canvas tents to the heavily used Glen Aulin backpackers' camp, complete with bear-proof food-storage boxes. (Note that the bridge across Conness Creek was destroyed by floodwaters in 2017, but it should be repaired in 2018.)

Many people will walk only as far as Glen Aulin—some for a day hike, others as an overnight destination. Others will choose to camp two nights at Glen Aulin and continue downcanyon on the middle day without the burden of their large packs. However, if you wish to continue with your pack, there are additional campsites downstream. Just note that different wilderness permits are required for camping at the Glen Aulin backpackers' camp versus camping farther downcanyon, so you must make the choice of where to stay in advance of your trip. Whether you continue with or without your pack, if the cascades and waterfalls you've seen so far have whetted your appetite for surging, tumbling spray, then you ought to continue 3.4 miles down to California and Waterwheel Falls for even more spectacular displays of the dashing waters of the Tuolumne River at high volume.

Just 40 feet past the Glen Aulin High Sierra Camp bridge and spur trail, the Tuolumne Canyon Trail leaves the northbound Pacific Crest Trail (5.41 miles) ▶9 and heads left to climb over a low knoll that sports rust-stained metamorphic rocks. From the knoll is an excellent view west down the flat-floored, steep-walled canyon. You switchback quickly down into Glen Aulin proper, and paralleling the Tuolumne River walk through a decidedly marshy (early summer) lodgepole pine forest. Abundant downed trees, the aftermath of the 1987 Glen Aulin Fire, provide useful, if narrow and zigzagging, boardwalks; otherwise it is best to accept wet shoes during June and early July, for the river can lap at the trail, even rearranging the trailside logs at the highest flows. Well-used campsites are about 0.5 mile from the last trail junction and again at 0.85 mile, about halfway along Glen Aulin where the cliff face extends right to the trail. The campsites are north of the trail at the base of the cliffs and small—big groups should plan to camp at the High Sierra Camp. Continuing down to Waterwheel Falls, the campsites become ever more dwarfish and cryptic: Keep your eyes open on the river side of the trail when passing glades of trees or rocky knobs, and remember to camp only in previously used sites along this heavily traveled corridor.

At the far end of the glen, you cross the outlet creek from Mattie Lake, which at times disperses to cover 300 feet of trail. Beyond, you arrive at the brink of cascading California Falls (7.0 miles), ▶10 perched at the base of towering Wildcat Point. Be cautious around these falls and other falls downstream because the bedrock is polished and slippery, even when dry. Switchbacking down beside the cascade, you leave behind the glen's thick forest of predominantly lodgepole pines with associated red firs and descend past scattered Jeffrey pines and junipers and through lots of brush. At the base of the cascade, lodgepoles, western white pines, and red firs return once more as you make a gentle descent north. Near the end of this short stretch, you parallel a long pool, which is a good spot to break for lunch or perhaps take a swim. However, stay away from the pool's outlet, where the Tuolumne River plunges over a brink.

The trail parallels the cascading river as it generally descends through brush and open forest. The water flow composes your experience—at high flows it seems to engulf the entire canyon, lapping at the forest's edge, the thundering noise reverberating off giant boulders through which the trail weaves; with every step you remember that you are following the course of an impressive river. In late summer—or drought years— you eagerly await the trail's bends carrying you back to the river's edge to experience the river. As you descend ever deeper into the Tuolumne River canyon, temperatures increase, undoubtedly noticeable to a hiker and also reflected in the gradual change in conifer species. On this descent, red firs have yielded to white firs, their generally lower-elevation conge- ner, and sugar pines put in their first appearance as you reach the brink of broad Le Conte Falls.

Returning your attention to the waterfalls, Le Conte cascades down fairly open granite slabs with good, safe break spots to the side; this is actually my favorite of the cascades to sit next to, for you can share the

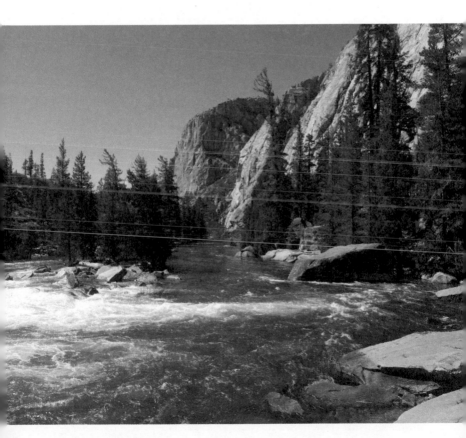

Water churning *beneath Glen Aulin Cascade*

granite slabs with the tumbling water, giving you a good vantage point of some smaller waterwheels. In the forest below, you reach your fifth and final cascade, extensive Waterwheel Falls (8.8 miles). ▶11 This cascade gets its name from the curving sprays of water tossed into the air that occur when the river is flowing with sufficient force. The cascade's classic views are from midway between its brink and its base, at the end of the second zigzag down—a long descent of an increasingly hot slope—but the falls are unfortunately mostly hidden at their brink. You'll probably spot a use trail out to this vicinity. On the slabs that the falls descend, use extreme caution even where the rock is dry. And then you must retrace your steps up, up, up, first to Glen Aulin and then on to the trailhead (17.6 miles). ▶12

🚶	**MILESTONES**	
▶1	0.0	Start at Glen Aulin Trailhead
▶2	0.38	Right on the PCT toward Soda Springs
▶3	1.25	Left at junction with stables spur trail
▶4	1.65	Left at junction to Young Lakes
▶5	2.75	Cross Dingley Creek
▶6	4.1	Tuolumne River bridge
▶7	5.25	Right at junction to McGee and May Lakes
▶8	5.40	Straight at Glen Aulin High Sierra Camp junction
▶9	5.41	Left at Cold Canyon–Tuolumne River Canyon junction
▶10	7.0	California Falls
▶11	8.8	Waterwheel Falls
▶12	17.6	Return to Glen Aulin Trailhead

Vogelsang High Sierra Camp and Lyell Canyon

At about 10,130 feet, subalpine Vogelsang is the highest of the park's High Sierra Camps. At such a high elevation, nights and mornings can be brisk. A plus of high elevation is that you are treated to very starry nights, especially around the time of a new moon, when a section of our Milky Way galaxy is visible streaming across the sky. While a few lucky people win lottery spots for the pricey High Sierra Camp (see "Camping and Lodging," page 20), most folks camp overnight at one of the nearby lakes. All summer, the camping quota fills quickly, so plan ahead and reserve your permit months in advance or be prepared to wait in line for first-come, first-served permits the day before your trip. Alternatively, strong hikers can day hike to and from this camp and its adjacent lakes, though few people will choose to hike the entire 19.3-mile circuit as a day hike.

Permits

Overnight visitors require a wilderness permit for the Rafferty Creek to Vogelsang Trailhead (loop as described) or Lyell Canyon Trailhead (loop in reverse), issued by Yosemite National Park. Pick up your permit at the Tuolumne Meadows Wilderness Center, located in the parking lot a short way down Tuolumne Meadows Lodge Road.

Maps

This trail is covered by the Tom Harrison *Tuolumne Meadows* map (1:42,240 scale), the National Geographic Trails Illustrated *#309 Yosemite SE* map

TRAIL USE
Day Hike, Backpack, Horse
LENGTH
19.3 miles, 8–14 hours (over 1–4 days)
VERTICAL FEET
One-way: +1,590', −140'
Round-trip: ±2,400'
DIFFICULTY
− 1 2 3 **4** 5 +
TRAIL TYPE
Balloon

FEATURES
Lake
Stream
Wildflowers
Great Views
Camping
Swimming
Granite Slabs

FACILITIES
Bear Boxes
Campground
Horse Staging
Restrooms
Shuttle Stop
Store
Visitor Center
Water

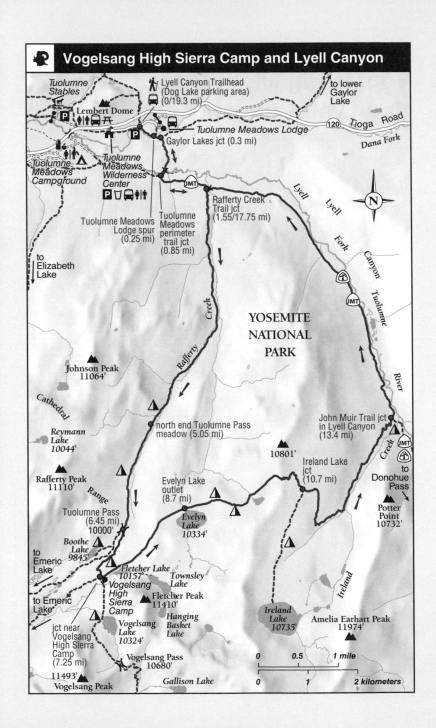

Vogelsang High Sierra Camp and Lyell Canyon

Tuolumne Stables

Lyell Canyon Trailhead
(Dog Lake parking area)
(0/19.3 mi)

to lower
Gaylor
Lake

Lembert Dome

120 Tioga Road

Tuolumne Meadows Lodge

Dana Fork

Gaylor Lakes jct (0.3 mi)

Tuolumne
Meadows
Campground

Tuolumne
Meadows
Wilderness
Center

JMT

Lyell

Lyell

N

Rafferty Creek
Trail jct
(1.55/17.75 mi)

Fork

Canyon

Tuolumne

to Elizabeth
Lake

Tuolumne Meadows
Lodge spur
(0.25 mi)

Tuolumne
Meadows
perimeter
trail jct
(0.85 mi)

Creek

YOSEMITE
NATIONAL
PARK

JMT

Rafferty

Johnson Peak
11064'

Cathedral

River

John Muir Trail jct
in Lyell Canyon
(13.4 mi)

JMT

Reymann
Lake
10044'

north end Tuolumne Pass
meadow (5.05 mi)

10801'

Ireland Lake
jct
(10.7 mi)

to
Donohue
Pass

Rafferty Peak
11110'

Range

Evelyn Lake
outlet
(8.7 mi)

Potter
Point
10732'

Tuolumne Pass
(6.45 mi)
10000'

Evelyn
Lake
10334'

Boothe
Lake
9845'

to
Emeric
Lake

Fletcher Lake
10157'

Townsley
Lake

Vogelsang
High
Sierra
Camp

Fletcher Peak
11410'

Ireland

to Emeric
Lake

Hanging
Basket
Lake

Vogelsang
Lake
10324'

jct near
Vogelsang
High
Sierra
Camp
(7.25 mi)

Ireland
Lake
10735'

Amelia Earhart Peak
11974'

Vogelsang Pass
10680'

11493'
Vogelsang Peak

Gallison Lake

0   0.5   1 mile

0   1   2 kilometers

(1:40,000 scale), and the USGS 7.5-minute series *Vogelsang Peak* map (1:24,000 scale).

Best Time

Though Tioga Road usually opens by late May (to late June in high snow years), this hike is likely to have snow patches until early July, making parts of the trail hard to follow. Be forewarned that mosquitoes can be very abundant through July along the entire route. Of course, the spectacular alpine wildflowers also peak in late June–July. August lacks the vibrant greens and colorful hues of early summer, but the bugs are also gone. The choice is yours! Permits are easier to come by after the Labor Day weekend, and September can be a fine time to hike the trail, often accompanied by brilliant blue skies—but be prepared for subfreezing nights and mornings.

The Vogelsang High Sierra Camp environs are well worth a layover day to explore the diverse lakes nearby, from slab-ringed Vogelsang Lake to meadow-fringed Evelyn Lake, more-forested Boothe Lake, and starkly alpine Townsley Lake.

Finding the Trail

Start from the large parking lot for hikers and backpackers, on the left, 0.4 mile along Tuolumne Meadows Lodge Road. To reach this lot from Tuolumne Meadows Campground (the only campground in the area), drive 0.6 mile northeast on Tioga Road, turning right onto Tuolumne

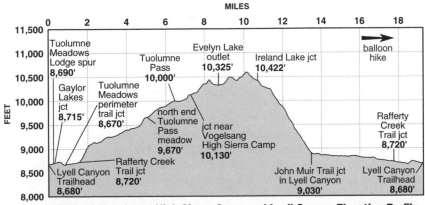

TRAIL 12 Vogelsang High Sierra Camp and Lyell Canyon Elevation Profile

OPTION: Emeric Lake

If you camp in the Vogelsang area and have some spare time to explore nearby, you might also take the time to visit several nearby lakes, including Vogelsang Lake, Fletcher Lake, Boothe Lake, or Emeric Lake (see the map on page 163). Each is different—indeed a visit to all is warranted if you have time or make repeat visits. To reach Emeric Lake, from Vogelsang High Sierra Camp ►7, descend 2.3 miles southwest, most of it along Fletcher Creek, to a scissors junction. At this junction you cross the main trail (which leads from Tuolumne Pass via Boothe Lake to your current location and continues down Emeric Creek to Lewis Creek), following the signpost to Emeric Lake. Vaulting a low bedrock ridge between the junction and the lake, an additional 0.3-mile walk takes you to the east shore of Emeric Lake. You could now follow the trail along the eastern shore or cross the marshy meadow at the lake's head to the western side. At 9,338 feet, this somewhat isolated lake is the lowest one mentioned along this hike, and from about mid-July through early August, swimming is quite pleasant. Should you camp here, look for sites above the lake's northeast or northwest shore in clusters of trees that rise slightly above the marshy meadow. Along the descent to this lake you've lost about 800 feet, which you'll now have to make up on the way out.

Meadows Lodge Road. If you are descending from Tioga Pass, drive 6.4 miles southwest to the only road that branches left before you reach Tuolumne Meadows; you pass it just beyond a pedestrian crossing and reduced speed limit signs. Along Tuolumne Meadows Lodge Road, pass the Tuolumne Meadows Wilderness Center parking area and a collection of employee houses before reaching the parking lot. The closest water and toilets are at the Tuolumne Meadows Wilderness Center. Note that the parking lot near Tuolumne Meadows Lodge is only for lodge guests.

Trail Description

Start on the Pacific Crest Trail (PCT), concurrent with the John Muir Trail (JMT). ►1 The trail runs beside the Dana Fork of the Tuolumne River, slowly diverging from Tuolumne Meadows Lodge Road. You hike east to a junction with a spur trail that goes to the west end of the lodge's parking lot (0.25 mile). ►2 Turning right (south) at this junction, you cross the Dana Fork on a bridge and, after a brief walk upstream, reach a junction ►3 with a trail signposted to the Gaylor Lakes (0.3 mile).

Veering right, away from the Dana Fork, the PCT leads over a slight rise and descends to the Lyell Fork, where two bridges span the river as it churns down polished granite at the west end of a long meadow.

At the southwestern corner of the meadow, you meet a trail that heads 0.9 mile west down the river to the east end of the Tuolumne Meadows Campground (0.85 mile). ►4 The PCT turns left (east), traveling parallel to the Lyell Fork Tuolumne River. Some decades ago, you skirted the edge of the long, lovely meadow bordering the river, but lodgepole pine encroachment means that trees now shield your view, with just brief glimpses to the meadow where slabs extend right to the meadow's edge. Your route leads to a junction on the west bank of Rafferty Creek (1.55 miles), from which the PCT/JMT continues its traverse east, the route on which you will return if you complete the full loop. ►5

Your route, the Rafferty Creek Trail, turns right and immediately begins an often-warm climb at moderate grade through scattered lodgepole pines. The climb eases after 0.5 mile, with the trail assuming a gentler grade to match a change in topography. Paralleling Rafferty Creek upward, you walk across slabs interspersed with sandy patches, hosting colorful blooms for only a few weeks after snowmelt before the ground becomes a rather monotonous gray-beige. In places the landscape is open and offers good views eastward to reddish-brown Mount Dana and Mount Gibbs, as well as gray-white Mammoth Peak, rising northeast of Lyell Canyon. At 3.4 miles the trail slightly changes course and you parallel the now rather diminutive Rafferty Creek upward, crossing a few small tributaries that have rocks to balance on at high flows, becoming trivial as the flow diminishes (or even ceases). You pass a meadow with a few mediocre camping options in the forests that ring it, and soon reenter the thinning lodgepole forest.

Crossing additional seasonal creeks, you exit the last stand of lodgepoles and find yourself in an even larger meadow (5.05 miles). ►6 Through this, you ascend easily upcanyon, having backward views north to the Sierra Crest between Tioga Pass and Mount Conness, and views ahead to cliff-bound, dark-banded Fletcher Peak and Vogelsang Peak to the right of it. This boulder-strewn, marmot-rich meadow leads remarkably gradually to Tuolumne Pass, a major gap in the Cathedral Range (6.45 miles). ►7 At the pass, some lodgepole pines and a few whitebark pines diminish the force of winds that often sweep through it. If your goal is to swim, you would take the right (southwesterly) trail that descends 0.5 mile to Boothe Lake, a slightly warmer alternative to the lakes adjacent to Vogelsang High Sierra Camp. There is a selection of small campsites around the lake.

To reach the Vogelsang area, take the left (slightly more easterly) trail that traverses gradually upward across a moderately steep slope above

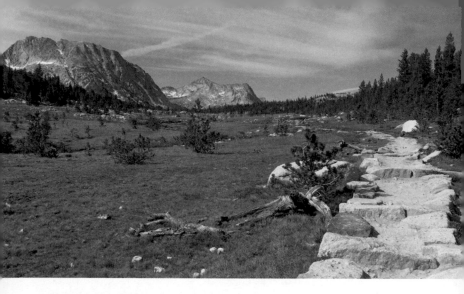

Approaching *Tuolumne Pass*

Boothe Lake. The trail makes a short climb, and as it bends slightly south, the tents of Vogelsang High Sierra Camp are immediately in view, spread out at the foot of Fletcher Peak's rock glacier (7.25 miles). ▶8 At Vogelsang High Sierra Camp, you may buy a few snacks, or even enjoy dinner or breakfast if you have a reservation. Camping on the shores of Fletcher Lake is not allowed. Rather, use a designated camping area just to the northwest of Fletcher Lake, complete with animal-proof food-storage boxes; note there is no longer a pit toilet or potable water for backpackers at Vogelsang. Additional, starker camping options are available among slabs at Vogelsang Lake, 0.6 mile along the trail to Vogelsang Pass (often with fewer early-summer mosquitoes), or at Townsley Lake, 0.4 mile along a use trail from the eastern side of Fletcher Lake (often with horrific mosquitoes and spectacular wildflowers due to surrounding wet meadows). Those wishing to visit Emeric Lake follow Fletcher Creek downstream from the High Sierra Camp (see the Option on page 134).

Many people will choose to explore the Vogelsang environs for a day and then retrace their steps the 7.25 miles to Tuolumne Meadows. Those with additional time (or excess energy) may be interested in a longer alternative: a loop past Evelyn Lake, the Ireland Lake junction, and down to Lyell Canyon, a distance of 12.05 miles to the trailhead. If this appeals to you, follow the northern shore of Fletcher Lake across sparse gravelly meadows, climbing gently to the northeast once you reach the lake's east end. The landscape remains open, with scattered crooked lodgepoles growing in small clusters broken by larger expanses of meadow, as well as polished slab ribs and grassy benches. In early summer moisture trickles across the trail, bringing bright flushes of wildflowers.

At the top of the rise, you walk along a meadowy channel and then turn east as you enter the expansive meadow filling the shelf to the north of Evelyn Lake (8.7 miles at outlet). ►9 Sleeping atop the meadow grasses itself is forbidden—except by the abundant Belding's ground squirrels and marmots—but some lovely sites exist in the sandy patches among slabs both to the west and east of the lake. The views from here are outstanding—in addition to the open views to the north, the Kuna Crest and Koip Peak are now visible to the east, and Fletcher and Parsons Peaks remain dominant to the southwest. Perhaps the best campsites are as you continue eastward, climbing gently toward the next saddle, where you will stumble across multiple picturesque sites partially sheltered by whitebark pines, all with memorable views. Descending, you pass additional campsites and a smaller unnamed lake that you skirt well to the north to avoid its marshy shores. More campsites are found as you ascend the next knob, but the terrain is steeper here and the campsites less ideal. With views to the east, the trail zigzags down between rock benches—the going is slower—leading to the first continuous forest cover in many miles and the junction to Ireland Lake (10.7 miles). ►10 A 1.5-mile track leads to Ireland Lake, a big, deep lake at the rear of an enormous moist meadow. It's worth a detour for the views, but searching for camping near the lake itself is not recommended as it is all grass! Instead, there are a few options about halfway there, near a small stream.

The trail now descends ever more steeply, leading to Lyell Canyon through a dense lodgepole forest just north of Ireland Creek. It is, in places, a surprisingly steep, narrow track—surprising, given the popularity of this route. This is the moistest forest you have walked through on this hike, and the understory is notably denser, with a collection of heath species creating near continuous ground cover. Meanwhile, mixed flocks of small songbirds flit about the trees. The forest starts to thin during the final mile into Lyell Canyon—first because stretches of forest have suffered recent blowdowns, identifiable by the tangle of trees lying about the forest floor, and later because the slabs are closer to the surface, so the soils are thin and the trees are more spaced apart. Marching along, you quite suddenly reach a large camping area and a junction with the PCT/ JMT corridor (13.4 miles). ►11

Turning left, you begin a quicker-paced walk north along Lyell Canyon. Take a break at one of the divine riverside slabs you pass during the first mile along the river. In early summer, listen to the tumbling water and later splay yourself out on the warm slabs for a quick nap—or take a chilly swim. If you plan to spend another night on the trail, do so at the campsite near the last junction or within the next mile of trail because you will soon be back within the 4-trail-mile radius of Tuolumne Meadows, where camping is prohibited. You continue your trot along the river corridor, occasionally near its banks but mostly well to the west to avoid damaging the riparian meadows. At 16.1 miles you skirt away from the river's edge a final time and pass through a notch between some small bluffs, and the trail then turns decisively to the west. Passing through some meadow that is infamously marshy early summer, step carefully or accept wet shoes, but take care not to walk off the trail and damage the surrounding vegetation. Then turning back into dry lodgepole forest, you soon reach a sturdy bridge spanning Rafferty Creek. Just beyond is the junction with the trail ascending Rafferty Creek (17.75 miles), ▶12 where you headed near the beginning of your walk. Now trending right, retrace your steps to the trailhead (19.3 miles). ▶13

🚶	**MILESTONES**	
▶1	0.0	Start at Lyell Canyon Trailhead (Dog Lake parking area)
▶2	0.25	Right at Tuolumne Meadows Lodge junction
▶3	0.3	Right at Gaylor Lakes junction
▶4	0.85	Left at Tuolumne Meadows perimeter trail junction
▶5	1.55	Right onto Rafferty Creek Trail
▶6	5.05	North end Tuolumne Pass meadow
▶7	6.45	Left at Tuolumne Pass junction
▶8	7.25	Left at junction near Vogelsang High Sierra Camp
▶9	8.7	Evelyn Lake outlet
▶10	10.7	Straight at Ireland Lake junction
▶11	13.4	Left at John Muir Trail junction in Lyell Canyon
▶12	17.75	Right at Rafferty Creek Trail junction
▶13	19.3	Return to Lyell Canyon Trailhead

Elizabeth Lake

Due to its accessibility, Elizabeth Lake ranks with Dog Lake (Trail 8) in popularity as a day hike. Dog Lake is certainly better for swimming, Elizabeth Lake for scenery.

Maps

This trail is covered by the Tom Harrison *Tuolumne Meadows* map (1:42,240 scale), the National Geographic Trails Illustrated *#309 Yosemite SE* map (1:40,000 scale), and the USGS 7.5-minute series *Vogelsang Peak* map (1:24,000 scale).

Best Time

Though Tioga Road usually opens by late May (late June in high snow years), this hike is likely to have snow patches through late June, making parts of the trail difficult to follow. Be forewarned that mosquitoes can be very abundant through July along the entire route, and most people seeking a relaxing picnic destination will prefer an August visit. Crowds are usually gone after the Labor Day weekend, and September is a fine time to hike the trail, with cooler temperatures and yellow and red autumn hues replacing the July wildflowers in meadows.

Finding the Trail

If you are driving up Tioga Road, drive east through Tuolumne Meadows toward its east end, passing the store and then reaching the entrance to the Tuolumne Meadows Campground, the only campground in the area. If you are not staying at the campground, you will need to explain to the campground kiosk clerk your reason for entering

TRAIL USE
Day Hike,
Child-Friendly

LENGTH
4.6 miles; 2–4 hours

VERTICAL FEET
One-way: +870', –5'
Round-trip: ±875'

DIFFICULTY
– 1 **2** 3 4 5 +

TRAIL TYPE
Out-and-Back

FEATURES
Lake
Wildflowers
Great Views

FACILITIES
Bear Boxes
Campground
Store
Restrooms
Shuttle Stop
Visitor Center
Water

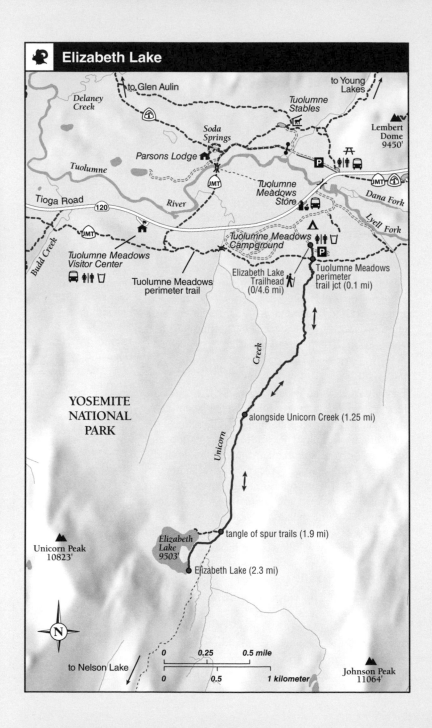

Elizabeth Lake

to Glen Aulin

to Young Lakes

Delaney Creek

Tuolumne Stables

Soda Springs

Lembert Dome 9450'

Parsons Lodge

Tuolumne

P

Tuolumne Meadows Store

Tioga Road

River

JMT

Dana Fork

120

Lyell Fork

JMT

Tuolumne Meadows Campground

Budd Creek

JMT

Tuolumne Meadows Visitor Center

P

Tuolumne Meadows perimeter trail jct (0.1 mi)

Elizabeth Lake Trailhead (0/4.6 mi)

Tuolumne Meadows perimeter trail

Creek

YOSEMITE NATIONAL PARK

alongside Unicorn Creek (1.25 mi)

Unicorn

tangle of spur trails (1.9 mi)

Unicorn Peak 10823'

Elizabeth Lake 9503

Elizabeth Lake (2.3 mi)

N

0   0.25   0.5 mile

to Nelson Lake

0   0.5   1 kilometer

Johnson Peak 11064'

and should then be given a map showing the trailhead location (just past campsite B49). If the trailhead parking is full, you must park outside the campground entrance, adding 0.5 mile each direction to your walk. The campground entrance has a map to help you navigate to the trailhead. If you are staying at the campground, please leave your car at your campsite, as trailhead parking is quite limited. The parking area has toilets and water faucets.

If you wish to camp, consider Nelson Lake, about 6 miles from the trailhead, reached by an unofficial, yet somewhat popular, trail that continues south from the Elizabeth Lake environs.

Trail Description

From the campground trailhead, ▶1 the signed Elizabeth Lake Trail goes south and, after just 200 steps, crosses the well-used Tuolumne Meadows perimeter trail; the perimeter trail heads east to Lyell Canyon and west to Tenaya Lake (0.1 mile). ▶2 You continue straight ahead for a steady southward ascent; because you're above 9,000 feet, the walking requires more exertion than expected. Along this lodgepole pine–shaded climb, the trail crosses several seasonal runnels and slowly trends more southwesterly as it sidles over a small rise to reach the side of Unicorn Creek (1.25 miles). ▶3

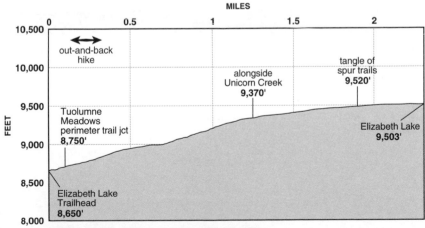

TRAIL 13 Elizabeth Lake Elevation Profile

The gradient now lessens and lodgepoles become both increasingly stunted and spaced farther apart. After an 800-foot climb, you emerge at the foot of a long meadow and are soon faced with a tangle of use trails (1.9 miles). ▶4 All lead to Elizabeth Lake's eastern shore—just make sure that you trend right within the next 5 minutes to avoid missing the lake. During early season, crossing Unicorn Creek—required to reach the lake—can be a wet affair; a long jump or shoes off is required at full flow, but the channel is only wide and deep, not swift-flowing. Picking one of the use trails, you will momentarily reach Elizabeth Lake (2.3 miles to southeast side). ▶5

Few places in Yosemite give so much for so little effort as this lovely subalpine lake, situated at 9,503 feet. Backdropped by Unicorn Peak, Elizabeth Lake faces the snow-topped peaks of the Sierra Crest north of Tuolumne Meadows. From the east and north sides of the lake, the views across the waters to Unicorn Peak are classic. The glacier-carved lake basin is indeed one of the most beautiful in the Tuolumne Meadows area. Though generally a bit cold for swimming, this lake is perfect for a family picnic with some shallow shoreline for splashing. If you have spare time, peruse the meadow wildflowers—pink shooting stars give way to purple asters and yellow monkeyflowers as the season matures. Note that camping is not permitted in this entire drainage, as it all lies within 4 trail miles of Tuolumne Meadows. After a relaxing break, retrace your steps to the campground trailhead (4.6 miles). ▶6

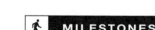

▶1	0.0	Start at Elizabeth Lake Trailhead (in Tuolumne Meadows Campground)
▶2	0.1	Straight at Tuolumne Meadows perimeter trail junction
▶3	1.25	Alongside Unicorn Creek
▶4	1.9	Tangle of spur trails near Elizabeth Lake
▶5	2.3	Elizabeth Lake
▶6	4.6	Return to Elizabeth Lake Trailhead

Lower Cathedral Lake

Justifiably popular lower Cathedral Lake receives much use by backpackers and day hikers alike. Unless you plan your summer far in advance (or are fortunate to score a first-come, first-served permit the day before), you might have to be satisfied with a day hike—a perfectly satisfying alternative for this relatively short walk. You can extend your excursion with a visit to Medlicott and Mariuolumne Domes, worthy goals in themselves. Because shuttle buses operate between Tuolumne Meadows and Tenaya Lake, strong day hikers have another option: after visiting the lower Cathedral Lake, follow the John Muir Trail 4.55 miles to Sunrise High Sierra Camp, then head out and down 5.15 miles to Tenaya Lake, for a grand total of about 15 miles. Then take the shuttle bus back to your trailhead. The trail from Sunrise High Sierra Camp to Tenaya Lake is described beginning on page 182 (Trail 17).

Permits

Overnight visitors require a wilderness permit for the Cathedral Lakes Trailhead, issued by Yosemite National Park. Pick up your permit at the Tuolumne Meadows Wilderness Center, located in the parking lot a short way down Tuolumne Meadows Lodge Road.

Maps

This trail is covered by the Tom Harrison *Tuolumne Meadows* map (1:42,240 scale), the National Geographic Trails Illustrated *#309 Yosemite SE* map (1:40,000 scale), and the USGS 7.5-minute series *Tenaya Lake* map (1:24,000 scale).

TRAIL USE
Day Hike, Backpack,
Run, Child-Friendly

LENGTH
7.2 miles, 3–5 hours
(over 1–2 days)

VERTICAL FEET
One-way: +1,050', –335'
Round-trip: ±1,385'

DIFFICULTY
– 1 **2** 3 4 5 +

TRAIL TYPE
Out-and-Back

FEATURES
Lake
Great Views
Camping
Swimming
Granite Slabs

FACILITIES
Bear Boxes
Campground
Restrooms
Shuttle Stop
Store
Visitor Center

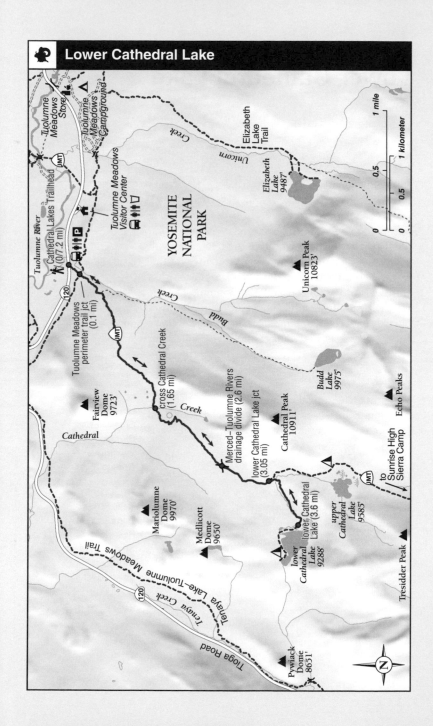

Lower Cathedral Lake

Tuolumne Meadows Store

Tuolumne Meadows Campground

Elizabeth Lake Trail

1 mile

1 kilometer

Unicorn Creek

Elizabeth Lake 9487'

0.5

0.5

JMT

Tuolumne Meadows Visitor Center

YOSEMITE NATIONAL PARK

Unicorn Peak 10823'

0

0

Tuolumne River

Cathedral Lakes Trailhead (0/7.2 mi)

P

120

Tuolumne Meadows perimeter trail jct (0.1 mi)

Budd Creek

JMT

cross Cathedral Creek (1.65 mi)

Budd Lake 9975'

Fairview Dome 9723'

Cathedral

Creek

Merced-Tuolumne Rivers drainage divide (2.6 mi)

lower Cathedral Lake jct (3.05 mi)

Cathedral Peak 10911'

Echo Peaks

to Sunrise High Sierra Camp

JMT

Mariolumne Dome 9970'

Medlicott Dome 9650'

Tenaya Lake-Tuolumne Meadows Trail

120

Tenaya Creek

upper Cathedral Lake 9585'

lower Cathedral Lake (3.6 mi)

lower Cathedral Lake 9288'

Tresidder Peak

Tioga Road

Pywiack Dome 8651'

N

Best Time

Though Tioga Road usually opens by late May (to late June in high snow years), the aspect of the trail means that some big patches of snow usually remain in shaded areas until late June (or beyond). Meanwhile, mosquitoes may detract from your experience—especially in early mornings and evenings—through July, making August the most relaxing time for a visit. September is beautiful as well, with crisp, cool air; fewer visitors; and beautiful yellow and red leaves on some ground cover plants.

Finding the Trail

In Tuolumne Meadows, drive 1.5 miles west on Tioga Road from the entrance to the Tuolumne Meadows Campground, which is the only campground in the area. Or drive about 0.75 mile east on Tioga Road from the Pothole Dome parking area, the westernmost trailhead in Tuolumne Meadows. The "parking lot" is the dirt shoulder on either side of CA 120, and on most summer days, vehicles are parked along quite a lengthy stretch of Tioga Road, adding a little to your hiking distance; get an early start to ensure the best parking. There are pit toilets at the trailhead, but the closest flush toilets and water are at the Tuolumne Meadows Visitor Center.

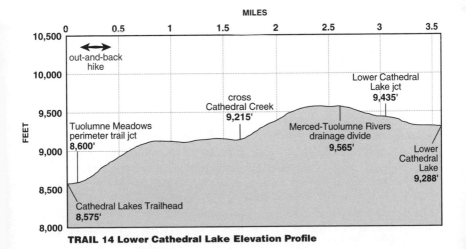

TRAIL 14 Lower Cathedral Lake Elevation Profile

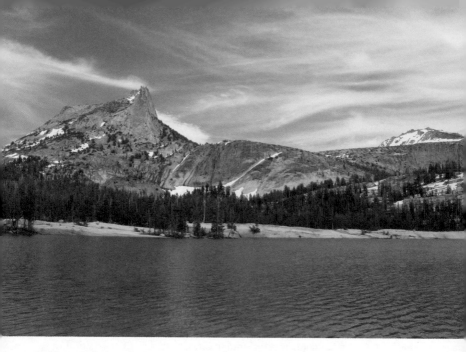

Cathedral Peak *viewed from the lower Cathedral Lake*

Trail Description

From behind the long row of food-storage boxes, ▶1 walk southwest 0.1 mile to a junction with the Tuolumne Meadows–Tenaya Lake Trail (also known as the Tuolumne Meadows perimeter trail). ▶2 East, this trail goes 1.2 miles to the southwest corner of Tuolumne Meadows Campground. West, it traverses 7.8 miles down to the Sunrise Lakes Trailhead at the southwest corner of Tenaya Lake.

Now on the John Muir Trail, you climb moderately on a stretch that can, at times, be objectionably dusty as thousands of humans and equines churn up the forest floor humus and abundant glacial deposits. The trail switchbacks diligently, stepping endlessly over and around the boulders embedded in these moraine deposits. Lodgepole pines dominate your 0.75-mile ascent to the crest of a lateral moraine, from which the trail briefly descends west before turning southwest.

With glades of dense hemlocks replacing the lodgepole pines, the John Muir Trail now traverses boggier terrain, at times cumbersome in the month following snowmelt, as you are torn between the obligation to remain on the trail to avoid damaging the surrounding vegetation and your deep-seated desire to keep your feet dry; please force your feet to vote in favor of protecting the plants. A collection of heath species, including dwarf bilberry, provide a thick ground cover, shifting from a vibrant green in June to an attractive glowing red in late summer. Boggy meadows, cleared of trees by past avalanches, afford a vista to Fairview Dome. You step across nascent Cathedral Creek on rocks (1.65 miles) ►3 and then ascend short, moderate to steep switchbacks beneath the shady cover of lodgepole pines and mountain hemlocks. After 300 feet of climbing, your trail's gradient eases and you traverse along the base of Cathedral Peak, a mass of granodiorite towering 1,400 feet above you that slowly enters your view. You leave the Tuolumne River drainage for that of the Merced River at an unmarked pass as you traverse what appears to be a completely flat, dry, sandy expanse (2.6 miles); ►4 it is hard to believe a drop of water on one side descends to the Tuolumne River and that on the other heads for Yosemite Valley. A brief descent through wetter lodgepole forest leads to a junction with a spur trail to the lower Cathedral Lake (3.05 miles). ►5 Keep right on the spur trail.

This spur trail soon crosses the Cathedral Lake inlet stream. At times of high flow, search for a steady fallen log across the channel to avoid a wet-shoe crossing; you will likely have to walk a short stretch above or below the trail, but options usually abound. Descending through lodgepole pines, the trail emerges in a large meadow—or perhaps a shallow lake—which is best encircled on its south side. A rust-stained waterline on the side of bedrock slabs marks the high-water level to which the meadow floods in early summer; granite slabs underlie the shallow soils, and as the snow melts, it pools in the bowllike depression, taking many weeks to evaporate and seep out. Across the meadow you reach the bedrock slabs lining the east shore of lower Cathedral Lake (3.6 miles). ►6 Campsites exist on both the north and south shores, the northern ones being roomier. Campfires are not allowed. Due to high angler use, fishing for brook trout is likely to be poor. Because of the relative shallowness of this fairly large lake, swimming in it is tolerable despite its nearly 9,300-foot altitude.

If you want to explore further, it is an additional 0.5 mile to the lake's outlet, reached by following the lakeshore in a counterclockwise direction. You cross back over the inlet creek just above the lakeshore and then follow the lake's perimeter west. From the lake's outlet you can look across to Polly Dome, standing on the skyline across Tioga Road, while Pywiack Dome lies at the head of Tenaya Lake. Also visible are Mount Hoffmann and a bit of Tenaya Lake, nestled between Tenaya Peak and Polly Dome. And the aforementioned Medlicott and Mariuolumne

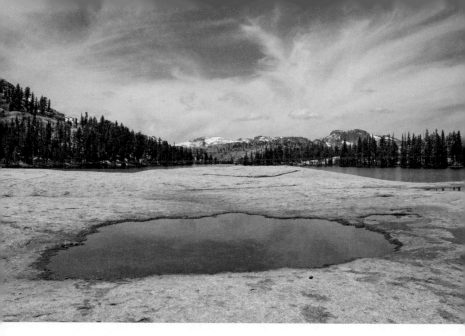

Lower *Cathedral Lake*

Domes? Those are the two domes due north of the lower Cathedral Lake, which people comfortable with off-trail navigation could visit on their return, as both have quite gentle eastern slopes that are straightforward to ascend. Afterward, trend back to the trail near the previously described flat pass. As your day or weekend away comes to a close, retrace your route to the trailhead (7.2 miles). ▶7

🚶 MILESTONES

▶1	0.0	Start at Cathedral Lakes Trailhead
▶2	0.1	Straight ahead at Tuolumne Meadows perimeter trail
▶3	1.65	Cross Cathedral Creek
▶4	2.6	Merced–Tuolumne Rivers drainage divide
▶5	3.05	Right on spur trail to the lower Cathedral Lake
▶6	3.6	Lower Cathedral Lake
▶7	7.2	Return to Cathedral Lakes Trailhead

High Sierra Camps Loop, Northwest Section

The High Sierra Camps Loop hike is very popular, not surprisingly, because the five backcountry camps are spaced 6–10 miles apart, distances that are about right for most backpackers. If you can get reservations to stay at these camps (see "Camping and Lodging," page 20), then your food and bedding will be provided, which allows you to hike with a light pack. In reality, your chances of getting reservations are poor (and the camps are expensive), so most people settle for staying in the backpackers' camps adjacent to each site.

I've broken the loop into two parts for two reasons. First, most hikers don't have the luxury of spending six days in the backcountry. Second, by being out fewer days, you will have a lighter pack because you carry less food.

I prefer hiking the loop in a counterclockwise direction because, this way, on your first day, when your pack is heaviest and you are the least acclimated to high elevation, your hike is mostly level and downhill. Energetic hikers sometimes day hike this section of the High Sierra Camps Loop, which takes about as much energy as does the popular Half Dome hike (Trail 34). Easy traverses dominate over ups and downs, making this route a great one for serious runners.

Permits

Overnight visitors require a wilderness permit for the Glen Aulin Trailhead (first night at Glen Aulin backpackers' camp), Glen Aulin Pass Thru (first night beyond Glen Aulin backpackers' camp), or May Lake Trailhead (hiking in reverse of description),

TRAIL USE
Day Hike, Backpack, Horse, Run

LENGTH
16.8 miles, 8–12 hours (over 1–3 days)

VERTICAL FEET
One-way:
+2,320', –2,750'

DIFFICULTY
– 1 2 3 **4** 5 +

TRAIL TYPE
Point-to-Point

FEATURES
Canyon
Lake
Stream
Waterfall
Wildflowers
Great Views
Camping
Granite Slabs

FACILITIES
Bear Boxes
Campground
Horse Staging
Picnic Tables
Restrooms
Shuttle Stop
Store
Visitor Center
Water

(continued on page 152)

149

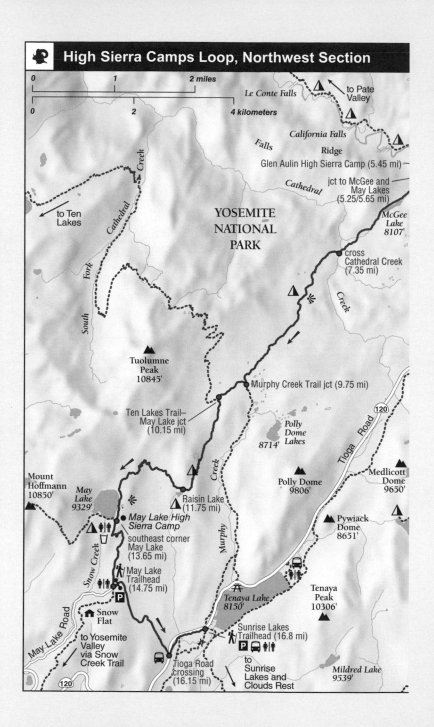

0   1   2 miles

0   2   4 kilometers

Le Conte Falls

to Pate Valley

California Falls

Falls   Ridge

Glen Aulin High Sierra Camp (5.45 mi)

Cathedral   jct to McGee and May Lakes (5.25/5.65 mi)

to Ten Lakes

YOSEMITE NATIONAL PARK

McGee Lake 8107'

Creek

cross Cathedral Creek (7.35 mi)

Cathedral

South Fork

Tuolumne Peak 10845'

Murphy Creek Trail jct (9.75 mi)

Tioga Road 120

Ten Lakes Trail– May Lake jct (10.15 mi)

Polly Dome Lakes 8714'

Mount Hoffmann 10850'

May Lake 9329'

Medlicott Dome 9650'

Polly Dome 9806'

Raisin Lake (11.75 mi)

Creek

May Lake High Sierra Camp

Pywiack Dome 8651'

southeast corner May Lake (13.65 mi)

Murphy

May Lake Trailhead (14.75 mi)

Snow Creek

Tenaya Lake 8150'

Tenaya Peak 10306'

Snow Flat

May Lake Road

to Yosemite Valley via Snow Creek Trail

Sunrise Lakes Trailhead (16.8 mi)

120

Tioga Road crossing (16.15 mi)

to Sunrise Lakes and Clouds Rest

Mildred Lake 9539'

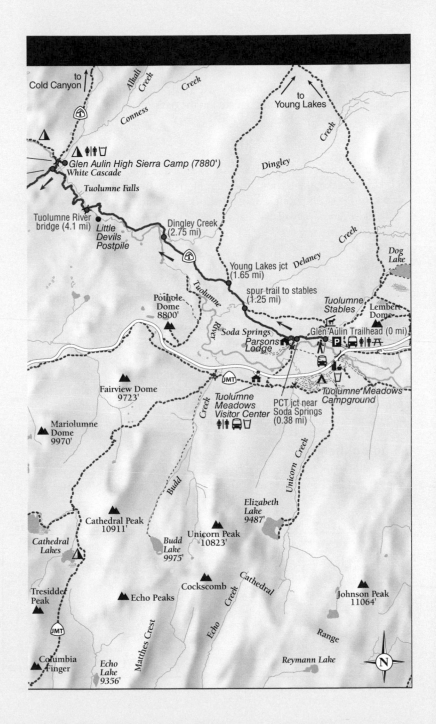

to Cold Canyon

Alkali Creek

Creek

Conness Creek

to Young Lakes

Dingley Creek

Glen Aulin High Sierra Camp (7880')
White Cascade

Tuolumne Falls

Tuolumne River
bridge (4.1 mi)

*Little
Devils
Postpile*

Dingley Creek
(2.75 mi)

Delaney Creek

Dog
Lake

Tuolumne River

Young Lakes jct
(1.65 mi)

spur trail to stables
(1.25 mi)

*Pothole
Dome
8800'*

*Tuolumne
Stables*

Lembert
Dome

Soda Springs

Glen Aulin Trailhead (0 mi)

Parsons
Lodge

P

JMT

*Fairview Dome
9723'*

*Tuolumne
Meadows
Visitor Center*

PCT jct near
Soda Springs
(0.38 mi)

*Tuolumne Meadows
Campground*

*Mariolumne
Dome
9970'*

Budd Creek

Unicorn Creek

*Elizabeth
Lake
9487'*

*Cathedral Peak
10911'*

*Budd
Lake
9975'*

*Unicorn Peak
10823'*

*Cathedral
Lakes*

*Tresidder
Peak*

Echo Peaks

Cockscomb

Cathedral Creek

*Johnson Peak
11064'*

JMT

*Columbia
Finger*

*Echo
Lake
9356'*

Matthes Crest

Echo Creek

Range

Reymann Lake

N

(continued from page 149)

issued by Yosemite National Park. Pick up your permit at the Tuolumne Meadows Wilderness Center, located in the parking lot a short way down Tuolumne Meadows Lodge Road.

Maps

This trail is covered by the Tom Harrison *Tuolumne Meadows* map (1:42,240 scale), the National Geographic Trails Illustrated #308 *Yosemite NE* map (1:40,000 scale), and the USGS 7.5-minute series *Tioga Pass, Falls Ridge,* and *Tenaya Lake* maps (1:24,000 scale).

Best Time

If you plan to stay at the camps or eat your meals at them, note that they are only open from around mid-July through mid-September. For others, you will want to begin your hike after the snow has melted—the beginning of July is generally a safe bet, though mid-June is fine in lower snow years. During June and July the mosquitoes can be quite prevalent, and if you want to avoid them, wait until August. Lakes are near their optimal temperatures mid-July–mid-August, so if you want to minimize mosquitoes and snow and enjoy dips in the lakes, then early August is best—but of course, don't expect solitude during these peak backpacking weeks. September is cooler but still a beautiful month for hiking; just bring warmer clothes and check the forecast to ensure no early snow is expected.

Finding the Trail

Drive along Tioga Road to a dirt road starting west from the base of Lembert Dome, at a spot located at the east end of Tuolumne Meadows and

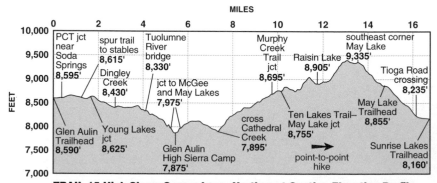

TRAIL 15 High Sierra Camps Loop, Northwest Section Elevation Profile

OPTION: **Mount Hoffmann**

If you have the time, you might take the 1.75-mile trail (each way) from May Lake ►12 to the top of Mount Hoffmann, which is located at the geographic center of Yosemite National Park and offers a 360-degree view of much of the park's lands. Bring a map of the park to identify dozens of features. See Trail 19 for details.

immediately northeast of the Tuolumne River. You will have passed the entrance to Tuolumne Meadows Campground, the only campground in the area, just before the river. This road immediately leads to the small Lembert Dome parking area and then continues 0.3 mile to a locked gate; parking is allowed on the verge along this stretch. If there is no available parking, just before the locked gate, turn right (north) to the Tuolumne Stables, where there is a large parking area. You can retrace your steps to the official trailhead, or use the connecting trails fanning out from the stables parking area; both are a similar hiking distance. The mileage is measured from the locked gate.

The route ends at the Sunrise Lakes Trailhead, along Tioga Road near Tenaya Lake's southwest corner. Though the trailheads are some 9 miles apart, a shuttle bus makes it possible to get a ride back to your original trailhead. During the summer season, these buses run every half hour, plying between Olmsted Point and Tuolumne Meadows and stopping at all the popular trailheads in between. Before starting your hike, check the schedule for the shuttle's last run; you don't want to walk the 9.6 miles back to your starting point. Note that the shuttle buses charge a fee, so be sure to carry cash.

Trail Description

From the locked gate ►1 you walk along an old road that skirts the northern edge of Tuolumne Meadows, traipsing through meadow interspersed with clusters of lodgepole pines. On it you are treated to fine views south toward Unicorn Peak, Cathedral Peak, and some of the knobby Echo Peaks. You may also see an occasional marmot foraging for food or Belding's ground squirrels standing upright by their holes. After 0.25 mile you meet a smaller trail heading northeast to the horse stables and soon thereafter the main trail splits (0.38 mile). ►2 The left branch heads to a bridge across the nearby Tuolumne River and inspiring views. Your route, still

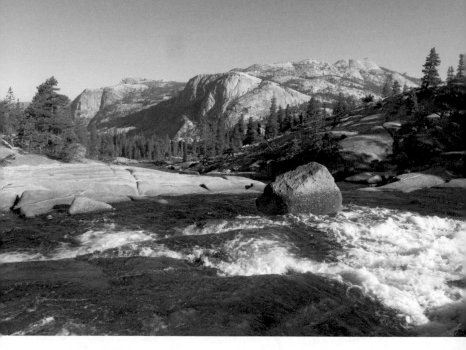

The Tuolumne River *starts its plunge toward Glen Aulin.*

on an old road, veers right, slightly uphill, and quickly encounters a spur trail to the bubbling natural Soda Springs. You can follow the spur trail west across this vicinity or continue on the main trail, which arcs counterclockwise; the two reconnect just 0.1 mile to the north. The main trail passes the site of the old Soda Springs Campground, open 1912–1976.

From the effervescent Soda Springs, your westbound trail passes a reed-filled lake and then traverses open sandy flats interspersed with lodgepole pine patches, where large-scale rock fractures allow deeper soils to accumulate. Another spur trail from the stables merges from the southwest (right) (1.25 miles), ►3 and just beyond you descend to cross Delaney Creek. With significant flow during June and early July, you will want to search for a log to balance across; later on, boulder-hopping will do. High spring runoff in 2017 dislodged the previously used logs, making this crossing dangerous in the afternoons of the highest-flow periods—usually in mid-June. Stepping across a second, smaller tributary you soon reach the junction to Young Lakes (1.65 miles), ►4 on which those taking Trail 10 will branch right, north.

You instead veer left (northwest), winding through scattered lodgepoles and then descending some bare granite slabs and entering a flat-floored forest. You are now northwest of Tuolumne Meadows. The unseen Tuolumne River is cascading down slabs just 0.2 mile to your south. A glimpse at a satellite photo would show that your route is carefully chosen: your rambling traverse across the granite slabs picks a route that follows a series of shallow, forested depressions, making for easier walking. A mile's pleasant walking brings you to the west end of a huge meadow near the bank of the Tuolumne River and then to three branches of Dingley Creek (2.75 miles). ▶5 The channels are broad with cobble underfoot; without conveniently located logs, they are a wade during high flows, albeit an easy one, so make sure to stay in your water shoes (or barefoot) until you've passed all three. From here, the nearly level trail often runs along the river, and in these stretches by the stream, there are numerous glacier-smoothed granite slabs on which to take a break—or dip, if the river's current is slow.

After a mile-long winding traverse, the trail leaves the last slabs to climb briefly on a granite outcrop to get around the river's gorge. You can leave the trail and walk toward a brink, from where you'll see, on the south side of the gorge below you, Little Devils Postpile, a small outcrop of columnar basalt. Back on the trail you wind down, soon reaching a sturdy Tuolumne River bridge (4.1 miles), ▶6 and immediately beyond it you can look north up long Cold Canyon to Matterhorn Peak and Whorl Mountain and, to their right, Mount Conness.

The river now flows rapidly down a series of sparkling rapids separated by large pools and wide sheets of water spread out across more slightly inclined granite slopes. The trail alongside this beautiful stretch of river also descends more steeply; you will find the walking rockier, slower, and most certainly harder on the knees. As you descend, give yourself time to gaze at Tuolumne Falls in particular. The trail trends away from the creek to one moister glen, skirts back to the riverbank, and then enters a second glade where you reach a junction with the trail to McGee Lake and May Lake (5.25 miles) ▶7; you will head along this route after a detour to Glen Aulin. Below you, watch White Cascade tumbling into a circular pool and cross another bridge high above the churning Tuolumne River. During high runoff, you may have to wade just to reach this bridge—note the expanse of rounded river cobble and boulders strewn across the trail.

From here it is only a few minutes' walk to the junction to Glen Aulin High Sierra Camp, reached on a spur trail by crossing a bridge over Conness Creek. From the camp (5.45 miles) ▶8 a short spur trail leads north past the High Sierra Camp's canvas tents to the heavily used Glen Aulin backpackers' camp, complete with bear-proof food-storage boxes. If you will be camping at Glen Aulin and have spare hours before nightfall, you could detour down the Tuolumne River to see California, Le Conte, and/or Waterwheel Falls (see Trail 11, page 122).

The second day's hike is to the May Lake High Sierra Camp. You retrace your steps for 0.2 mile, across the Conness Creek bridge and the bridge across the Tuolumne River, to again reach the junction to McGee Lake and May Lake (5.65 miles). ▶9 Heading west (right), you briefly curve northwest through a notch, and then your trail ascends gently southwest, crossing and recrossing McGee Lake's northeast-flowing ephemeral outlet. Where the trail levels off, McGee Lake, long and narrow and bordered on the southwest by a granite cliff, comes into view through the lodgepole trees. The dead snags and dense thickets of western Labrador tea along the shallow margin, as well as the fallen limbs and downed trees in the lake, limit shoreline access and enjoyment. Moreover, in late summer the lake, perched on a saddle and receiving no incoming water, may dwindle to a stale pond and is not too attractive. Adept campers can find isolated, level spots, some with views, on slopes north of the lake, beneath the east end of Falls Ridge.

Beyond the lake your trail descends along its southwest-flowing outlet (yes, it has two outlets during high flow!) for 0.75 mile, and then you cross it. Passing a collection of seasonal tarns and meadow patches thick with corn lilies, you soon have a view northwest through the shallow Cathedral Creek canyon to hulking Falls Ridge, which Cathedral Creek has to detour around in order to join the Tuolumne River. After several minutes you reach 20-foot-wide Cathedral Creek (7.35 miles), ▶10 which can be a ford in early summer and a boulder hop later on. Starting a moderate ascent beyond the creek, you soon reach a stand of tall, healthy red firs set between two granite ribs. Seeing the contrast between these sturdy-trunked, dispersed trees and the straggly overcrowded lodgepoles is inescapable.

The trail continues its ascent, never steep, never flat. You mount a few brief switchbacks to take you to the top of an open bluff and suddenly the panorama emerges to the northeast, most welcome after several miles of walking through moderate and dense forest. In the distant northeast stand Sheep Peak, North Peak, and Mount Conness, encircling the basin of Roosevelt Lake. In the near north, Falls Ridge is a mountain of pinkish granite that contrasts with the white and gray granite of the other peaks, while Wildcat Point is visible across the Tuolumne River canyon. When you look back toward McGee Lake, the route appears to be entirely carpeted with lodgepole pines. Near here are a few small campsites, lacking water by late summer as ephemeral tarns and rivulets dry up.

The trail continues up a moderate slope on gravel and granite shelves through a forest cover of hemlock, red fir, and lodgepole. Stepping across a branch of Cathedral Creek, you have one more stretch of uphill under dense hemlock cover to reach the Murphy Creek Trail junction (9.75 miles). ►11 The Murphy Creek Trail departs left from this junction to go down to Tenaya Lake. Meanwhile, you turn right.

Skirting to the south of lush forest and seasonally boggy meadows (beware of mosquitoes!), the nearly flat trail soon leads to a junction with the Ten Lakes Trail (10.15 miles), ►12 which trends northwest (right) to traverse slabs and bluffs beneath the quite steep face of Tuolumne Peak. You branch left and ascend briefly to a long, narrow, shallow, forested saddle, beyond which large Tenaya Lake is visible to the south. In early summer this is a favorite break spot of mine because you are on dry slab and have left the swarms of mosquitoes behind. After traversing somewhat open slopes of sagebrush, huckleberry oak, and lupine, you reach a spring, followed by a series of switchbacks. A profusion of wildflowers decorates these slopes, fed by the subterranean (and aboveground) moisture. The gradient of these zigzags is mostly gentle, truncated by intermittent stairs, but the path is rockier underfoot than the forest paths you've been pad- ding along, so as requested by your feet, take breaks and enjoy the striking views of Mount Conness, Mount Dana, and the other peaks on the Sierra Crest, which delineates the Yosemite border. The trail then passes through a little saddle just north of a glacier-smoothed peak, and ahead, suddenly, is another Yosemite landmark, Clouds Rest, rising grandly in the south. Though there is no water just here, this saddle sports sandy campsites dis- tinguished by the outstanding views; it is well worth carrying water to this location and relaxing on the surrounding polished slabs.

Now the trail descends gradually over fairly open granite to a forested flat and bends west above the north shore of Raisin Lake (11.75 miles), ►13 a notably warm lake. It has few obvious campsites, but there are some waterless, isolated ones with views, located on slabs about 0.25 mile south of the lake. From the lake's vicinity, the trail continues beside a flower-lined seasonally flowing streambed under a sparse forest cover of mountain hemlock and western white and lodgepole pines, and it then swings west to cross three unnamed, seasonal streams.

Finally the trail makes a 0.5-mile-long steep ascent across a conifer-dotted slope. Views improve constantly, and presently you have again

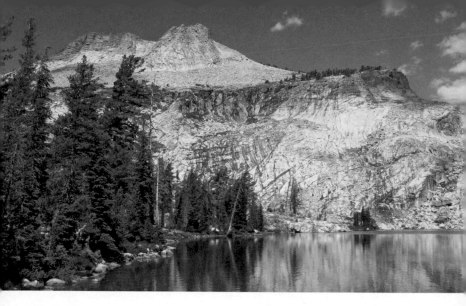

May Lake

earned the panorama of peaks on the Sierra Crest from North Peak south to the obvious Tioga Pass notch and onward to Mount Gibbs. At the top of this climb is a gentle upland where several small meadows are strung along the trail. Corn lilies grow at an almost perceptible rate in early summer, while aromatic lupine commands your attention later. In the west, Mount Hoffmann dominates. Now you swing south, descend gently, and reach the northeast corner of May Lake and parallel its east shore to reach

first the May Lake High Sierra Camp and then, at the southeast corner, the backpackers' camp. Note that swimming is prohibited at May Lake. At May Lake's southeast corner, you'll see a junction with a trail striking west—this is the trail to Mount Hoffmann (13.65 miles). ▶14 If you have a few hours to spare, an ascent of Mount Hoffmann is highly recommended. See page 194 (Trail 19) for a description of the route.

You begin the third day's hike, a mere 3.15 miles long and virtually all downhill, by taking the trail south from the junction at the southeast corner of May Lake to the trailhead at Snow Flat. This trail winds briefly down broken slabs and then reenters open forest cover as it follows a passageway nearly due south between two shallow ridges. The tree cover shifts between sparse and sparser, reflecting the shallowness of the soils. Passing a shallow, often-buggy tarn, you reach the Snow Flat (May Lake) Trailhead (14.75 miles). ▶15

Your continuing route is at the far back of the parking area (northeast end) behind a locked gate. You will now follow this closed road, old Tioga Road, down to a crossing of the current CA 120, Tioga Road. The walking is fast and uneventful, with broken views and limited enticing scenery. Quite soon you reach Tioga Road and cross it (16.15 miles). ►16 On the east side of the road is a shuttle stop, but shuttles seem to sometimes miss this stop, so I recommend continuing to the larger stop at the Sunrise Lakes Trailhead. To do so, you follow the trail that parallels the road downhill, toward Tenaya Lake. At a junction with a wooden sign simply declaring TRAIL JUNCTION, remain to the left adjacent to the road, and cross a small creek. If the water is high, simply detour to the road for an easy crossing. Flat, sandy walking through open lodgepole forest quickly leads to a T-junction with a more prominent trail. Turn left (west) and you are almost immediately at the Sunrise Lakes Trailhead (16.8 miles). ►17 There are pit toilets but no water faucet here. The Tuolumne Meadows–bound shuttle bus will pull into the parking area just in front of the toilets.

🚶 MILESTONES

►1	0.0	Start at Glen Aulin Trailhead
►2	0.38	Right on the PCT toward Soda Springs
►3	1.25	Left at junction with stables spur trail
►4	1.65	Left at junction to Young Lakes
►5	2.75	Cross Dingley Creek
►6	4.1	Tuolumne River bridge
►7	5.25	Right at trail junction to McGee and May Lakes
►8	5.45	Left to Glen Aulin High Sierra Camp
►9	5.65	Right at trail to McGee and May Lakes
►10	7.35	Cross Cathedral Creek
►11	9.75	Right at junction with Murphy Creek Trail
►12	10.15	Left at Ten Lakes Trail–May Lake junction
►13	11.75	Raisin Lake
►14	13.65	Southeast corner May Lake
►15	14.75	May Lake Trailhead
►16	16.15	Cross Tioga Road
►17	16.8	Finish at Sunrise Lakes Trailhead

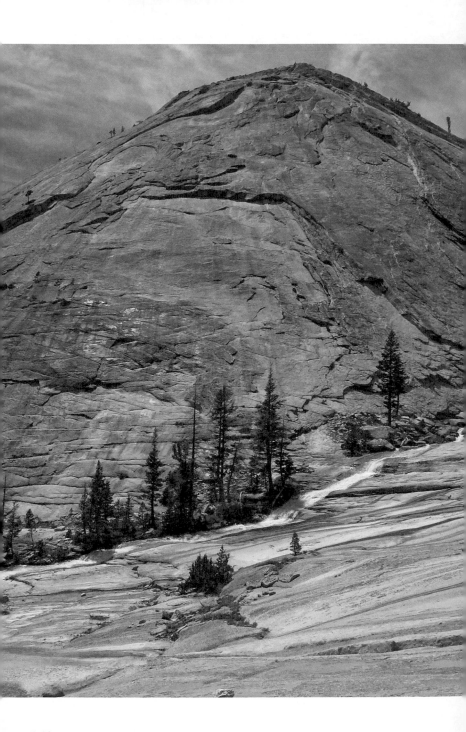

High Sierra Camps Loop, Southeast Section

The High Sierra Camps Loop hike is very popular, not surprisingly, because the five backcountry camps are spaced 6–10 miles apart, distances that are about right for most backpackers. If you can get reservations to stay at these camps (see "Camping and Lodging," page 20), then your food and bedding will be provided, which allows you to hike with a light pack. In reality, your chances of getting reservations are poor (and the camps are expensive), so most people settle for staying in the backpackers' camps adjacent to each site.

I've broken the loop into two parts for two reasons. First, most hikers don't have the luxury of spending six days in the backcountry. Second, by being out fewer days, you will have a lighter pack because you carry less food. An advantage of the high camps is the bear-proof food-storage boxes at each site, allowing you to carry slightly bulkier food than might fit into a bear canister—although regulations still dictate you must have a canister—as well as drinking water and pit toilets at some camps. However, you can camp at endless alternative locations—many equally scenic—between the High Sierra Camps. If you wish to complete the entire loop, you will hike the final day of Trail 15 and the first 5.15 miles of this hike as your third day.

I prefer hiking the loop in a counterclockwise direction because, this way, on your first day, when your pack is heaviest, your hike is along the

(continued on page 165)

TRAIL USE
Backpack, Horse

LENGTH
30.1 miles, 15–24 hours
(over 2–4 days)

VERTICAL FEET
One-way:
+5,700', –5,180'

DIFFICULTY
– 1 2 3 4 **5** +

TRAIL TYPE
Point-to-Point

FEATURES
Canyon
Lake
Stream
Wildflowers
Great Views
Camping
Swimming
Steep
Granite Slabs

FACILITIES
Bear Boxes
Restrooms
Shuttle Stop

Opposite: *Cascades below Emeric Lake*

161

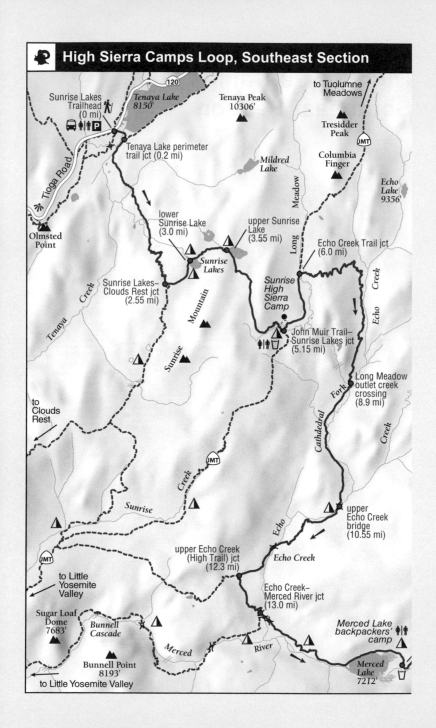

to Tuolumne
Meadows

Sunrise Lakes
Trailhead
(0 mi)

*Tenaya Lake
8150'*

Tenaya Peak
10306'

Tresidder
Peak

Columbia
Finger

JMT

Tioga Road

Tenaya Lake perimeter
trail jct (0.2 mi)

*Mildred
Lake*

*Echo
Lake
9356'*

Long

Olmsted
Point

lower
Sunrise Lake
(3.0 mi)

upper Sunrise
Lake
(3.55 mi)

Echo Creek Trail jct
(6.0 mi)

Meadow

Echo

Creek

Sunrise Lakes–
Clouds Rest jct
(2.55 mi)

Tenaya

Creek

*Sunrise
Lakes*

*Sunrise
High
Sierra
Camp*

John Muir Trail–
Sunrise Lakes jct
(5.15 mi)

Echo

Mountain

Fork

Long Meadow
outlet creek
crossing
(8.9 mi)

Creek

to
Clouds
Rest

Sunrise

JMT

Cathedral

Creek

JMT

to Little
Yosemite
Valley

Sunrise

Echo

upper
Echo Creek
bridge
(10.55 mi)

upper Echo Creek
(High Trail) jct
(12.3 mi)

Echo Creek

Echo Creek–
Merced River jct
(13.0 mi)

Sugar Loaf
Dome
7683'

*Bunnell
Cascade*

*Merced Lake
backpackers'
camp*

Bunnell Point
8193'
to Little Yosemite Valley

Merced

River

*Merced
Lake
7212'*

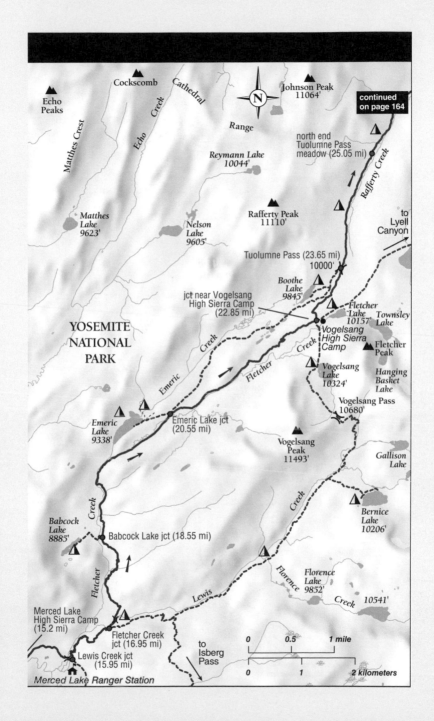

Echo
Peaks

Cockscomb

Echo Creek

Cathedral

Johnson Peak
11064'

continued
on page 164

Range

Matthes Crest

Reymann Lake
10044'

north end
Tuolumne Pass
meadow (25.05 mi)

Rafferty Creek

Matthes
Lake
9623'

Nelson
Lake
9605'

Rafferty Peak
111'10'

to
Lyell
Canyon

Tuolumne Pass (23.65 mi)
10000'

YOSEMITE
NATIONAL
PARK

jct near Vogelsang
High Sierra Camp
(22.85 mi)

Boothe
Lake
9845'

Fletcher
Lake
10157'

Townsley
Lake

Emeric

Creek

Fletcher

Creek

Vogelsang
High Sierra
Camp

Fletcher
Peak

Vogelsang
Lake
10324'

Hanging
Basket
Lake

Emeric Lake jct
(20.55 mi)

Emeric
Lake
9338'

Vogelsang Pass
10680'

Vogelsang
Peak
11493'

Gallison
Lake

Creek

Creek

Bernice
Lake
10206'

Babcock
Lake
8885'

Babcock Lake jct (18.55 mi)

Fletcher

Lewis

Florence

Creek

Florence
Lake
9852'

Creek

10541'

Merced Lake
High Sierra Camp
(15.2 mi)

Fletcher Creek
jct (16.95 mi)

Lewis Creek jct
(15.95 mi)

Merced Lake Ranger Station

to Isberg
Pass

0		0.5		1 mile

0		1		2 kilometers

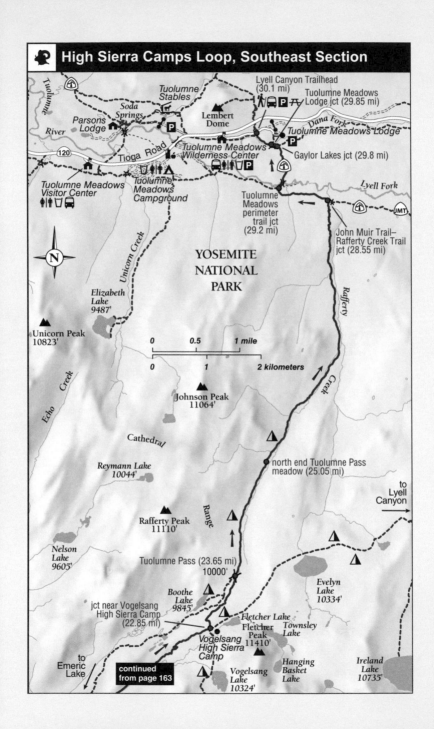

High Sierra Camps Loop, Southeast Section

Tuolumne River

Tuolumne Stables

Lyell Canyon Trailhead (30.1 mi)

Tuolumne Meadows Lodge jct (29.85 mi)

Soda Springs

Parsons Lodge

Lembert Dome

Dana Fork

Tuolumne Meadows Lodge

River

120

Tioga Road

Tuolumne Meadows Wilderness Center

Gaylor Lakes jct (29.8 mi)

Lyell Fork

Tuolumne Meadows Visitor Center

Tuolumne Meadows Campground

Tuolumne Meadows perimeter trail jct (29.2 mi)

JMT

John Muir Trail–Rafferty Creek Trail jct (28.55 mi)

N

Unicorn Creek

YOSEMITE NATIONAL PARK

Elizabeth Lake 9487'

Rafferty Creek

▲ Unicorn Peak 10823'

0   0.5   1 mile

0   1   2 kilometers

Echo Creek

▲ Johnson Peak 11064'

Cathedral

△

Reymann Lake 10044'

north end Tuolumne Pass meadow (25.05 mi)

to Lyell Canyon

Range

▲ Rafferty Peak 11110'

△

△

Nelson Lake 9605'

△

Tuolumne Pass (23.65 mi) 10000'

Boothe Lake 9845'

△

Evelyn Lake 10334'

jct near Vogelsang High Sierra Camp (22.85 mi)

△

Fletcher Lake

Fletcher Peak 11410'

Townsley Lake

to Emeric Lake

Vogelsang High Sierra Camp

Hanging Basket Lake

Ireland Lake 10735'

continued from page 163

△

Vogelsang Lake 10324'

(continued from page 161)

shortest stretch, 5.15 miles to Sunrise High Sierra Camp (versus 7.2 miles to Vogelsang High Sierra Camp) and you are at lower elevations. However, the grade to Vogelsang is more gradual. If you are short on time but are a strong backpacker, you could cut out a day by spending your first night at Merced Lake High Sierra Camp, a lengthy 15.1 miles, but the 10 miles past Sunrise High Sierra Camp are relatively easy, having only about 600 feet of gain and about 2,700 feet of loss.

Permits

Overnight visitors require a wilderness permit for the Sunrise Lakes Trailhead (as described) or Rafferty Creek to Vogelsang Trailhead (walk in reverse of description), issued by Yosemite National Park. Pick up your permit at the Tuolumne Meadows Wilderness Center, located in the parking lot a short way down Tuolumne Meadows Lodge Road or at another of the Yosemite permit-issuing stations (see "Permits," page 21).

Maps

This trail is covered by the Tom Harrison *Tuolumne Meadows* map (1:42,240 scale), the National Geographic Trails Illustrated #309 *Yosemite SE* map (1:40,000 scale), and the USGS 7.5-minute series *Tenaya Lake, Merced Peak,* and *Vogelsang Peak* maps (1:24,000 scale).

Best Time

If you plan to stay at the camps or eat your meals at them, note that they are only open from around mid-July through mid-September. Those camping will want to take this hike after the snow has melted—the beginning of July is generally a safe bet, though late June is fine in lower snow years. During June and July the mosquitoes can be quite prevalent, and if you want to avoid them, wait until August. Lakes are near their optimal temperatures mid-July–mid-August, so if you want to minimize mosquitoes and snow and enjoy dips in the lakes, then early August is best—but of course, don't expect solitude during these peak backpacking weeks. September is cooler but still a beautiful month for hiking, and permits are considerably easier to obtain once Labor Day weekend passes; just bring warmer clothes and check the forecast to ensure no early snow is expected.

Finding the Trail

The trail begins on Tioga Road at the Sunrise Lakes Trailhead, a large pullout at a highway bend near Tenaya Lake's southwest shore. It is located 30.7 miles northeast of Crane Flat and 8.7 miles southwest of the Tuolumne Meadows Campground.

You will complete your hike at a trailhead parking area along Tuolumne Meadows Lodge Road. To reach this lot from Tuolumne Meadows Campground (the only campground in the area), drive 0.6 mile northeast on Tioga Road, turning right onto Tuolumne Meadows Lodge Road. Follow this road 0.4 mile—the parking area is on the left and the trailhead is obvious just to the right of the road.

If your party has only one car, a shuttle bus makes it possible to get a ride back to your original trailhead. During the summer season, these buses run every half hour, plying between Olmsted Point and Tuolumne Meadows and stopping at all the popular trailheads in between, including the aforementioned parking areas. Before starting your hike, check the schedule for the shuttle's last run; you don't want to walk the approximately 10 miles back to your vehicle. Note that the shuttle buses charge a fee, so be sure to carry cash. There are pit toilets at the trailhead, but the closest water faucets and flush toilets are at the Tuolumne Meadows

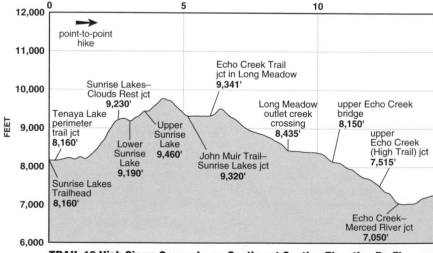

TRAIL 16 High Sierra Camps Loop, Southeast Section Elevation Profile

Visitor Center (for those coming from the east) or at the Crane Flat store or White Wolf Campground (for those coming from the west), so be sure to fill your water bottle before reaching the trailhead.

Trail Description

From the trailhead parking area, ▶1 take a trail that heads east, passes two small spur trails that depart to the right (south), and soon crosses the usually flowing outlet of Tenaya Lake. Just beyond this crossing you reach a trail junction. The trail left goes northeast along Tenaya Lake's eastern shore (0.2 mile). ▶2

You veer right on a trail that heads south for an additional 0.25 mile along Tenaya Creek before turning to the southeast as the trail gently ascends in sparse forest over a little rise and drops to a ford of Mildred Lake's outlet. Like the other

At 180 feet, Tenaya Lake is the park's deepest, and it has only been filled with a few feet of sediments since the last glacier retreated about 15,000 years ago.

streams over the next 2 miles, this crossing can dry up in late summer or early fall but requires a sandy wade (or wobbly log balance) in early summer. Beyond the Mildred Lake stream, the trail undulates and winds

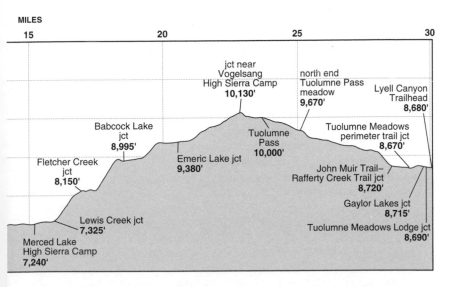

MILES

| 15 | 20 | 25 | 30 |

jct near
Vogelsang
High Sierra Camp
10,130'

north end
Tuolumne Pass
meadow
9,670'

Lyell Canyon
Trailhead
8,680'

Babcock Lake
jct
8,995'

Tuolumne
Pass
10,000'

Tuolumne Meadows
perimeter trail jct
8,670'

Fletcher Creek
jct
8,150'

Emeric Lake jct
9,380'

John Muir Trail–
Rafferty Creek Trail jct
8,720'

Lewis Creek jct
7,325'

Gaylor Lakes jct
8,715'

Tuolumne Meadows Lodge jct
8,690'

Merced Lake
High Sierra Camp
7,240'

generally south, passing several pocket meadows browsed by mule deer. At 1.4 miles, the trail then begins to climb in earnest through a thinning cover of lodgepole pine and occasional red fir, western white pine, and mountain hemlock. As your trail rises above Tenaya Canyon, you pass several vantage points from which you can look back on its smooth, steep granite walls, though you never see Tenaya Lake. To the east the canyon is bounded by Tenaya Peak; in the northwest are the cliffs of Mount Hoffmann and Tuolumne Peak.

Now on switchbacks, you see Tioga Road across the canyon and can even hear vehicles, but these annoyances are infinitesimal compared to the pleasures of polished granite expanses all around. Your route ahead is steep—few Sierra trails ascend 1,000 feet in just 1.1 miles. The trail is also, in places, annoyingly rocky, reflecting the many half-buried boulders and partially submerged slabs with which the trail construction crew had to contend. At least these switchbacks are, for the most part, mercifully shaded, and where they become steepest, requiring a great output of energy, they give back with the beauty of a fine flower display, including lupine, penstemon, paintbrush, larkspur, buttercup, and sunflowers such as aster and senecio. Finally the switchbacks end and the trail levels as it arrives at a junction on a shallow, forested saddle (2.55 miles). ▶3

Straight ahead leads to Clouds Rest and beyond (Trail 18), but you turn left and first contour east, cross a low gap, and descend north through broken forest to lower Sunrise Lake (3.0 miles). ▶4 The western shore of this lake sports a number of small campsites, the first under forest cover, the latter smaller and more open in flat patches between slabs. Steep exfoliating slabs dominate the cross-lake view, while heath species, including red mountain heather and western Labrador tea, decorate the lakeshore. Climbing from this lake, you reach a crest in several minutes, and from it you could descend cross-country an equally short distance north to more isolated, island-dotted middle Sunrise Lake. The trail, however, veers east and gains a very noticeable 150 feet as it climbs to upper Sunrise Lake, the largest and most popular lake of the trio (3.55 miles). ▶5 Campsites are plentiful along its north shore, away from the trail and reached by crossing the lake at its outlet.

With 1.6 miles remaining to Sunrise High Sierra Camp, you skirt the edge of the flower-filled meadow ringing the lake, diagonal up a slope, and soon find yourself in a shallow gully that you follow south across dry, gravelly soils. At a broad pass you can look back to Mount Hoffmann or ahead to see the Clark Range head-on, piercing the southern sky. From the gap, which is sparsely clothed with mountain hemlocks, whitebark pines, and western white pines, you begin a shallow descent, still on decomposing granite and hopefully catching a glimpse of a Clark's nutcracker, the gray-and-white relative of blue jays that frequents the timberline country. The grade increases and you descend south into denser cover. Veer east and then north to make a steep descent to the Sunrise backpackers' camp, complete with a water faucet, pit toilet, food-storage boxes, and ample (if crowded) campsites. From near the pit toilet, a use trail leads northeast to the Sunrise High Sierra Camp. An overnight stay at either camp gives you an inspiring sunrise over Matthes Crest and the Cathedral Range.

Continuing down the main trail below the campsite leads to a T-junction with the John Muir Trail (JMT) (5.15 miles). ►6 Turning right takes you to Yosemite Valley, while you head left to traipse the length of L-shaped Long Meadow. A verdant green early summer, the grasses assume a yellow hue as the water table drops and the grasses dry. As the meadow pinches to a close, you reach the next junction, with the Echo Creek Trail. Here, the JMT continues straight ahead to the Cathedral Lakes and on to Tuolumne Meadows, while you turn right on the trail signposted to Merced Lake (6.0 miles). ►7 You immediately ford Long Meadow's creek, a sandy-cobbly wade at high water, when all good balancing rocks can be submerged. This trail quickly switchbacks up to the top of a forested ridge, about 200 feet above the meadow. It then descends, mostly through moist, dense hemlock-and-lodgepole forest alongside a small seasonal tributary of Echo Creek. Crossing this twice, you emerge onto expansive slabs and then momentarily reach the west bank of Echo Creek's Cathedral Fork (7.2 miles).

From your trail beside the Cathedral Fork, you have fine views of the creek's water gliding down a series of granite slabs. The sloping landscape limits camping options, but a determined small party will certainly find some sandy patches that suffice for a night's sleep. After nearly a mile of delightful streamside walking (though slow because the trail is quite rocky), the trail veers away from the creek at 8.05 miles and descends gently along a shelf well above it. Even in late summer these shaded slopes are watered by numerous rills, which are bordered by still-blooming flowers. On this downgrade the trail crosses the Long Meadow creek (8.9 miles), ►8 which has found an escape from that meadow through a gap between two small domes high above your trail. The creek fans out where it crosses the trail, leading to three separate crossings at high water; the first and last can be navigated via logs, while the middle one is a cobble-bottomed wade under high flows, yielding to a rock hop later on. All three will have insignificant flows in late summer. The route then levels out in a mile-long flat, in part burned, section of this valley, where the wet ground yields wildflowers all summer but also many mosquitoes in early to mid-July. Beyond this flat "park" the trail descends more open slopes, and eventually you can see across the valley the steep course of the main fork of Echo Creek plunging down to its rendezvous with its western Cathedral Fork. Still along the Cathedral Fork, your trail levels off and passes good campsites immediately before you take a bridge over Echo Creek (10.55 miles). ▶9 Note that the largest campsites are some distance south of the trail and not visible until you trend southwest off the trail.

Beyond the bridge, your trail leads down the forested valley and easily fords a tributary stream, staying well above the main creek. This pleasant, shaded descent soon becomes more open and steep, and it encounters fibrous-barked juniper trees and butterscotch-scented Jeffrey pines, while the river cascades and plummets steadily downslope in the gorge below. After briefly diverging from the river, the trail drops to another bridge (11.7 miles), beyond which it rises slightly and the creek drops precipitously, so that you are soon far above it. Then the sandy tread swings west and heads diagonally down a slope, where a dense growth of huckleberry oak, chinquapin, greenleaf manzanita, and whitethorn merge together to form a continuous expanse of "brush." Across it the views are excellent of Echo Valley, a flat interruption in the otherwise descending Merced River canyon below. On this slope you arrive at a T-junction (12.3 miles), ▶10 where right takes you 2.7 miles west to a junction with the JMT along the so-called High Trail, while your route turns to the left.

You immediately drop into a lush forest draw, replete with beautiful big red firs decorated with vibrant chartreuse lichen. A short while later, you return to dry, brushy slopes and complete your descent to the Merced Lake Trail junction in Echo Valley, 450 feet below your last junction (13.0 miles). ▶11 A few quite small campsites are near the junction, but the abundance of downed trees from past fires severely limits options; it is best to hold out and continue at least partway to Merced Lake.

You go east (left), immediately crossing the many-tentacled Echo Creek on a trio of bridges, and then pass through a lengthy burned-but-boggy area. Ascending on slabs, the trail continues east above the Merced River's gushing cascades and pools. If you were to head north to explore some areas with gently sloping slabs and small glades of lodgepole pine, you will find delightful camping for a small group, but note that you won't be terribly close to water. Continuing along a stretch of trail immediately above the roiling river, you shortly reach Merced Lake's west shore (14.3 miles). Don't camp here because there is no flat ground 100 feet from trail and water, but rather continue along the north shore. You reach the large camping area a little beyond the end of the lake (15.0 miles) and the Merced Lake High Sierra Camp buildings soon thereafter (15.2 miles). ▶12

While day three isn't the longest, it easily has the most elevation to gain, about 3,075 feet. Fortunately, by now your pack is lighter and you will be feeling a little more acclimated to the high elevation. You begin with an easy warm-up by hiking level east, often beneath stately Jeffrey pines, soon reaching the Merced Lake Ranger Station and an adjacent trail junction (15.95 miles). ▶13 Note that there are camping options in the direction of the river as you traverse these flats. At the junction you turn left and abruptly exit forest cover and labor up a decidedly rocky trail, broken by only short, forested stretches. The mostly unseen creek descends a gorge to the north; you rarely even have the tumbling water to distract you as you struggle upward, ascending 850 feet in the mile to the next junction, where you leave Lewis Creek and turn left onto the Fletcher Creek Trail (16.95 miles). ▶14

From the junction you descend on short switchbacks to a bridge over Lewis Creek. Just 150 feet past the bridge is a reasonably good campsite, although toppled trees occupy some of the flat real estate. The trail then enters more open slopes as it climbs moderately on a cobbled path bordered with proliferating bushes of whitethorn and huckleberry oak. Just past a tributary 0.5 mile from Lewis Creek, you have fine views of Fletcher Creek chuting and cascading down from a notch at the base of a granite dome before it leaps off a ledge in free fall. The few solitary pine

OPTION: Alpine Alternative

▶14 An alternate route to Vogelsang High Sierra Camp is to continue straight on the Lewis Creek Trail. It is 0.7 mile longer and has about an additional 600 feet of gain and 600 feet of loss. In addition, it is a more forested walk, lacking both the arrestingly expansive slabs lining stretches of Fletcher Creek as well as the meadows you encounter near the Emeric Lake junction. On the plus side, both Bernice Lake (reached by a 0.5-mile spur trail) and Vogelsang Lake sit at the boundary of the alpine zone, with view-rich, but smaller and often windswept, campsites nestled among timberline trees.

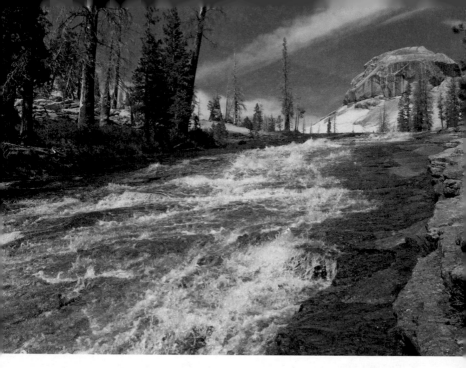

Cascades *along Fletcher Creek*

trees on this otherwise blank dome testify to nature's extraordinary persistence. You switchback up at the eastern edge of these slabs, but, time permitting, you should drop your pack and seat yourself for a break in the middle of this never-ending rock. At the notch your trail levels off and you soon reach the Babcock Lake Trail (18.55 miles), ▶15 which leads to the deep, forest-ringed lake in 0.5 mile; for most people this lake, often buggy and with an abundance of dead trees due to recent bark beetle attacks, won't be worth the detour.

Onward, you walk 0.6 mile through flat, marshy forest, passing springs and small meadow patches brightly colored with flowers. Turning a little west, the Fletcher Creek Trail breaks out into the open and begins to rise more steeply via rocky switchbacks. From these one can see a little to the north the outlet stream of Emeric Lake—though not the lake itself, which is behind a dome just to the right of the outlet's notch. If you choose not to take the alternate route up the inlet to Emeric Lake (see the Option on page 173), at least pop briefly to the river's edge and imbibe the beauty of the stream-polished rock and smoothly flowing water. The trail continues along Fletcher Creek, soon reaching a long meadow guarded in the west by a highly polished knoll and presided over in the east by huge Vogelsang Peak. Fletcher Creek runs through the meadow in a reasonably broad, deep channel—a narrow log is present for nimble hikers, while others will prefer to wade through the sandy creek.

When you come to a scissors junction (20.55 miles) ►**16** at the north end of the meadow, you can detour along it 0.45 mile to Emeric Lake and its collection of campsites or veer right, the route to Vogelsang High Sierra Camp. Straight ahead leads to Boothe Lake and Tuolumne Pass; campsites at Boothe Lake are the most sheltered in this vicinity, sporting lodgepole pine clusters. The trail to Vogelsang (the route described here) ascends a shallow trough beside the much-diminished Fletcher Creek. Forest walking yields to increasing slabs and small meadow openings as the elevation increases; a few final switchbacks across an open slope take you to a junction at the edge of the High Sierra Camp (22.85 miles). ►**17** The backpackers' camping area is straight ahead, in the direction signposted for Lyell Canyon and Ireland Lake; you will see the use trail to the left after just 0.1 mile. You could alternatively detour to Vogelsang, Townsley, or Evelyn Lakes for additional camping options. Vogelsang lies nearly in the alpine, with campsites in sandy patches between slabs and stunted whitebark pines, while Townsley sports barely a tree. At Evelyn Lake, you can camp beneath whitebark pines at the edge of the expansive lakeside meadow.

Day four, your last day, is the easiest; it's one of the shortest legs, and almost all of it is downhill or level. You begin by dropping slightly as you traverse north across slopes to Tuolumne Pass (23.65 miles). ►**18** From the pass you head north 1.4 miles through a large, linear meadow,

OPTION: Emeric Lake

If you wish to camp at Emeric Lake—and it's a fine place—there is an off-trail shortcut to the lake, following the outlet creek's west side upward from its confluence with Fletcher Creek. First cross Fletcher Creek at a safe spot (do not attempt this in high water), and then climb along the outlet creek's west side and camp above the lake's northwest or northeast shore; camping is prohibited in the lakeside meadows—instead head to the flat patches of trees you spy because these proclaim that the ground is slightly higher and drier. The next morning circle the head of the lake and find a trail at the base of the low granite ridge at the northeast corner of the lake. Follow this trail 0.4 mile northeast to a scissors junction alongside Fletcher Creek, at which point you'll rejoin the main route at ►**16**. If you prefer to remain on trails, you can follow Fletcher Lake Trail to this junction and then follow the spur trail to the lake.

speckled with boulders and home to a healthy population of lumbering marmots and ever-alert Belding's ground squirrels. I must always laugh at the "fledgling" ground squirrels—the young old enough to be allowed outside their burrows but still far too curious, only remembering to be scared and retreat when you are a step away; they then nearly trip themselves in their hurry to disappear underground. You have views north to the Sierra Crest between Tioga Pass and Mount Conness and views back to cliff-bound, dark-banded Fletcher Peak and Vogelsang Peak cradling the Vogelsang area. Where the meadow pinches to a close (25.05 miles), ►19 the Rafferty Creek Trail enters an open lodgepole forest and continues a viewless 0.5 mile to a second, smaller meadow, which you skirt on its western perimeter. Beyond the meadow the trail descends its namesake creek, crossing a few small tributaries; you are almost always walking in open, dry lodgepole pine forest interspersed with broken slabs. Only the larger cones from a western white pine occasionally shake you to attention as you amble down to a junction with the JMT (28.55 miles). ►20

Turning left, the route ahead is almost flat as you traverse west to another junction (29.2 miles). ►21 Here, straight ahead continues around the southern perimeter of Tuolumne Meadows, including access to the Tuolumne Meadows Campground, while you branch north (right) on the route of the John Muir Trail. Walking at the edge of a narrow meadow, you reach two bridges across branches of the Lyell Fork of the Tuolumne River, a wonderful place to spend the last hour of your hike. If it is late in the day, Mounts Dana and Gibbs glow on the eastern horizon, catching the late sun, while trout dart along the wide Lyell Fork.

Past the second bridge, the JMT leads over a slight rise and descends to a junction with a trail, to the right, that ascends parallel to CA 120, eventually leading to the Gaylor Lakes (29.8 miles). ►22 You stay to the left, and after a brief walk downstream, you bridge the Dana Fork and reach a T-junction with a spur trail that trends north (right) to the Tuolumne Meadows Lodge parking lot (29.85 miles). ►23 Rather, you turn left and continue downstream, paralleling the Dana Fork until your path sidles back toward a road (30.1 miles). ►24 A 70-foot-long spur trail leads across the meadow to the road and a large parking area, where you may have left your car and from where you can catch the Tuolumne Meadows shuttle bus. Of course, if you are a purist and wish to truly complete the High Sierra Camps Loop, then continue west to a crossing of Tioga Road, immediately beyond which is a parking area at the base of Lembert Dome and the Glen Aulin Trailhead, an additional 1.05 miles.

⚑ MILESTONES

►1	0.0	Start at Sunrise Lakes Trailhead
►2	0.2	Right at junction with Tenaya Lake perimeter trail
►3	2.55	Left at Sunrise Lakes–Clouds Rest junction
►4	3.0	Lower Sunrise Lake
►5	3.55	Upper Sunrise Lake
►6	5.15	Left at John Muir Trail–Sunrise Lakes junction
►7	6.0	Right onto Echo Creek Trail in Long Meadow
►8	8.9	Long Meadow outlet creek crossing
►9	10.55	Upper bridge along Echo Creek
►10	12.3	Left at upper Echo Creek (High Trail) junction
►11	13.0	Left at junction in Merced canyon at base of Echo Creek
►12	15.2	Merced Lake High Sierra Camp
►13	15.95	Left onto Lewis Creek Trail
►14	16.95	Left onto Fletcher Creek Trail
►15	18.55	Right at Babcock Lake Trail
►16	20.55	Right at scissors junction near Emeric Lake
►17	22.85	Left at junction near Vogelsang High Sierra Camp
►18	23.65	Tuolumne Pass
►19	25.05	North end Tuolumne Pass meadow
►20	28.55	Left at John Muir Trail–Rafferty Creek Trail junction
►21	29.2	Right at Tuolumne Meadows perimeter trail junction
►22	29.8	Left at junction with trail to Gaylor Lakes
►23	29.85	Left at junction with trail to Tuolumne Meadows Lodge
►24	30.1	Finish at Lyell Canyon Trailhead (Dog Lake parking area)

CHAPTER 3

Central Yosemite

The most conspicuous and perhaps most photographed feature of Central Yosemite is Tenaya Lake, which is skirted by the heavily traveled Tioga Road (also known as CA 120). On a windless day the sandy beach on the northeast shore is sublime, while on a cooler day, the more bouldery southwest shore is much more pleasant. The sandy beach of the northeast shore is lacking here, but so too are the strong upcanyon winds that were needed to form it. Instead, you can wade in smaller sandy bays or find a few small boulder islands worth swimming or wading to.

From Tenaya Lake's southwest shore, southeast of Tioga Road, this chapter's first two trails begin, bound for very different destinations: the three Sunrise Lakes and aptly named Sunrise High Sierra Camp versus the summit of Clouds Rest.

To view all of Central Yosemite, and indeed, most of the park, make the safe, relatively easy ascent to the area's highest peak, Mount Hoffmann. From it you'll see dozens of features identifiable with a topographic map of the park. Walks to lakes are always popular, and the three subalpine lake clusters described in this chapter are all popular—the very-easy-to-reach May Lake on the way to Mount Hoffmann, the trio of Sunrise Lakes en route to Sunrise High Sierra Camp, and the longer walk to the charming Ten Lakes. Too many folks visit only the three most easily reached Ten Lakes, leaving the other four with only moderate to light use (not to mention the three that are tiny tarns).

North Dome is an unmistakable feature rising above the east end of Yosemite Valley, opposite from Half Dome. While rock climbers can reach its summit by first climbing vertical Washington Column and then the near-vertical south face of the dome, the vast majority of folks prefer to take a relatively short and easy trail heading south from Tioga Road. As atop Mount Hoffmann, the summit of North Dome provides panoramic, remunerative views, especially across Yosemite Valley and to Half Dome.

Finally, the Central Yosemite chapter ends with an ordinary looking, but quite unique and rare lake, Harden Lake. Whereas the vast majority of

Opposite: *Lake 2 in the Ten Lakes Basin (see Trail 21, page 207)*

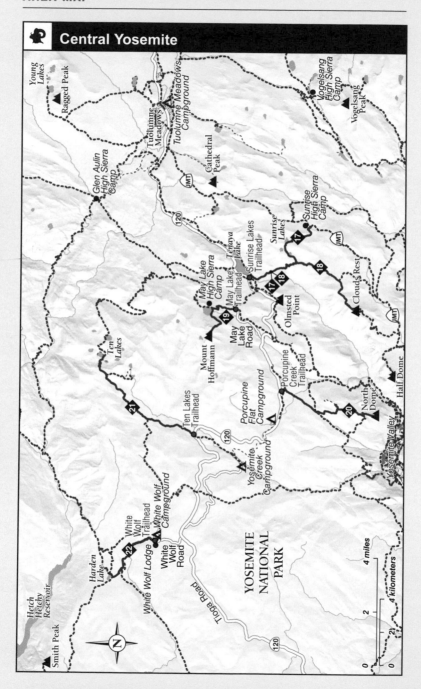

Central Yosemite

Central Yosemite

Trail	Difficulty	Length	Type	USES & ACCESS	TERRAIN	NATURE	OTHER
17	3	10.3					
18	3–4	12.6					
19	3	5.7					
20	3	9.2					
21	3	12.3					
22	2	5.7					

TYPE	USES & ACCESS	TERRAIN	NATURE	FEATURES
Point-to-Point	Day Hiking	Canyon	Autumn Colors	Great Views
Loop	Backpacking	Summit	Wildflowers	Camping
Out-and-Back	Horses	Lake	Giant Sequoias	Swimming
Balloon	Running	Stream		Secluded
	Wheelchair Access	Waterfall		Steep
DIFFICULTY	Stroller Access			Granite Slabs
– 1 2 3 4 5 +	Child-Friendly			Historical Interest
less more	Caution			Geological Interest

Sierran lakes owe their existence to glaciers excavating basins out of weathered and fractured bedrock, Harden Lake (and nearby Lukens Lake) owes its existence to water ponded up behind glacial deposits known as lateral moraines. In the case of Harden, the deposits are thin and the lake leaks, so that by midsummer it is quite shallow, whereas Lukens Lake, reached by a choice of easy trails from the White Wolf area, retains its depth all summer.

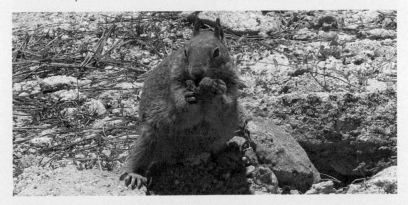

California ground squirrel

Central Yosemite

**Sunrise Lakes and
Sunrise High Sierra Camp 182**
The terrain passed on this quite short hike is varied
and scenic, with two superb camping possibilities,
the upper Sunrise Lake and Sunrise High Sierra
Camp. Those who choose the latter are rewarded
with a beautiful sunrise—the reason the camp is situated where it is. Hikers pursuing this route must,
however, be prepared for a steep climb as you rise
above the Tenaya Creek drainage: you ascend 1,000
feet in just 1.1 miles, an unusually sharp climb for
a Sierra trail. You can't avoid this climb, but if you
wish to make it a shorter day, the hike to upper
Sunrise Lake is just 3.55 miles each way.

Clouds Rest. 188
Though Clouds Rest is higher than Half Dome, it is
easier and safer to climb, and it provides far better
views of the park than does the more popular Half
Dome. Except for its last 0.1 mile, the Clouds Rest
Trail lacks the terrifying, potentially lethal drop-
offs found along Half Dome's shoulder and back
side, thereby making it a good trail for acrophobic
photographers.

May Lake and Mount Hoffmann. . . . 194
May Lake is a very popular destination because it is
such a short hike. Day hikers can reach it in about
a half hour, and all but the slowest backpackers in
under an hour. At a distance of 1.2 miles, May Lake
has the most easily accessible backcountry campsites
in the park, so it is ideal for novice backpackers or
for those with young children. Meanwhile, Mount

Hoffmann, easily reached in an afternoon from the May Lake campsites, is one of the park's most satisfying short day hikes—a beautiful, not-too-long, but tough walk, with a little scrambling near the summit and views in all directions.

North Dome 200

North Dome, which looks so inaccessible from the Yosemite Valley floor, can be reached in a couple of hours by this route. From the dome you get perhaps the best views of the expansive faces of Half Dome and Clouds Rest, as well as excellent views of Yosemite Valley. Along this hike you can also visit one of Yosemite's few known natural arches, colloquially referred to as Indian Rock arch, and also visit the true Indian Rock, a summit to the north that provides a broad panorama.

TRAIL 20

Day Hike, Backpack, Child-Friendly
9.2 miles,
Out-and-Back
Difficulty: 1 2 **3** 4 5

Ten Lakes Basin 207

The Ten Lakes Basin is extremely popular with weekend backpackers because with only a few hours' hiking effort, you can attain any of its seven major lakes. The three most accessible receive moderate to heavy use, but the other four, off the beaten track, are worth the effort for those who want relatively secluded camping.

TRAIL 21

Day Hike, Backpack, Horse
12.3 miles,
Out-and-Back
Difficulty: 1 2 **3** 4 5

Harden Lake 216

Just over an hour's hike from White Wolf Campground, this lake attracts quite a number of summer visitors, virtually all of them day hikers. Mid-June–July this shallow lake can be fine for swimming, but the lake lies in a leaky basin, and by mid-August it usually has dwindled to an oversize wading pool. Don't expect to catch any fish because the lake becomes far too shallow by late summer to support any. The moist forests the trail traverses sport colorful early summer flowers—as does the slope north of Harden Lake, a possible extension to your day.

TRAIL 22

Day Hike, Backpack, Horse, Run, Child-Friendly
5.7 miles,
Out-and-Back
Difficulty: 1 **2** 3 4 5

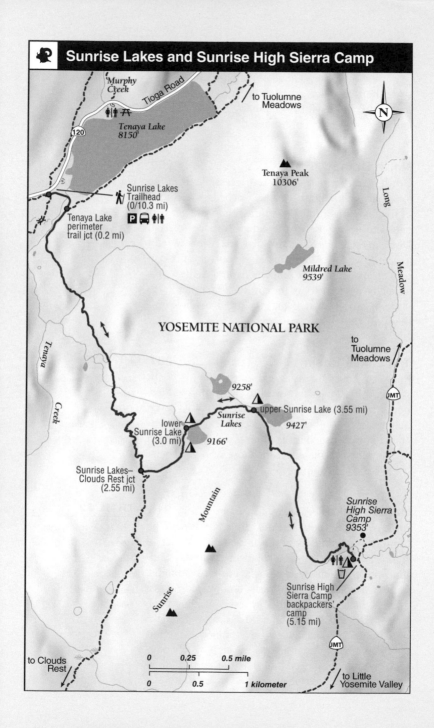

Sunrise Lakes and Sunrise High Sierra Camp

Murphy Creek

Tioga Road

Tenaya Lake
8150'

120

to Tuolumne
Meadows

N

Tenaya Peak
10306'

Sunrise Lakes
Trailhead
(0/10.3 mi)

P 🚌 ♦♦

Tenaya Lake
perimeter
trail jct (0.2 mi)

Mildred Lake
9539'

Tenaya Creek

YOSEMITE NATIONAL PARK

to
Tuolumne
Meadows

JMT

9258'

upper Sunrise Lake (3.55 mi)

lower
Sunrise Lake
(3.0 mi)

Sunrise
Lakes

9427'

9166'

Sunrise Lakes–
Clouds Rest jct
(2.55 mi)

Sunrise
High Sierra
Camp
9353'

Mountain

Sunrise High
Sierra Camp
backpackers'
camp
(5.15 mi)

Sunrise

to Clouds
Rest

0   0.25   0.5 mile

0   0.5   1 kilometer

JMT

to Little
Yosemite Valley

Sunrise Lakes and Sunrise High Sierra Camp

The terrain passed on this quite short hike is varied and scenic, with two superb camping possibilities, the upper Sunrise Lake and Sunrise High Sierra Camp. Those at the latter are rewarded with a beautiful sunrise—the reason the camp is situated where it is. Hikers pursuing this route must, however, be prepared for a steep climb as you rise above the Tenaya Creek drainage: you ascend 1,000 feet in just 1.1 miles, an unusually sharp climb for a Sierra trail. You can't avoid this climb, but if you wish to make it a shorter day, the hike to upper Sunrise Lake is just 3.55 miles each way.

Permits

Overnight visitors require a wilderness permit for the Sunrise Lakes Trailhead, issued by Yosemite National Park. Pick up your permit at the Tuolumne Meadows Wilderness Center, located in the parking lot a short way down Tuolumne Meadows Lodge Road or at another of the Yosemite permit-issuing stations (see "Permits," page 21).

Maps

This trail is covered by the Tom Harrison *Tuolumne Meadows* map (1:42,240 scale), the National Geographic Trails Illustrated *#309 Yosemite SE* map (1:40,000 scale), and the USGS 7.5-minute series *Tenaya Lake* map (1:24,000 scale).

Best Time

Because of fairly high elevations and some northerly aspects, the pass between upper Sunrise Lake and the High Sierra Camp can have snow patches into

TRAIL USE
Day Hike, Backpack, Horse
LENGTH
10.3 miles, 4–8 hours (over 1–2 days)
VERTICAL FEET
One-way: +1,800', –640'
Round-trip: ±2,440'
DIFFICULTY
– 1 2 **3** 4 5 +
TRAIL TYPE
Out-and-Back

FEATURES
Lake
Wildflowers
Great Views
Camping
Swimming
Steep

FACILITIES
Bear Boxes
Restrooms
Shuttle Stop

July; only in lower snow years will you want to take this route in June. Lakes are near their optimal temperatures mid-July–August, and mosquitoes have tapered by late July, making August the favorite month of many backpackers. To avoid crowds, consider a September trip, though nights will be notably cooler. You can even go in early and mid-October, though then be prepared for cool days and subfreezing nights to complement the yellow grasses and often bright blue skies.

> Sunrise is the only High Sierra Camp not located by a lake or river, but what sunrises!

Finding the Trail

The trail begins on Tioga Road at the Sunrise Lakes Trailhead, a large pullout at a highway bend near Tenaya Lake's southwest shore. It is located 30.7 miles northeast of Crane Flat and 8.7 miles southwest of the Tuolumne Meadows Campground. There are pit toilets at the trailhead, but the closest flush toilets and drinking water are located at the Tuolumne Meadows Visitor Center (to the east) or at the White Wolf Campground or Crane Flat store (to the west), so fill your water bottles before heading to the trailhead.

Trail Description

From the trailhead parking area, ▶1 take a trail that heads east, passes two small spur trails that depart to the right (south), and soon crosses the usually flowing outlet of Tenaya Lake. Just beyond this crossing you

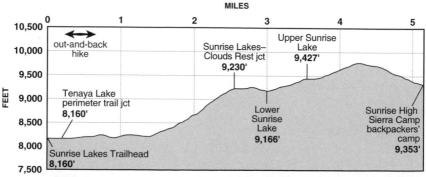

TRAIL 17 Sunrise Lakes and Sunrise High Sierra Camp Elevation Profile

reach a trail junction. The trail left goes northeast along Tenaya Lake's southeastern shore (0.2 mile). ►2

You, however, veer right on a trail that heads south for an additional 0.25 mile along Tenaya Creek before turning to the southeast as the trail gently ascends in sparse forest over a little rise and drops to a ford of Mildred Lake's outlet. Like the other streams over the next 2 miles, it can dry up in late summer or early autumn but requires a sandy wade (or wobbly log balance) in early summer. Beyond the Mildred Lake stream the trail undulates and winds generally south, passing several pocket meadows browsed by mule deer and crossing additional seasonal tributaries, the outlets of the Sunrise Lakes. At 1.4 miles, the trail then begins to climb in earnest, through a thinning cover of lodgepole pine and occasional red fir, western white pine, and mountain hemlock. As the trail rises above Tenaya Canyon, you pass several vantage points from which you can look north to the polished granite walls rising above Tenaya Creek, though you never see Tenaya Lake. To the east the canyon is bounded by Tenaya Peak; in the northwest are the cliffs of Mount Hoffmann and Tuolumne Peak.

Now on switchbacks, you see Tioga Road across the canyon and can even hear vehicles, but these annoyances are infinitesimal compared to the pleasures of polished granite expanses all around. Your route ahead is steep—few Sierra trails ascend 1,000 feet in just 1.1 miles. The trail is also, in places, annoyingly rocky, reflecting the many half-buried boulders and partially submerged slabs with which the trail construction crew had to contend. At least these switchbacks are, for the most part, mercifully shaded, and where they become steepest, requiring a great output of energy, they give back with the beauty of a fine flower display, including lupine, penstemon, paintbrush, larkspur, buttercup, and sunflowers such as aster and senecio. Finally the switchbacks end and the trail levels as it arrives at a junction on a shallow, forested saddle (2.55 miles). ►3

Straight ahead leads to Clouds Rest and beyond (Trail 18), but you turn left and first contour east, cross a low gap, and descend north through broken forest to lower Sunrise Lake (3.0 miles). ►4 The western shore of this lake sports a number of small campsites, the first under forest cover, the latter smaller and more open in flat patches between slabs. Steep exfoliating slabs dominate the cross-lake view, while heath species, including red mountain heather and western Labrador tea, decorate the lakeshore. Climbing from this lake, you reach a crest in several minutes, and from it you could descend cross-country an equally short distance north to more isolated, island-dotted middle Sunrise Lake. Your trail, however, veers east and gains a very noticeable 150 feet as it climbs to upper Sunrise Lake, the largest and most popular lake of the trio (3.55 miles). ▶5 Campsites are plentiful along its north shore, away from the trail and reached by crossing the lake at its outlet.

With 1.6 miles remaining to your day's goal, you skirt the edge of the flower-filled meadow ringing the lake, diagonal up a slope, and soon find yourself in a shallow gully that you follow south across dry gravelly soils. At a broad pass you can look back to Mount Hoffmann or ahead to see the Clark Range head-on, piercing the southern sky. From the gap, which is sparsely clothed with mountain hemlocks, whitebark pines, and western white pines, you begin a shallow descent, still on decomposing granite and hopefully catching a glimpse of a Clark's nutcracker, the gray-and-white relative of blue jays that frequents the timberline country. The

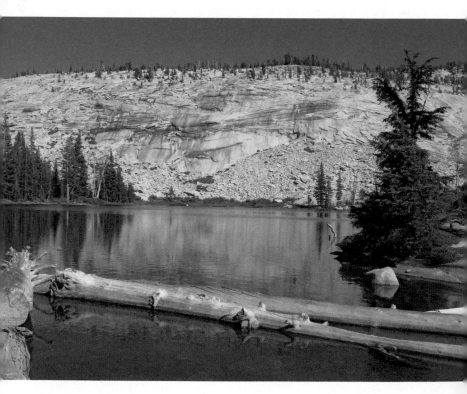

Lower *Sunrise Lake*

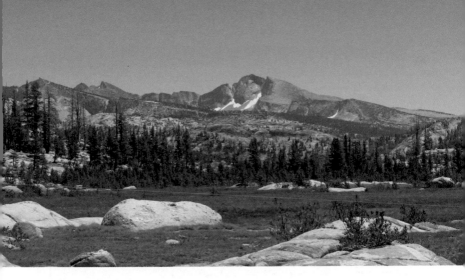

Vista to Mount Florence *from Sunrise High Sierra Camp*

grade increases and you descend south into denser cover, veer east, and
then north to make a steep descent to the Sunrise backpackers' camp,
complete with a water faucet, pit toilet, food storage boxes, and ample (if
crowded) campsites. From near the pit toilet, a use trail leads northeast
to the Sunrise High Sierra Camp. An overnight stay at either camp gives
you an inspiring sunrise over Matthes Crest and the Cathedral Range.
Continuing briefly down the main trail below the campsite leads to a
T-junction with the John Muir Trail, where turning right takes you to
Yosemite Valley and left (north) takes you along L-shaped Long Meadow
toward the Cathedral Lakes and Tuolumne Meadows (5.15 miles). ►6
After a beautiful night's sleep or picnic lunch, you then retrace your steps
to the trailhead (10.3 miles). ►7

🚶	MILESTONES	
►1	0.0	Start at Sunrise Lakes Trailhead
►2	0.2	Right at junction to Tenaya Lake perimeter trail
►3	2.55	Left at Sunrise Lakes–Clouds Rest junction
►4	3.0	Lower Sunrise Lake
►5	3.55	Upper Sunrise Lake
►6	5.15	Sunrise High Sierra Camp backpackers' campground
►7	10.3	Return to Sunrise Lakes Trailhead

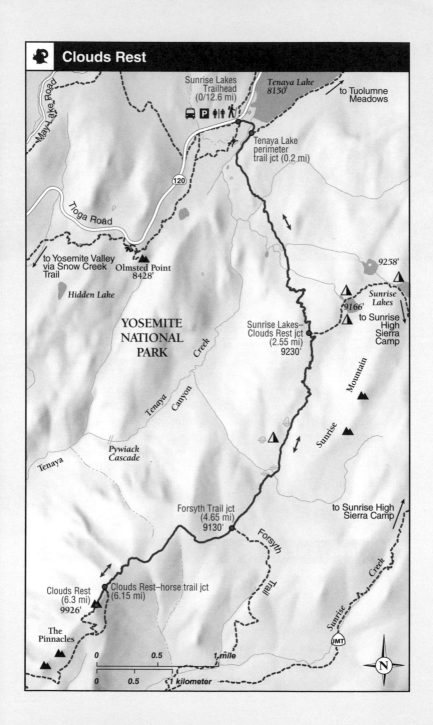

Clouds Rest

Sunrise Lakes
Trailhead
(0/12.6 mi)

Tenaya Lake
8150'

to Tuolumne
Meadows

Tenaya Lake
perimeter
trail jct (0.2 mi)

120

Tioga Road

to Yosemite Valley
via Snow Creek
Trail

Olmsted Point
8428'

Hidden Lake

9258'

Sunrise
Lakes

9166'

to Sunrise
High
Sierra
Camp

YOSEMITE
NATIONAL
PARK

Sunrise Lakes–
Clouds Rest jct
(2.55 mi)
9230'

Sunrise Mountain

Tenaya Canyon

Tenaya Creek

Pywiack
Cascade

Tenaya

Forsyth Trail jct
(4.65 mi)
9130'

to Sunrise High
Sierra Camp

Forsyth Trail

Sunrise Creek

Clouds Rest
(6.3 mi)
9926'

Clouds Rest–horse trail jct
(6.15 mi)

The
Pinnacles

JMT

0   0.5   1 mile

0   0.5   1 kilometer

N

Clouds Rest

Though Clouds Rest is higher than Half Dome, it is easier and safer to climb, and it provides far better views of the park than does the more popular, crowded Half Dome. Except for its last 0.1 mile, the Clouds Rest Trail lacks the terrifying exposure found along Half Dome's shoulder and back side, thereby making it a good trail for acrophobic photographers, especially because the views from just before the final narrow ridge to the summit are already superb and worth the trip. If you're an avid photographer, you'll want to start this trek at the crack of dawn to reach this summit before shadows become poor for photography. All hikers should strive to reach this summit by noon or thereabouts if thunderstorms are forecast for the afternoon.

Permits

Overnight visitors require a wilderness permit for the Sunrise Lakes Trailhead, issued by Yosemite National Park. Pick up your permit at the Tuolumne Meadows Wilderness Center, located in the parking lot a short way down Tuolumne Meadows Lodge Road or at another of the Yosemite permit-issuing stations (see "Permits," page 21).

Maps

This trail is covered by the Tom Harrison *Tuolumne Meadows* map (1:42,240 scale), the National Geographic Trails Illustrated *#309 Yosemite SE* map (1:40,000 scale), and the USGS 7.5-minute series *Tenaya Lake* map (1:24,000 scale).

TRAIL USE
Day Hike, Backpack, Horse

LENGTH
12.6 miles; 6–10 hours (over 1–2 days)

VERTICAL FEET
One-way: +2,440', –675'
Round-trip: ±3,115'

DIFFICULTY
– 1 2 **3 4** 5 +

TRAIL TYPE
Out-and-Back

FEATURES
Summit
Wildflowers
Great Views
Camping
Steep
Granite Slabs

FACILITIES
Bear Boxes
Restrooms
Shuttle Stop

Best Time

This trail is most popular late July–early September, when you are ensured a snow-free trail and fewer mosquitoes. However, the trail is usually snow-free by early July and the wildflower display peaks soon thereafter, starting to dwindle by late July. Because the mosquitoes are only prevalent along short stretches of this trail—and absent near the summit—you can avoid most of them if you don't dawdle. As always, the crowds disappear after Labor Day, and if you like hiking in cooler weather, you often can take this trail through mid- and late October.

Finding the Trail

The trail begins on Tioga Road at the Sunrise Lakes Trailhead, a large pullout at a highway bend near Tenaya Lake's southwest shore. It is located 30.7 miles northeast of Crane Flat and 8.7 miles southwest of the Tuolumne Meadows Campground. There are pit toilets at the trailhead, but the closest flush toilets and drinking water are located at the Tuolumne Meadows Visitor Center (to the east) or at the White Wolf Campground or Crane Flat store (to the west), so fill your water bottles before heading to the trailhead.

Trail Description

From the trailhead parking area, ▶1 take a trail that heads east, passes two small spur trails that depart to the right (south), and soon crosses the usually flowing outlet of Tenaya Lake. Just beyond this crossing you

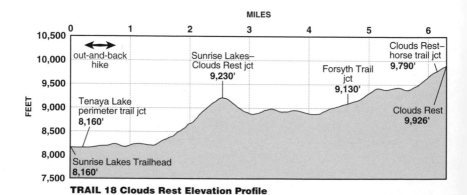

TRAIL 18 Clouds Rest Elevation Profile

reach a trail junction. The trail left goes northeast along Tenaya Lake's southeastern shore (0.2 mile). ▶2

You, however, veer right on a trail that parallels Tenaya Creek south for an additional 0.25 mile before turning to the southeast as the trail gently ascends in sparse forest over a little rise and drops to a ford of Mildred Lake's outlet. Like the other streams over the next 2 miles, it can dry up in late summer or early autumn but requires a sandy wade (or wobbly log balance) in early summer. Beyond the Mildred Lake stream the trail undulates and winds generally south, passing several pocket meadows browsed by mule deer and crossing additional seasonal tributaries, the outlets of the Sunrise Lakes. At 1.4 miles, the trail then begins to climb in earnest, through a thinning cover of lodgepole pine and occasional red fir, western white pine, and mountain hemlock. As the trail rises above Tenaya Canyon, you pass several vantage points from which you can look north to the polished granite walls rising above Tenaya Creek, though you never see Tenaya Lake. To the east the canyon is bounded by Tenaya Peak; in the northwest are the cliffs of Mount Hoffmann and Tuolumne Peak.

Now on switchbacks, you see Tioga Road across the canyon and can even hear vehicles, but these annoyances are infinitesimal compared to the pleasures of polished granite expanses all around. Your route ahead is steep—few Sierra trails ascend 1,000 feet in just 1.1 miles. The trail is also, in places, annoyingly rocky, reflecting the many half-buried boulders and partially submerged slabs with which the trail construction crew had to contend. At least these switchbacks are, for the most part, mercifully shaded, and where they become steepest, requiring a great output of energy, they give back with the beauty of a fine flower display, including lupine, penstemon, paintbrush, larkspur, buttercup, and sunflowers such as aster and senecio. Finally the switchbacks end and the trail levels as it arrives at a junction on a shallow, forested saddle (2.55 miles). ▶3 Here the High Sierra Camps Loop veers left, bound for Sunrise High Sierra Camp (Trail 17). If you were to head 0.45 mile along this trail, you would reach lower Sunrise Lake, sporting campsites, some forested, others in sandy flats, around the lake's western shore. Though a bit of a detour off your main route, these campsites are better than the only watered campsites along the trail to Clouds Rest.

Assuming you are beelining for the summit, with the initial hard climb behind you, trend right, descending south, bound for Clouds Rest. Your trail switchbacks for a relatively minor descent to a shady, sometimes damp, flat, then climbs to a block-strewn ridge that sprouts dense

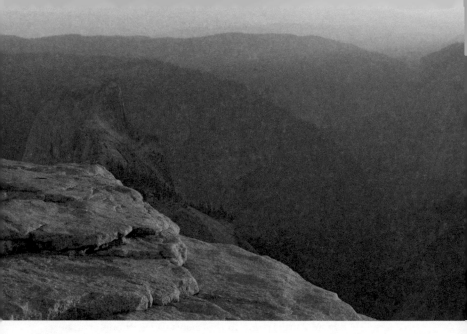

Sunset view *to Half Dome and Yosemite Valley from the summit of Clouds Rest*

clumps of chinquapin and aspen. Beyond it the trail descends briefly to a tree-fringed pond—adequate for nearby camping —then wanders south before reaching an often-boggy (and buggy) meadow. You cross three creeklets in rapid succession, your last usually reliable sources of water. After you cross the first creeklet, follow the trail briefly downstream, then veer left to cross the second creeklet before climbing to the third. Beyond that, the trail rapidly eases its gradient and soon reaches a quite flat, sandy shoulder, adequate for a campsite if you carry water from below. At 4.65 miles it reaches the Forsyth Trail junction, ▶4 which approximately marks the northeastern boundary of forest damaged by the 2014 Meadow Fire; downslope the once-dense conifer forest is mostly destroyed.

The Forsyth Trail forks left, headed for the John Muir Trail and Merced River canyon, but you keep right and, for about a mile, ascend the Clouds Rest Trail west to a gravelly crest and then follow it down to a shallow saddle. The final ascent begins here. After a moderate ascent of 0.25 mile, you emerge from the forest cover—what remains of it following the fire—to get your first excellent views of the endless slabs defining Tenaya Canyon and the country west and north of it. After another 0.25 mile along the crest you come to a junction with a horse trail (6.15 miles). ▶5 If you're riding a horse from Tenaya Lake to Yosemite Valley via the Clouds Rest Trail, you'll take this left-trending trail after first walking to the summit without your equine companion.

The Clouds Rest foot trail, the right ridge option, now becomes exposed, and you scramble a few feet up to the narrow and potentially dangerous crest. One wishes there were a hand railing in spots. Acrophobes and klutzes should not continue, but luckily you already have spectacular views of Tenaya Canyon, Half Dome, and Yosemite Valley that are nearly identical with those seen from the summit. Spreading below is the expansive 4,500-foot-high face of Clouds Rest—the largest granite face in the park. Those who follow the now steeper, narrow, almost trailless crest 0.1 mile to the summit (6.3 miles) ►6 are further rewarded with views of the Clark Range and the Merced River canyon west toward Yosemite Valley. Growing on the rocky summit are a few knee-high Jeffrey pines and whitebark pines, plus assorted bushes and wildflowers. Note that if you wish to reach the summit but are unwilling to follow this crest, a considerably longer but less exposed alternative exists. You follow the horse trail west to a junction with the Clouds Rest Trail from Yosemite Valley and proceed up this trail to the summit (head right). It adds 0.9 mile each direction, but for some will be worth the extra distance. When you are finished imbibing the view, return the way you came (12.6 miles). ►7

MILESTONES

►1	0.0	Start at Sunrise Lakes Trailhead
►2	0.2	Right at junction to Tenaya Lake perimeter trail
►3	2.55	Right at Sunrise Lakes–Clouds Rest junction
►4	4.65	Right at Forsyth Trail junction
►5	6.15	Right at horse trail junction
►6	6.3	Clouds Rest summit
►7	12.6	Return to Sunrise Lakes Trailhead

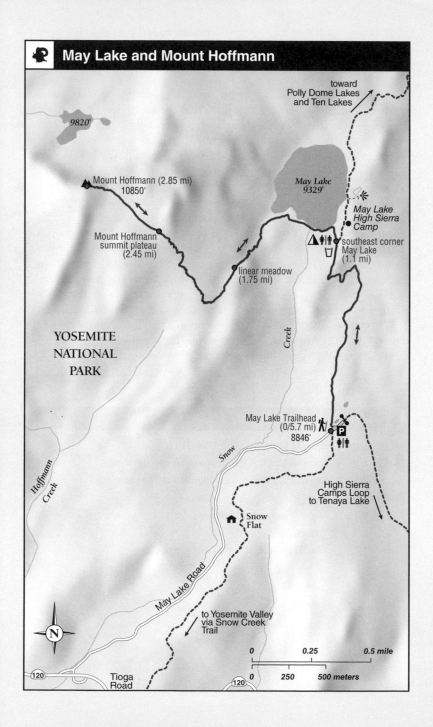

May Lake and Mount Hoffmann

9820'

Mount Hoffmann (2.85 mi)
10850'

May Lake
9329'

Mount Hoffmann
summit plateau
(2.45 mi)

May Lake
High Sierra
Camp

southeast corner
May Lake
(1.1 mi)

linear meadow
(1.75 mi)

toward
Polly Dome Lakes
and Ten Lakes

Creek

YOSEMITE
NATIONAL
PARK

May Lake Trailhead
(0/5.7 mi)
8846'

High Sierra
Camps Loop
to Tenaya Lake

Snow

Hoffmann

Creek

Snow
Flat

May Lake Road

to Yosemite Valley
via Snow Creek
Trail

N

120

Tioga
Road

120

| 0 | 0.25 | 0.5 mile |

| 0 | 250 | 500 meters |

May Lake and Mount Hoffmann

May Lake is a very popular destination because it is such a short hike. Day hikers can reach it in a half hour and most backpackers in under an hour. At 1.2 miles from the trailhead, May Lake has the most easily accessible backcountry campsites in the park, so it is ideal for novice backpackers or for those with young children. Additionally, these are good base-camp sites for an ascent of Mount Hoffmann, to which most hikers dedicate a half day. Mount Hoffmann, centrally located in Yosemite National Park, provides the best all-around views of this park's varied landscapes. This summit is reached by at least 50 day hikers on sunny mid-summer days, as well as a good proportion of the backpackers staying at May Lake overnight.

Permits

Overnight visitors require a wilderness permit for the May Lake Trailhead, issued by Yosemite National Park. Pick up your permit at the Tuolumne Meadows Wilderness Center, located in the parking lot a short way down Tuolumne Meadows Lodge Road; at the Big Oak Flat Information Center; or at another of the Yosemite permit-issuing stations (see "Permits," page 21).

Maps

This trail is covered by the Tom Harrison *Yosemite High Country* map (1:63,360 scale), the National Geographic Trails Illustrated *#308 Yosemite NE* map (1:40,000 scale), and the USGS 7.5-minute series *Tenaya Lake* and *Yosemite Falls* maps (1:24,000 scale).

TRAIL USE
Day Hike, Backpack,
Horse, Child-Friendly
LENGTH
5.7 miles, 3–6 hours
(over 1–2 days)
VERTICAL FEET
One-way: +2,025', −30'
Round-trip: ±2,055'
DIFFICULTY
− 1 2 **3** 4 5 +
TRAIL TYPE
Out-and-Back

FEATURES
Summit
Lake
Wildflowers
Great Views
Camping

FACILITIES
Bear Boxes
Restrooms

Best Time

Snow lingers long at the trailhead's Snow Flat, making this hike impractical until late June in all but the lowest snow years. This is especially true because the 1.8-mile spur road leading from CA 120 (Tioga Road) to the trailhead often remains closed for several weeks after the highway opens, adding distance and elevation to your walk. In June and July, mosquitoes are notoriously bad at the trailhead but tend to be much diminished by the lake; just pack quickly and don't despair that the bugs will be this bothersome at May Lake itself! August is probably the most popular month, but virtually all the snow is gone from the landscape and so the surrounding terrain is less photogenic. September–mid-October also are good times because the crowds are gone. Overall, for best photography with patches of snow and bright patches of flowers, fight the mosquitoes on the first stretch and hike around early to mid-July. Because swimming is prohibited in May Lake, water temperature isn't a consideration.

Finding the Trail

From the Tioga Road–Big Oak Flat Road junction in Crane Flat, drive northeast 27.0 miles up Tioga Road to May Lake Road, a segment of old CA 120. (This turn is 3.2 miles east of the Porcupine Flat Campground.) If you are driving from the east, the turn is 12.6 miles west of the Tuolumne Meadows Campground or 2.3 miles west of the Olmsted Point vista pullout. Follow May Lake Road 1.8 miles to its end; the trailhead is on the left near the toilets. Note that this road may be closed for several

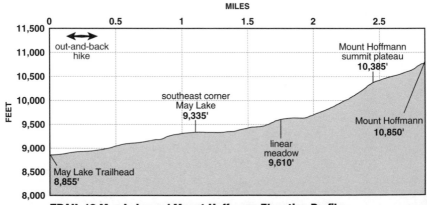

TRAIL 19 May Lake and Mount Hoffmann Elevation Profile

weeks after Tioga Road (CA 120) opens for the summer. There are pit toilets at the trailhead, but the closest flush toilets and drinking water are located at the Tuolumne Meadows Visitor Center (to the east) or at the White Wolf Campground or Crane Flat store (to the west), so fill your water bottles before heading to the trailhead.

May Lake was named for Lucy Mayotta Browne, who married Charles Hoffmann of the California State Geological Survey in 1870.

Trail Description

The trail begins by the southwest side of a small pond ►1 in a moderately dense stand of hemlock, red fir, and western white and lodgepole pines. This vale remains boggy well into summer, permitting corn lilies to bloom into August and mosquitoes to thrive just as long. Your sandy trail ascends gently through forest cover, where you recognize western white pines by their long, narrow cones and checkerboard bark pattern, and red firs by the rich burgundy color of their bark and by their cones, which grow upright on the branches near the tops of these trees, unlike the hanging cones of pines and hemlocks. Moreover, fir cones disintegrate before falling from the tree, so you will never find them on the ground.

The initial ascent leads to a shallow trench among broken granite slabs dotted with lodgepoles. Then, as you switchback west up a short, open, steep slope, you have fine views of Cathedral Peak in the east, Mount Clark in the southeast, and Clouds Rest and Half Dome in the south. Near the top of the slope, the forest cover thickens and the western white pines become larger and more handsome. Just beyond the crest, you find yourself in a flat beneath a half dozen superb hemlocks by deep, chilly May Lake and the nearby High Sierra Camp (to the right) and backpackers' campground (to the left, spread out along the lake's southern shore, set back a little into the forest; 1.1 miles). ►2 As at most other High Sierra backpackers' camping areas, you'll find bear-proof food storage boxes, a water faucet, and toilets. Swimming is not allowed, but you may try your luck at catching the lake's brook or rainbow trout while contemplating the lake's beautiful backdrop of the east slopes of massive Mount Hoffmann.

Perhaps more hikers ascend Mount Hoffmann than any other 10,000-plus-foot peak in the park, with only Mount Dana (Trail 6) challenging its popularity. As with any high-peak ascent, wear dark glasses and lots of sunscreen because there is one-third less atmosphere on the summit than at sea level, so the ultraviolet rays come on strong. Also, take steps

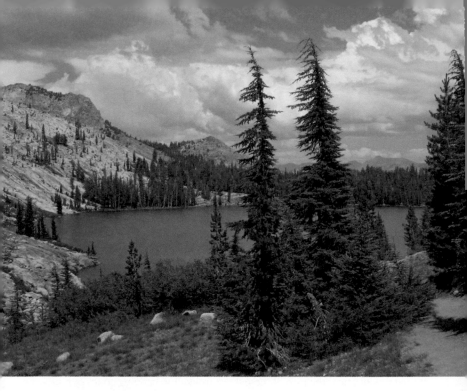

Mountain hemlocks *along the shore of May Lake*

to minimize altitude sickness, which is more likely to occur with exertion and fatigue. If you are prone to altitude sickness, camp overnight at May Lake to get partly acclimatized before climbing the peak the next day. And remember, abandon your attempt if a thunderstorm is approaching.

From the aforementioned junction, to reach Mount Hoffmann strike west along May Lake's southern shore and then, from the lake's southwest corner, begin a gradual climb across metasedimentary rocks cropping out above the lake's southwest shore. You now follow the trail southwest, first through a small gap, then through a steeper, boulder-strewn wildflower garden, resplendent with bright colors from the columbines, Jacob's ladder, monkeyflowers, penstemon, and much more. The wildflower gully leads to a small, linear meadow occupying a broad saddle (1.75 miles). ▶3 Encircling the meadow along its eastern edge, the trail continues 300 feet past the meadow's southwestern end and then climbs northwest, switchbacking up a dry, sandy slope dotted with whitebark pines. You climb persistently, absorbing the expanding views and mercifully distracted by colorful flowers, until you reach the lower end of the broad, sloping summit area decked with dense patches of lupine and Bolander's milkvetch (2.45 miles). ▶4 A well-trod use trail takes you across this summit plateau to a saddle at its northern end. Mount Hoffmann boasts numerous summits, of which the western summit is the highest, at 10,850 feet, and, turning left, you have an easy, safe scramble to its top (2.85 miles). ▶5 Using a topo map of the park, you can identify almost every major peak in it because most are visible from here. After a relaxing summit break, return to the May Lake Trailhead (5.7 miles), ▶6 but don't be tempted to take a more direct route to May Lake, as the terrain is much steeper.

🚶 MILESTONES

▶1	0.0	Start at May Lake Trailhead
▶2	1.1	Left at southeast corner May Lake
▶3	1.75	Linear meadow
▶4	2.45	Mount Hoffmann summit plateau
▶5	2.85	Mount Hoffmann
▶6	5.7	Return to May Lake Trailhead

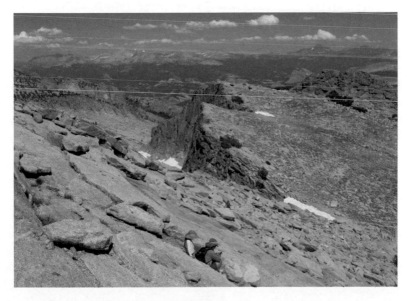

Just below *the summit of Mount Hoffmann*

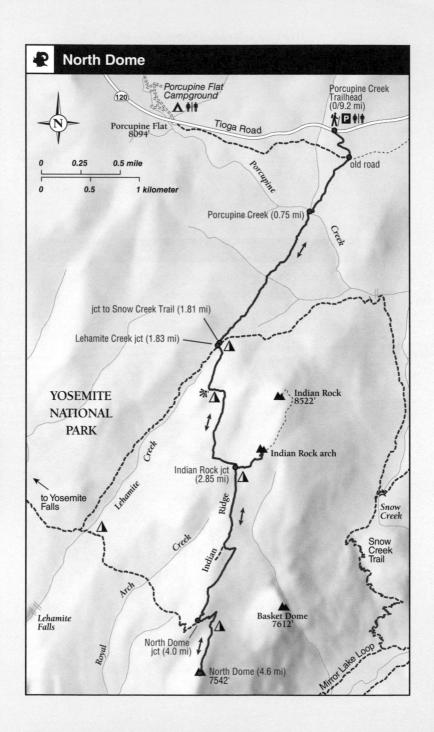

North Dome

Porcupine Flat
Campground

120

Porcupine Flat
8094'

Tioga Road

Porcupine Creek
Trailhead
(0/9.2 mi)

old road

N

0   0.25   0.5 mile

0   0.5   1 kilometer

Porcupine

Creek

Porcupine Creek (0.75 mi)

jct to Snow Creek Trail (1.81 mi)

Lehamite Creek jct (1.83 mi)

YOSEMITE
NATIONAL
PARK

Indian Rock
8522'

Indian Rock arch

Indian Rock jct
(2.85 mi)

to Yosemite
Falls

Lehamite

Creek

Snow
Creek

Snow
Creek
Trail

Indian

Ridge

Arch

Lehamite
Falls

Royal

Basket Dome
7612'

North Dome
jct (4.0 mi)

North Dome (4.6 mi)
7542'

Mirror Lake Loop

North Dome

North Dome, which looks so inaccessible from the Yosemite Valley floor, can be reached in a couple of hours by this route. From the dome you get perhaps the best views of the expansive faces of Half Dome and Clouds Rest, as well as excellent views of Yosemite Valley. Along this hike you can also visit one of Yosemite's few known natural arches, colloquially known as Indian Rock. (Another one is, surprisingly, underwater, near Tuolumne Meadows Lodge.) Additionally, you can visit the true Indian Rock, a tiny summit that provides a panorama of the valley's eastern uplands.

Permits

Overnight visitors require a wilderness permit for the Porcupine Creek Trailhead, issued by Yosemite National Park. Pick up your permit at the Tuolumne Meadows Wilderness Center, located in the parking lot a short way down Tuolumne Meadows Lodge Road; at the Big Oak Flat Information Center; or at another of the Yosemite permit-issuing stations (see "Permits," page 21).

Maps

This trail is covered by the Tom Harrison *Yosemite High Country* map (1:63,360 scale), the National Geographic Trails Illustrated *#306 Yosemite SW* map (1:40,000 scale), and the USGS 7.5-minute series *Yosemite Falls* map (1:24,000 scale).

Best Time

Of trails above 8,000 feet, this is one of the first to become mostly snow-free, so you can take it by

TRAIL USE
Day Hike, Backpack,
Child-Friendly

LENGTH
9.2 miles, 4–7 hours
(over 1–2 days)

VERTICAL FEET
One-way: +680', –1,280'
Round-trip: ±1,960'

DIFFICULTY
– 1 2 **3** 4 5 +

TRAIL TYPE
Out-and-Back

FEATURES
Summit
Wildflowers
Great Views
Camping
Granite Slabs
Geological Interest

FACILITIES
Bear Boxes
Restrooms

mid-June. On the shady, moist first 1.8 miles, mosquitoes may be prevalent through mid-July, but bugs will not interfere with your walk along most of its length and shouldn't be a major consideration for this hike. Tioga Road is usually open through late October, and day hiking until then is great. I particularly enjoy walking in September after Labor Day, when trail use is light and temperatures are just about right, neither too hot nor too cold, but I am also partial to the early July flowers, especially enjoying the red-and-white-striped sugar sticks that are common along this trail.

Porcupine Creek and Porcupine Flat above it are well named because they are located in a nearly pure stand of lodgepole pines—and pines, rather than firs, are the favorite food of the park's porcupines. Sadly—and for unknown reasons—these large rodents have become quite rare in the park.

Finding the Trail

From the Tioga Road–Big Oak Flat Road junction in Crane Flat, drive northeast 23.7 miles up Tioga Road to the Porcupine Flat Campground, then an additional 1.1 miles to a large pullout on the right, complete with toilets and food storage boxes. If you're westbound, the trailhead is 4.4 miles west of the Olmsted Point vista pullout. There are no nearby water faucets—you must fill your water bottles at the Crane Flat store, the White Wolf Campground,

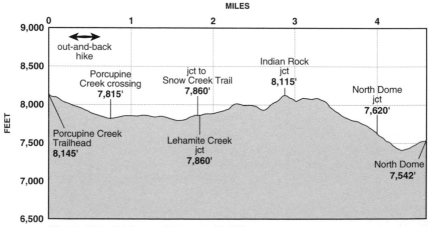

TRAIL 20 North Dome Elevation Profile

OPTIONS: **Campsites with Water**

A number of beautiful flat campsites, including those on the saddle just before the summit, are along the route to North Dome. Unfortunately, save for the sites near the Snow Creek junction, they are all dry and you need to carry your water from Porcupine Creek. An alternative is to take the trail descending southwest from ►4 along Lehamite Creek. This trail descends steeply for 1.55 miles to a T-junction alongside Lehamite Creek. There are some OK sites near the creek or, better, on more spacious (if dry) lands a few minutes east or west of it, located once you have ascended out of the drainage. Heading east from the T-junction is a 1.3-mile-long trail segment taking you back toward North Dome; you'll reintersect the described route at ►6. Midway along this undulating traverse you'll cross Royal Arch Creek, which can be dry before August, but nearby are some more acceptable campsites. This alternate route is 0.7 mile longer than the straight out-and-back route and involves about 250 more feet of ascent (and descent). My recommendation? Carry enough water from the trailhead for the night, and enjoy being able to camp so close to the summit of North Dome!

or the Tuolumne Meadows Campground or Visitor Center before heading to the trailhead.

Trail Description

Starting from the sign near the trailhead's pit toilets, ►1 a steep trail descends shortly to a nearby closed road. On it you descend to Porcupine Creek, along whose banks the Porcupine Creek Campground was located until it closed in 1977. In early summer the creek can be a wet ford or a narrow log crossing (0.75 mile). ►2 From its southwest bank your trail makes a rolling traverse. Through most of summer you may encounter creeks along this traverse, the last water you'll often encounter on the route. After a little over a mile you reach a junction atop a shady saddle dominated by red firs, where you trend to the right, while left leads to the Snow Creek drainage (1.81 miles). ►3 Just 0.2 mile down this track are some possible campsites.

Just 50 steps later, the trail to North Dome reaches another junction (1.83 miles), ►4 and here a trail forking right descends 1.55 miles down along Lehamite Creek to Yosemite Valley's North Rim Trail, an alternate route that is 0.7 mile longer but provides some mediocre campsites near

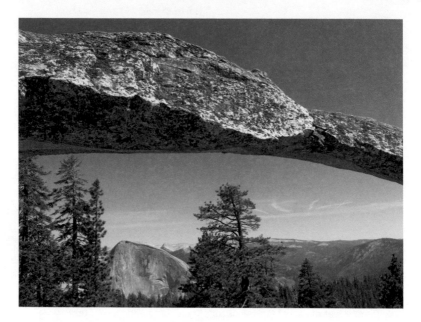

View of Half Dome *through Indian Rock arch*

water (see Options: Campsites with Water on page 203). You instead fork left and traverse 0.3 mile to a spur ridge with a large boulder on it—detour briefly to the right for a nice vista and picturesque but waterless campsites—then continue contouring across a dry, forested slope. Along this stretch is a large population of sugar sticks, a rare parasitic flowering plant whose stalks are red-and-white striped like candy canes. Take care not to trample their dispersed roots, but do take a moment to stare at the ground as you walk because many of the plants are within arms' reach of the trail. You drop to a sometimes moist gully before climbing steeply to a junction with the spur trail to Indian Rock (2.85 miles), ▶5 a worthy detour if you have spare energy on your return (see the Option on page 205).

Just beyond the junction you cross a shallow red-fir saddle and descend south, traversing across two low, broad ridge knolls that lie atop Indian Ridge. On a sandy flat, just beyond the second knob, the trail indistinctly veers east (left) off the now-descending ridge. While most folks take the trail, which descends a shallow trough east of the ridge, some merely walk down the view-blessed ridge. After about a 250-foot elevation loss, the trail heads southwest across granite slabs, from where those descending the ridge rejoin the trail. Walking down these trailless slabs is one of my favorite stretches of "trail" in Yosemite—artistic Jeffrey pines emerge from cracks in the rock and raised, erosion-resistant dykes create longitudinal stripes through the granite. The solitary trees have amazing shapes—some have lost their tops due to lightning, some are stunted bonsai due to insufficient soil, and others are tall trees with long, swaying limbs. To top it off, you already have a superb view toward Yosemite Valley.

Reaching a pine-shaded junction (4.0 miles), ►6 turn left and take the spur trail out to the bald, rounded summit of North Dome. Be careful on the first part of this trail, where you traverse down and east across broken slabs, because a slip on loose gravel could send you sliding down a dangerously steep slope. Descending this short headwall (which will feel much easier on the return) takes you to a broad saddle, a popular campsite for those willing to carry water out here. A short ascent of slabs and gravel leads to the top of the dome (4.6 miles). ►7

From the North Dome summit area, you have a superb view of Yosemite Valley and its adjacent uplands. Note that the views of the valley are even better from about 0.1 mile south of and below the summit area. Rising from the floor of Tenaya Canyon is the enormous 4,000-foot-high face of Clouds Rest, and to the south and west of it stands mighty Half Dome, perhaps Yosemite's best-remembered feature. Continuing your clockwise scan, you next recognize Mount Starr King, a steep-sided dome above Little Yosemite Valley. West of this unseen valley is Panorama Cliff, and then Illilouette Fall. Glacier Point stands west of the fall's gorge, and above and right of the point, bald Sentinel Dome bulges up into the sky. Looking down Yosemite Valley you see Sentinel Rock, with its near-vertical north face. Opposite the rock stand the Three Brothers, and

OPTION: Indian Rock

►5 Veering left is a trail signed for Indian Rock. The trail actually climbs very steeply 0.25 mile on brushy slopes to a delicate arch. About 1.5 feet thick at the thinnest part of its span, this 20-foot arch came into existence when the highly fractured rock beneath it broke away. This curious feature is best reached by looping counterclockwise around to its northwestern side, from which you can peek through the arch to Half Dome and the Glacier Point area. Most people now return to the main route, but you could continue north 0.5 mile up Indian Ridge to its north end, the true Indian Rock. This summit was one of the key points on the 1864 Yosemite Valley boundary. The summit area actually is two small—and I do mean small—summits of nearly equal elevation. If you are uncomfortable with scrambling up short cliffs without ropes, don't attempt either.

beyond them protrudes the brow of El Capitan. Farthest southwest lie the Cathedral Rocks, approximately opposite El Capitan. The view straight down illuminates meadows, forest, buildings, and traffic-choked roads—disappointingly you can even hear the car motors from this vantage point. After depleting your camera batteries, return the way you came, remembering to consider a detour to the arch on the ridge to Indian Rock en route to the trailhead (9.2 miles). ▶8

🚶	**MILESTONES**		
▶1	0.0	Start at Porcupine Creek Trailhead
▶2	0.75	Cross Porcupine Creek
▶3	1.81	Right at junction with Snow Creek Trail
▶4	1.83	Left at junction with Lehamite Creek Trail
▶5	2.85	Right at junction with Indian Rock spur
▶6	4.0	Left at North Dome junction (on slabs)
▶7	4.6	Summit of North Dome
▶8	9.2	Return to Porcupine Creek Trailhead

View up *Tenaya Canyon*

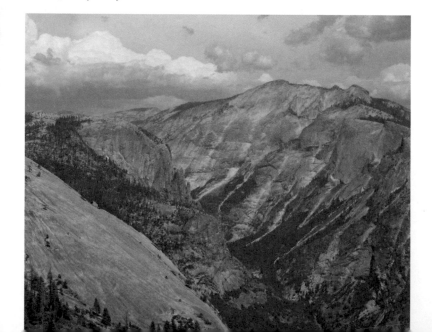

Ten Lakes Basin

The Ten Lakes Basin is extremely popular with weekend backpackers because with only a few hours' hiking effort, you can attain any of its seven major lakes. The three most accessible receive moderate to heavy use, but the other four, off the beaten track, are worth the effort for those who want relatively secluded camping. These lakes plus the two Grant Lakes are situated at about 8,950–9,400 feet, making them subalpine. At least the three lowest of the Ten Lakes Basin, situated on open shelves, get warm enough for enjoyable midsummer swimming.

Permits

Overnight visitors require a wilderness permit for the Ten Lakes Trailhead, issued by Yosemite National Park. Pick up your permit at the Tuolumne Meadows Wilderness Center, located in the parking lot a short way down Tuolumne Meadows Lodge Road; at the Big Oak Flat Information Center; or at another of the Yosemite permit-issuing stations (see "Permits," page 21).

Maps

This trail is covered by the Tom Harrison *Yosemite High Country* map (1:63,360 scale), the National Geographic Trails Illustrated *#307 Yosemite NW* map (1:40,000 scale), and the USGS 7.5-minute series *Yosemite Falls* and *Ten Lakes* maps (1:24,000 scale).

Best Time

Snow will linger in shaded patches through June, making July the start of the hiking season here. Should you like swimming, visit these lakes mid-July–early

TRAIL USE
Day Hike, Backpack, Horse

LENGTH
12.3 miles (plus extra to other lakes), 5–10 hours (over 1–3 days)

VERTICAL FEET
One-way: +2,260', –810'
Round-trip: ±3,070'

DIFFICULTY
– 1 2 **3** 4 5 +

TRAIL TYPE
Out-and-Back

FEATURES
Lake
Wildflowers
Great Views
Camping
Swimming
Secluded
Granite Slabs

FACILITIES
Bear Boxes
Restrooms

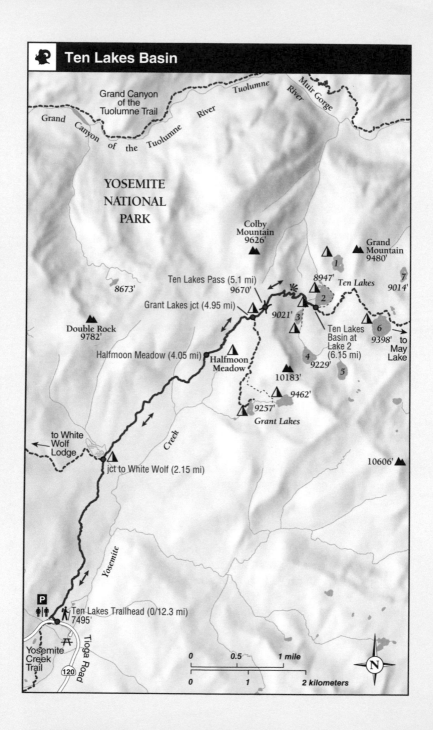

YOSEMITE
NATIONAL
PARK

Grand Canyon
of the
Tuolumne Trail

Grand Canyon of the Tuolumne

Tuolumne River

Muir Gorge

Colby
Mountain
9626'

Grand
Mountain
9480'

7
9014'

8947'

Ten Lakes

1

2

Ten Lakes Pass (5.1 mi)
9670'

Grant Lakes jct (4.95 mi)

9021'

3

Ten Lakes
Basin at
Lake 2
(6.15 mi)

6
9398'

to
May
Lake

8673'

Double Rock
9782'

Halfmoon Meadow (4.05 mi)

Halfmoon
Meadow

4

9229'

5

10183'

9462'

9257'

Grant Lakes

10606'

Creek

to White
Wolf
Lodge

jct to White Wolf (2.15 mi)

Yosemite

P

Ten Lakes Trailhead (0/12.3 mi)
7495'

Yosemite
Creek
Trail

Tioga Road

120

0   0.5   1 mile

0   1   2 kilometers

N

August. Be aware that mosquitoes—and beautiful wildflowers on the descent from Ten Lakes Pass—tend to be prevalent at all lakes through July. The lakes are pleasant destinations through September, after the crowds leave, but nights and mornings will be chilly.

Finding the Trail

The trailhead for Ten Lakes lies on Tioga Road exactly halfway between Crane Flat and the Tuolumne Meadows Campground—you have a 19.7-mile drive from either location. The trailhead is immediately across the street from the larger pullout signposted for the Yosemite Creek Trailhead; you may also park on either side of the road. These pullouts are immediately west of the highway bridges signed YOSEMITE CREEK. A picnic area is about 0.25 mile east of the trailhead parking area. There are pit toilets at the trailhead, but

By most people's count, Ten Lakes Basin has only seven lakes. When John Muir wrote of "a glacier basin with ten glassy lakes set all near together like eggs in a nest," he must have been including shallow tarns or lakes outside the basin.

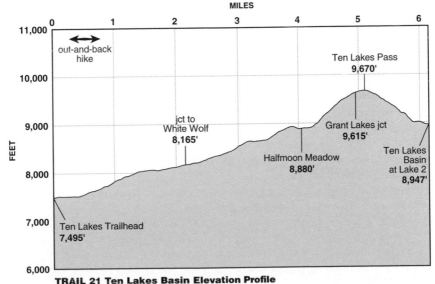

TRAIL 21 Ten Lakes Basin Elevation Profile

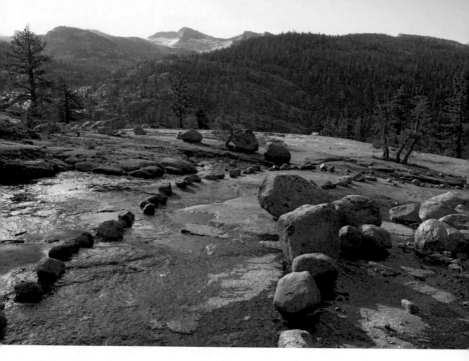

Endless slabs *in the Yosemite Creek drainage*

the closest flush toilets and drinking water are located at the Tuolumne Meadows Visitor Center (to the east) or the White Wolf Campground or the Crane Flat store (to the west), so fill your water bottles before heading to the trailhead.

Trail Description

From the west end of the highway's north parking lot, ▶1 a spur trail goes 0.1 mile northwest to a junction, where left (south) leads across CA 120 to follow Yosemite Creek to Yosemite Valley, while you turn right to hike upcanyon. Tramping through a lodgepole pine flat, the trail soon diverges from unseen Yosemite Creek and you encounter Jeffrey pines, huckleberry oaks, and western junipers as you climb moderately but relatively briefly to drier granitic slopes. The climb gives you views of the Yosemite Creek canyon, Mount Hoffmann, and the county line crest north of it. Soon after these views the trail levels, enters a forest, and eventually reaches a creekside junction with a trail that leads left to White Wolf, a campground and lodge lying 5.5 miles to the west (2.15

miles). ►2 You, however, turn right and from the junction boulder-hop
the creek and leave a nearby campsite to begin a moderate climb of a
well-forested moraine left after the retreat of a large glacier about 15,000
years ago. Your climb through a forest of red fir and western white pine
ends atop a moraine, behind which lies crescent-shaped, seasonally wet
Halfmoon Meadow (4.05 miles). ►3 The trail cuts across the meadow's
relatively dry north edge, and at its northeast corner lies a campsite. The
next stretch of ascent is steep and dry, so rest here and perhaps get a drink
from the nearby creek.

Roughly three dozen short, steep switchbacks guide you up, in sections dry with sagebrush underfoot, but elsewhere a delightful tangle
of dense flowers thriving in seasonal moisture—streamside bluebell,
miterwort, corn lilies, violets, and more. Almost reaching the Tuolumne–
Mariposa County line crest, the Tuolumne–Merced Rivers drainage divide,
you trend right, still in the Merced drainage, and parallel the ridge to a
junction with the trail to Grant Lakes (4.95 miles), ►4 a roughly built trail
heading 1.2 miles to lower Grant Lake and an additional 0.35 mile to the
upper slab-ringed lake. There are campsites at both lakes.

From the trail junction, the Ten Lakes Trail climbs gently across a
gravelly slope that can be covered in midsummer with large, deliciously
scented lupines. These taper off just before you cross the county line
crest, Ten Lakes Pass (5.1 miles). ►5 In early summer, when there is still
water in the meadows near the Grant Lake junction, sandy patches to the
side of Ten Lakes Pass make scenic, mosquito-sparse campsites near some
windblown whitebark pines. Now entering the Tuolumne River drainage
you descend briefly north to a shallow saddle. Just beyond it is a small
summit and to the left of it is flat-topped Colby Mountain, which crowns
the west rim of the Ten Lakes Basin.

As you start a descent from the shallow saddle, a panorama of steep-
sided, glaciated Ten Lakes Basin opens all around you, the three western
lakes clearly evident. On your descent of short switchbacks into Ten
Lakes Basin, the trail veers north far enough for you to get partial views
down into the upper part of the Grand Canyon of the Tuolumne River,
which is so deep that you can't see the canyon bottom. Beyond the canyon
you see parklands north to the Sierra Crest. In places sandy, but elsewhere rocky underfoot, the descent is not particularly fast walking; enjoy
the view and stare hard at the layout of the lakes, as it is so much easier
to decide where you'd like to spend the night (or the afternoon) from this
aerial perch—not to mention find the easiest way to get there.

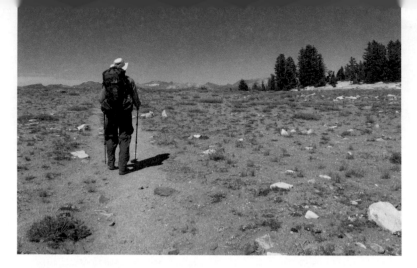

Crossing *Ten Lakes Pass*

The descent ends at a creek that flows from Lake 3 to Lake 2. The presence here of hemlock and lodgepole together with lakeside red heather and Labrador tea indicates prime mosquito country—at least before August. In September, dwarf bilberry makes its thumb-size presence known by turning to a blazing crimson color. From a boulder hop or log cross of the creek, you go just 250 feet east on the main trail to a use trail branching south (right) to Lakes 3 and 4, a route described later in this profile. Continuing straight, you approach the southwestern tip of Lake 2 and are soon just 40 feet above it. You will shortly encounter a maze of use trails descending toward the shore; indeed it is often difficult to discern which is the actual trail that continues east—worry not, the network of routes coalesces in a wet meadow at the lake's head and here I declare you've reached the Ten Lakes Basin, with Lake 2 just a few steps downslope (6.15 miles). ▶6 While some backpackers will be content to deposit their tents in the first legal patch of real estate, I recommend that you spend a little time exploring because the lakes have individual character and each person will want to find the perfect nook, by his or her definition.

Several ample campsites exist on the broad, low ridge above Lake 2's west shore, some smaller ones closer to its southern tip. Mid-July–mid-August, expect afternoon water temperatures to reach the mid- to high 60s. The northwest corner of the lake is almost cut off from the main part, and there are bedrock benches and small rock islands, and here is the warmest swimming, though it's mostly wadable. This is a great lake for basking on rocks but, given its popularity, a poor one for fishing. Just east of the outlet at Lake 2's north tip you may see a primitive trail climbing north to northeast toward Lake 1. This dies out amid bedrock, along which you may find more than one ducked (marked with stones) route. To reach Lake 1, just maintain a north-northeast bearing up to a minor gap in the crest, about 100 feet above Lake 2. (If you're heading north and suddenly realize you're headed downward, you're on your way to a treacherous drop into the Grand Canyon of the Tuolumne River.) From the crest Lake 1 is in plain view, and you drop about 70 feet to reach it. Lake 1 has a beautiful backdrop to the east—the cliffy west side of Grand Mountain. Small camps exist on a bench beside the north and northwest shores, and from them you have tree-filtered views across the Grand Canyon. Lake 1 competes with Lake 7 as the warmest lake. Afternoon water temperatures can reach 70°F or more. You can dive into the 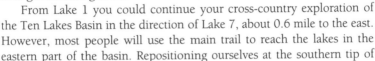 lake from its northeast shore or from a linear island along the east shore, near good basking rocks.

From Lake 1 you could continue your cross-country exploration of the Ten Lakes Basin in the direction of Lake 7, about 0.6 mile to the east. However, most people will use the main trail to reach the lakes in the eastern part of the basin. Repositioning ourselves at the southern tip of

OPTION: Ten Lakes Orientation

Ten Lakes Basin has seven prominent lakes that appear on the park's topographic map, and for the sake of easy reference, I refer to them by number, starting with the northwesternmost, Lake 1, and give distances to each lake via the most direct route from the trailhead. Lake 1 (6.8 miles) is situated just west of and below Grand Mountain. To its south is Lake 2 (6.15 miles), ▶6 which, being the first lake one reaches as well as being the largest of the western lakes (just north of and below the trail), is the most popular. (The elevation changes mentioned at the start of this trip are to Lake 2; all other lakes involve additional elevation changes.) Not much south of and above the trail is Lake 3 (6.3 miles), followed by Lake 4 (6.8 miles). Continuing counterclockwise you head east up to Lake 5 (7.3 miles), then northeast down to large, eastern Lake 6 (7.4 miles), also popular because it is along the trail. North of the trail and considerably below it is Lake 7 (7.6 miles). Overall, Lake 3 receives moderate use; Lake 1, lighter use; and Lakes 4, 5, and 7, very little use. All lakes have adjacent barren slopes or cliffs, making all photogenic, especially in evening and dawn light.

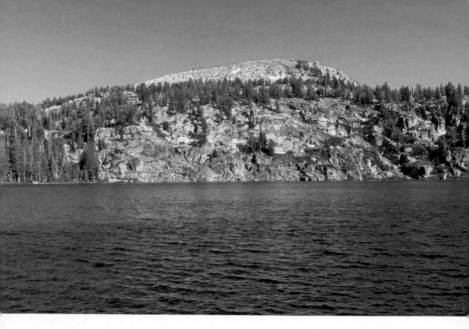

Lake 6 *in the Ten Lakes Basin*

Lake 2, ▶6 the main trail climbs about 500 feet in elevation to a divide south of Grand Mountain, then drops southeast, traversing broken slabs with scattered trees, including majestic junipers. The gradient nearly flattens to zero—this is where you depart to Lake 7—and then enters greater tree cover as you reach Lake 6's shore, 1.25 miles from Lake 2. Its northwest shore has quite a lot of flat land along it, a large camping area that can hold a couple dozen campers. It tends to be a bit cooler than Lake 2, but probably has better fishing, due to cooler water plus fewer anglers. From the west shore of this lake you have an easy cross-country hike southwest 0.5 mile to chilly Lake 5. (See directions in reverse just below.)

If your destination is Lake 7, from the open flats on the trail 0.25 mile west of Lake 6 (or 1.0 mile east of Lake 2), head east-northeast, reaching the lake in about 0.25 mile. Don't try to follow the outlet creek of Lake 6 because the slopes get steep along one stretch. This may be the least visited lake. It is shallow and grass lined, and though it may be the most mosquito prone, it also has a good swimming temperature. This lake rivals Lake 2 for camping area: there is about an acre of nearly flat land beyond the north shore, east of the outlet creek.

Positioning ourselves back at the junction just above Lake 2 yet again, if you were to head slightly to the west, where a cairn marks a use trail, you would reach the north end of Lake 3, just 0.1 mile from the main trail. While Lakes 1, 2, 6, and 7 are fanned out on the bench overlooking the Grand Canyon, where they receive abundant sunshine,

Lakes 3, 4, and 5 are set back against the escarpment, gathering more shade and later-lasting snowbanks; they are the coldest and the best for fishing but are less attractive swimming destinations. Lake 3 may have the most dramatic backdrop because an impressive crest looms high above it. It also has good camping above its north shore, as well as small sites along its east shore. The use trail continues south along the lake's east shore, then more or less follows the creek connecting Lakes 3 and 4. This part of the trail receives less use than the section below, and it becomes somewhat obscure for the last 0.1 mile before reaching Lake 4. Also dramatic, this lake is nestled in a very confining cirque. This lake probably is not popular because it is about 0.5 mile off the main trail with minimal camping possibilities.

To reach Lake 5 you go cross-country, walking up broken slabs on a ridge to the southeast of the meandering outlet creek; like Lake 4, Lake 5 is chilly and hemmed in. And like Lake 7, it is virtually unused, so it may have great fishing. Look for minimal-sized campsites on gentler slopes high above the northeast shore. From this lake you make a relatively easy cross-country jaunt over to Lake 6. From Lake 5's outlet you head north about 0.25 mile up to an ephemeral lakelet, then about 0.15 mile northeast to a minor gap in the lower part of a northwest-trending ridge, then descend 0.25 mile northeast to the northwest shore of Lake 6, the large, eastern trailside lake described a few paragraphs back. You can see that while it is just over 6 miles to reach the start of the basin, you might well want to give yourself a layover day to more fully explore the basin—and when time runs out, retrace your steps to the trailhead (12.3 miles). ▶7

🚶	**MILESTONES**	
▶1	0.0	Start at Ten Lakes Trailhead
▶2	2.15	Right at junction with trail to White Wolf
▶3	4.05	Halfmoon Meadow
▶4	4.95	Left at Grant Lakes junction
▶5	5.1	Ten Lakes Pass
▶6	6.15	Ten Lakes Basin at Lake 2
▶7	12.3	Return to Ten Lakes Trailhead

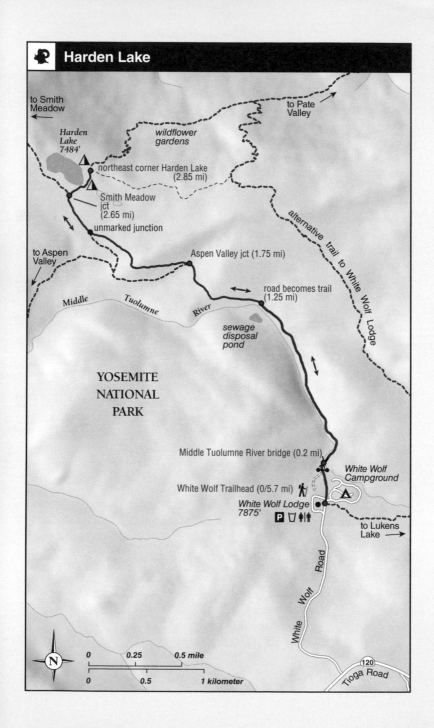

to Smith
Meadow

to Pate
Valley

Harden
Lake
7484'

wildflower
gardens

northeast corner Harden Lake
(2.85 mi)

Smith Meadow
jct
(2.65 mi)

unmarked junction

alternative trail to White Wolf Lodge

to Aspen
Valley

Aspen Valley jct (1.75 mi)

road becomes trail
(1.25 mi)

Middle *Tuolumne* *River*

sewage
disposal
pond

YOSEMITE
NATIONAL
PARK

Middle Tuolumne River bridge (0.2 mi)

White Wolf
Campground

White Wolf Trailhead (0/5.7 mi)

White Wolf Lodge
7875'

to Lukens
Lake

White *Wolf* *Road*

N

0   0.25   0.5 mile

0   0.5   1 kilometer

Tioga Road

120

Harden Lake

Only a little over an hour's hike from White Wolf Campground, this lake attracts quite a few summer visitors, virtually all of them day hikers, though there are some nice campsites near Harden Lake, perfect for an easy family backpacking trip. Mid-June–July this shallow lake can be fine for swimming, but the lake lies in a leaky basin, and by mid-August it usually has dwindled to an oversize wading pool. Don't expect to catch any fish because the lake becomes far too shallow by late summer to support any. The forests through which the trail traverses sport colorful early summer flowers, as does the slope north of Harden Lake, a possible extension to your day.

Permits

Overnight visitors require a wilderness permit for the White Wolf to Smith Meadow Trailhead, issued by Yosemite National Park. Pick up your permit at the Tuolumne Meadows Wilderness Center, located in the parking lot a short way down Tuolumne Meadows Lodge Road; at the Big Oak Flat Information Center; or at another of the Yosemite permit-issuing stations (see "Permits," page 21).

Maps

This trail is covered by the Tom Harrison *Yosemite High Country* map (1:63,360 scale), the National Geographic Trails Illustrated *#307 Yosemite NW* map (1:40,000 scale), and the USGS 7.5-minute series *Tamarack Flat* and *Hetch Hetchy Reservoir* maps (1:24,000 scale).

TRAIL USE
Day Hike, Backpack,
Horse, Run,
Child-Friendly

LENGTH
5.7 miles, 2–4 hours
(over 1–2 days)

VERTICAL FEET
One-way: +90', –470'
Round-trip: ±560'

DIFFICULTY
– 1 **2** 3 4 5 +

TRAIL TYPE
Out-and-Back

FEATURES
Lake
Autumn Colors
Wildflowers
Camping
Swimming
Geological Interest

FACILITIES
Bear Boxes
Campground
Horse Staging
Restrooms
Water

217

Except when Harden Lake is at its highest level, it is usually shallow enough to wade across. Be careful not to scrape your feet on the lake's many submerged glacier-transported boulders.

Best Time

This walk is accessible and pleasant virtually anytime the spur road to White Wolf is open, generally late June–mid-October. A few mosquitoes will demand your attention in the moist flats halfway to the lake, but they are never more than a minor nuisance near the lake. June and July are ideal for those seeking a wildflower walk—parts of the trail to Harden Lake and especially the 0.5 mile beyond the lake exhibit a full rainbow of petal shades, though the lake's shore itself is more barren. Swimming is a possibility at this warm lake until water levels drop in mid-July. Indeed, by fall there isn't even a lake to observe! September and October do provide great fall colors, particularly with the aspens and bracken ferns. Joggers may find September and October best, due to cooler temperatures.

Finding the Trail

From the Tioga Road–Big Oak Flat Road junction in Crane Flat, drive northeast 14.5 miles up Tioga Road to the White Wolf turnoff and follow that road 1.1 miles down to a parking area on the right, just before the entrance to White Wolf Campground. White Wolf Road is 24.8 miles west of the Tuolumne Meadows Store. When the spur road to White Wolf is closed, there is limited parking along the shoulder of Tioga Road,

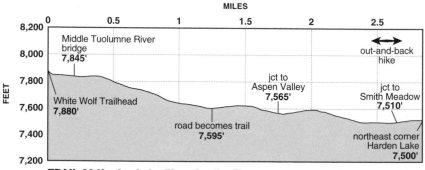

TRAIL 22 Harden Lake Elevation Profile

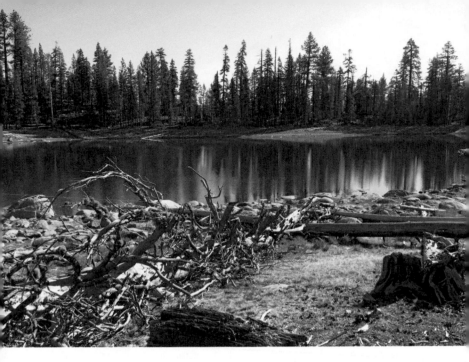

Harden Lake

adding 2.2 miles round-trip to your hike. There are toilets and a water faucet at the trailhead.

Trail Description

Your route, initially a closed service road, ►1 immediately passes the spur to the White Wolf Campground and continues past a collection of maintenance buildings to reach a locked gate and then bridges the infant Middle Tuolumne River (0.2 mile). ►2 The road then parallels the river's sometimes splashing course down unglaciated granitic terrain, through scattered stands of lodgepole pines. Easy descent along the road leads to a closed spur road that goes to a sewage treatment pond (1.25 miles). ►3 Beyond here, the road is in the process of being restored to a singletrack, allowing it to be classified as wilderness. The trail first climbs over a low ridge of glacial deposits before dipping slightly into a shady alcove of lodgepole pines and red firs that has a trail junction (1.75 miles). ►4

The left route, the old road, is the route of the original road from the western Sierra foothills to Tuolumne Meadows, here paralleling the Middle Tuolumne River for 8.1 miles downstream to Aspen Valley, a private inholding that was once the west entrance to Yosemite National Park. Today, that gently graded road is a pleasant riverside stroll for those looking for a lightly used creekside excursion or for distance running, though a growing number of large fir logs lying across the trail are turning it into more of a cross-training route with hurdles.

You take the right-branching narrower trail, which traverses the slope of a large glacial moraine. The well-drained sediments of this moraine support a different plant community than your generally rocky road descent, and on this moraine grows a forest of Jeffrey pines together with some firs and aspens. Thousands of bracken ferns seek the forest shade together with chinquapins, the bushes with spiny, seed-bearing spheres. In fall, the yellowing ferns and aspen leaves saturate your senses. Seeking the sun are snowbushes, which have spine-tipped branches. Many trees here bear fire scars, the consequence of a series of fires that have burned through this landscape over the past decades, including the Ackerson Fire in 1996, the Harden and Slope Fires in 2010, and the Rim Fire in 2013. The openings created by the fires provide perfect conditions for the regrowth of brush and outbursts of wildflowers, but ever less shade. Profusions of pink fireweed, yellow sneezeweed, and purple lupines greet you.

At the end of a long, moist flat a faint, unmarked trail departs to the southwest (left), while you continue straight ahead (north), now back on the route of an old road to Harden Lake. In a few minutes' time you arrive at a gravelly junction near the southwest corner of Harden Lake (2.65 miles). ▶5 The left fork goes around the southwest edge of Harden Lake and on to Smith Meadow on an often overgrown trail. You turn right, on the trail signposted to Pate Valley, and soon see the lake to your left. The walk officially ends on a sandy saddle at the northeast corner of Harden Lake (2.85 miles), ▶6 for here, to the left of the trail, are the best campsites. Seasonal Harden Lake has a rather uncommon origin because it occupies a small depression that formed between two lateral moraines. Most Sierran lakes have existed for only 13,000–16,000 years, but Harden could have originated earlier. This warm, shallow, 9-acre lake has no surface inlet or outlet, and not long after adjacent snow patches melt, the lake's level begins to drop, making it too shallow for trout.

An unmarked, abandoned trail departs east (right) from this saddle, while the main trail descends the north side of the saddle, beginning the long descent to the Tuolumne River at Pate Valley. For those with extra energy and time, continuing 0.5–1.0 mile along this trail leads to one of my favorite Yosemite wildflower gardens, where the water leaking out of Harden Lake—and the surrounding moraine-dammed soils—oozes out through the north side of the moraine throughout the summer, watering the landscape. After your foray to the lake—or beyond—return the way you came (5.7 miles). ▶7

🚶 MILESTONES

▶1   0.0   Start at White Wolf Trailhead
▶2   0.2   Middle Tuolumne River bridge
▶3   1.25   Straight ahead where road becomes trail
▶4   1.75   Right at Aspen Valley junction
▶5   2.65   Right at Smith Meadow junction
▶6   2.85   Northeast corner of Harden Lake
▶7   5.7   Return to White Wolf Trailhead

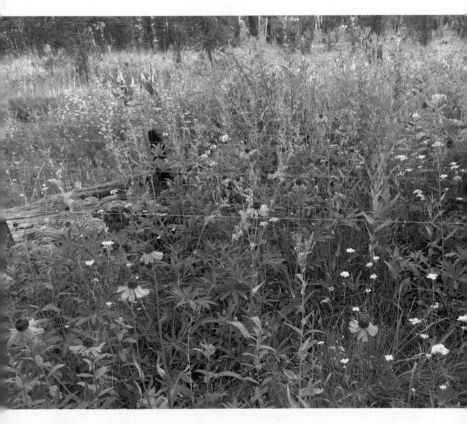

Abundant wildflowers *along the walk to Harden Lake*

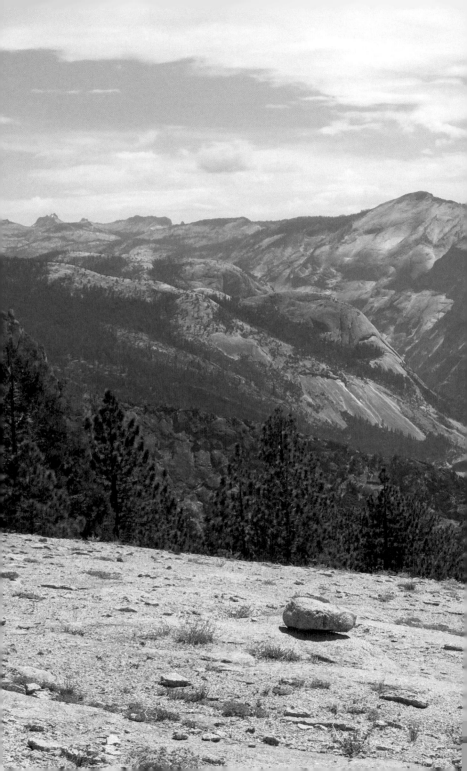

CHAPTER 4

Northwest Yosemite

These hikes give you just a slight flavor of the vast, less visited lands of Yosemite's northwest. Endless domes, lakes, sizeable rivers, and intricate topography define this region. A series of near-parallel river valleys, U-shaped in their upper reaches, drain this region and are notably exhausting to cross between. This and the long distances between "destinations" keep it much emptier than the park's other lands. As defined in this book, this region's southern perimeter are the steep-walled cliffs that make up the north wall of Yosemite Valley, forming an abrupt end to the mostly gentler, forested slopes.

Despite calling this a low- to moderate-use area, all but Trail 27 are heavily used. Why? Because there are several prized goals. The first, Kibbie Lake, lies just within the park and is reached by a hike that begins just west of the park. Two other popular lakes in the northwestern lands are Laurel Lake and Lake Vernon, and backpackers in good shape can visit both in a weekend. These midsize lakes, each with abundant campsites, are reached by starting across the dam that has flooded Hetch Hetchy Valley, which is second only to Yosemite Valley as Yosemite's most impressive U-shaped canyon. Along the north slopes of Hetch Hetchy Reservoir is a popular trail that takes you past vernal Tueeulala Falls to perennial Wapama Falls, whose voluminous water roars in May and June and soaks hikers with its spray. Later on, the falls still put on an impressive show. The trail, undulating as it follows the west side of the reservoir, continues east to Rancheria Falls Camp, a popular, spacious backcountry campground beside cascades and pools of Rancheria Creek.

South of Hetch Hetchy Valley the lakes disappear and the forests, except where burned, prevail. On these lands are two groves of giant sequoias, the Tuolumne Grove, just off the start of Tioga Road at Crane Flat, and the Merced Grove, a few miles west of Crane Flat and south from Big Oak Flat Road. I've included only the popular Tuolumne Grove because the closed road to it is shorter and because it has dozens of giant sequoias, some of them very impressive, but both locations are worth a visit.

Opposite: *View east from the summit of El Capitan (see Trail 27, page 255)*

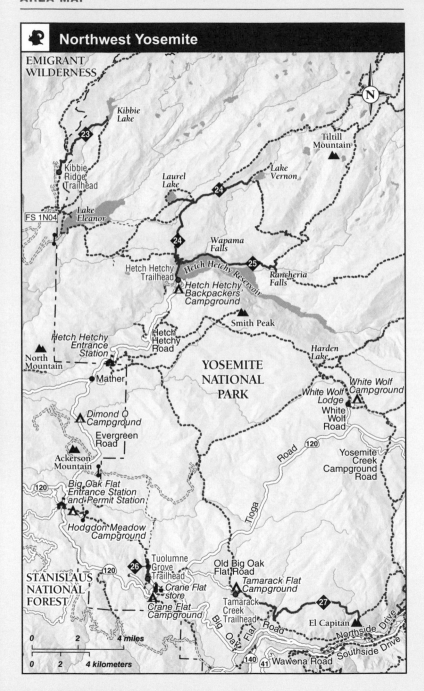

Northwest Yosemite

EMIGRANT
WILDERNESS

Kibbie
Lake

Tiltill
Mountain

23

Kibbie
Ridge
Trailhead

Laurel
Lake

Lake
Vernon

24

FS 1N04

Lake
Eleanor

24

Wapama
Falls

Hetch Hetchy Reservoir

25

Rancheria
Falls

Hetch Hetchy
Trailhead

Hetch Hetchy
Backpackers'
Campground

Hetch
Hetchy
Road

Smith Peak

Harden
Lake

Hetch Hetchy
Entrance
Station

North
Mountain

Mather

White Wolf
Campground

White Wolf
Lodge

White
Wolf
Road

Dimond O
Campground

YOSEMITE
NATIONAL
PARK

Evergreen
Road

Road

120

Yosemite
Creek
Campground
Road

Ackerson
Mountain

120

Big Oak Flat
Entrance Station
and Permit Station

Tioga

Hodgdon Meadow
Campground

120

26

Tuolumne
Grove
Trailhead

Old Big Oak
Flat Road

STANISLAUS
NATIONAL
FOREST

Crane Flat
store

Tamarack Flat
Campground

Crane Flat
Campground

Tamarack
Creek
Trailhead

27

El Capitan

Northside Drive

Big Oak Flat Road

0   2   4 miles

0   2   4 kilometers

140   41   Wawona Road   Southside Drive

Northwest Yosemite

Trail	Difficulty	Length	Type	USES & ACCESS	TERRAIN	NATURE	OTHER
23	2	8.2	↗	🚶‍♀️🥾🏇🚶🚶‍♀️👫	🌊 🏞️		⛺ 🏊 ⚓ 🗻
24	4	21.1	↗	🥾🏇🚶	🌊 🏞️	✳️	👁️ ⛺ 🏊 ⚓ 🗻 ⛏️
25	3	12.8	↗	🚶‍♀️🥾🏇🏃	🏔️ 🌊 🏞️ 🏞️	✳️	👁️ ⛺ 🗻 ⛏️
26	2	2.55	↻	🚶‍♀️⚓👫		✳️🌲	🏠
27	4	16.8	↗	🚶‍♀️🥾🏃	⛰️	✳️	👁️ 🗻 ⚓

TYPE	USES & ACCESS	TERRAIN	NATURE	FEATURES
↘ Point-to-Point	🚶‍♀️ Day Hiking	🔰 Canyon	✳️ Autumn Colors	👁️ Great Views
↻ Loop	🥾 Backpacking	🔺 Summit	✳️ Wildflowers	🔺 Camping
↗ Out-and-Back	🏇 Horses	🌊 Lake	🌲 Giant Sequoias	⚓ Swimming
↺ Balloon	🏃 Running	🏞️ Stream		🗻 Secluded
	🦽 Wheelchair Access	🏞️ Waterfall		🗻 Steep
DIFFICULTY	🦯 Stroller Access			🗻 Granite Slabs
− 1 2 3 4 5 +	👫 Child-Friendly			🏠 Historical Interest
less more	⚓ Caution			⛏️ Geological Interest

Finally, just as the previous chapter offers an easy route to the summit of North Dome (as opposed to scaling it from the floor of Yosemite Valley) this chapter offers a relatively easy route to the summit of El Capitan. OK, it is a bit lengthy, especially as a day hike, but it is a lot easier than scaling the face of El Cap.

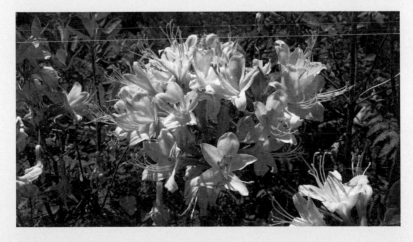

Western azaleas *at Laurel Lake (see Trail 24, page 235)*

Northwest Yosemite

Were it not for the long drive to the trailhead, Kibbie Lake would be a popular day hike. At 4.1 miles and only about 700 feet between its high and low points, the trail to Kibbie Lake is a good choice for beginning backpackers. Because Kibbie Lake is one of the lowest natural lakes reached by trail in and around the Yosemite National Park environs, it is one of the warmest and great for summer swimming. It is also a relatively large lake, so while it can be popular with weekend summer backpackers, there is plenty of shoreline on which to establish secluded camps.

This relatively low-elevation loop, a good early summer conditioner, visits two fairly large lakes—Laurel and Vernon—both good rainbow trout fisheries. These two lakes are popular on summer weekends, and most hikers go no farther, though these trails lead to several longer routes looping through northern Yosemite and into Emigrant Wilderness. At 6,490 feet, Laurel Lake is the lowest of any large natural lake in the park that is reached by trail, and it provides relatively warm swimming. Reaching Lake Vernon requires a longer walk; furthermore, you cross a low ridge and then drop 400 feet to the shores of the lake, lying at 6,564 feet. This is a more aesthetic lake, and it has plenty of slabs great for sunbathing, especially for warming up after a swim.

Wapama Falls and Rancheria Falls Camp............ 243

A stately grove of pines and incense cedars harboring a spacious camping area near Rancheria Falls marks the terminus of this hike. Its cascades and pools are the goals for some, but also rewarding are inspirational vistas of the cliffs and two waterfalls, Tueeulala and Wapama, seen along the undulating path on the north wall of Hetch Hetchy Reservoir. Because you are traversing above a reservoir, you might think this is a level hike. Instead, the route is anything but flat, as the trail navigates through cliff bands and you face gains and losses of hundreds of feet. Also, the route, being quite open and at a relatively low elevation, can be sunny and hot, so on a summer's day it is best begun in early morning.

Tuolumne Grove of Big Trees...... 250

The Tuolumne Grove has more than a dozen trees at least 10 feet in diameter near the base, and though this pales in comparison with the much larger Mariposa Grove's approximately 200 trees of similar or larger size, you'll certainly see fewer tourists. Much of the grove is observable from a paved road (closed to cars), making it a good choice for families with a stroller.

El Capitan from Tamarack Flat..... 255

The vertical walls of 3,000-foot-high El Capitan attract rock climbers from all over the world, and more than five dozen extremely difficult routes ascend it. For nonclimbers this hike provides a more practical means to attain El Capitan's summit. This walk is not particularly distinguished by its terrain or wildflowers and passes no lakes, but reaching the flat-topped El Capitan is sufficient reward for your efforts.

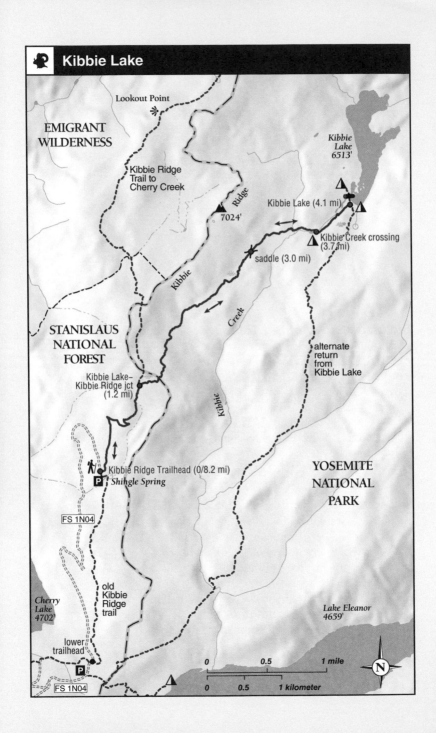

Kibbie Lake

EMIGRANT
WILDERNESS

Lookout Point

Kibbie Lake
6513'

Kibbie Ridge
Trail to
Cherry Creek

7024'

Kibbie Lake (4.1 mi)

Kibbie Creek crossing
(3.7 mi)

saddle (3.0 mi)

STANISLAUS
NATIONAL
FOREST

alternate
return
from
Kibbie Lake

Kibbie Lake–
Kibbie Ridge jct
(1.2 mi)

Kibbie Ridge Trailhead (0/8.2 mi)

Shingle Spring

YOSEMITE
NATIONAL
PARK

FS 1N04

old
Kibbie
Ridge
trail

Cherry
Lake
4702'

Lake Eleanor
4659'

lower
trailhead

FS 1N04

0   0.5   1 mile

0   0.5   1 kilometer

N

Kibbie Lake

Were it not for the long drive to the trailhead, Kibbie Lake would be a popular day hike. At 4.1 miles, the trail to Kibbie Lake is a good choice for beginning backpackers and families. Because it's one of the lowest natural lakes reached by trail in and around the Yosemite National Park environs, it is one of the warmest and great for swimming from about mid-June through mid-August. At just under 1 mile in length, the shoreline provides plenty of space for secluded camps, even with weekend crowds of summer backpackers. I particularly like Kibbie Lake as a destination because it has the feel of a lake close to 8,000 feet in elevation, making it a wonderful way to feel like I'm up high while the true high country is still snow covered.

Permits

Overnight visitors require a wilderness permit for the Kibbie Lake Trailhead, issued by Stanislaus National Forest. Pick up your permit at the Groveland Ranger District Station, located on CA 120 in Buck Meadows.

Maps

This trail is covered by the Tom Harrison *Emigrant Wilderness* or *Hetch Hetchy* maps (1:63,360 scale), the National Geographic Trails Illustrated *#307 Yosemite NW* map (1:40,000 scale), and the USGS 7.5-minute series *Cherry Lake North and Kibbie Lake* maps (1:24,000 scale).

TRAIL USE
Day Hike, Backpack, Horse, Child-Friendly

LENGTH
8.2 miles, 3–6 hours (over 1–2 days)

VERTICAL FEET
One-way: +1,035', –410'
Round-trip: ±1,445'

DIFFICULTY
– 1 **2** 3 4 5 +

TRAIL TYPE
Out-and-Back

FEATURES
Lake
Stream
Camping
Swimming
Secluded
Granite Slabs

FACILITIES
Bear Boxes
Horse Staging

Best Time

Situated at 6,513 feet, Kibbie Lake will usually be snow-free by Memorial Day weekend, making it a good late-spring or early-summer destination before temperatures heat up and while wildflowers are showy. July and August are perfect months for basking and swimming, with minimal mosquitoes and maximum summer temperatures, but the mostly unshaded walk is less appealing midsummer. With September come cooler temperatures and fewer backpackers, so solitude increases through the weeks of September. The road across Cherry Lake Dam is generally closed December 15–April 1, making the hike not worth the effort unless you want serious solitude. Check the Stanislaus National Forest website, as the road sometimes closes as early as the start of the fall hunting season in late September.

Finding the Trail

From Groveland drive east 13.6 miles on Tioga Road (CA 120) to paved Cherry Road 1N07, also known as Forest Service Road 17. This road starts just beyond the highway bridge over the South Fork Tuolumne River. (A spur road right, immediately before the bridge, leads briefly down to the popular Rainbow Pool day-use area—a refreshing spot to visit after your

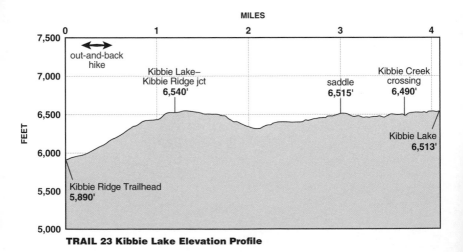

TRAIL 23 Kibbie Lake Elevation Profile

OPTION: **Return via Loop Trail**

A second, lesser-used trail accesses Kibbie Lake via a more easterly route. From Kibbie Lake to your car, this route is 7.8 miles in length and includes 1,680 feet of ascent and 2,260 feet of descent (or 5.85 miles and 680 feet of ascent and 2,260 feet of descent if you can convince one energetic hiker in your group to hike from the lower to upper trailheads to fetch the car). From the south end of the lake, where Kibbie Lake visitors leave the trail, the trail does a near U-turn, climbing briefly on a sand and slab slope to a broad trough bedecked with pine-mat manzanita and huckleberry oak. Climbing more steeply, you cross a saddle (1.35 miles) and descend equally steeply to the west bank of a Kibbie Creek tributary (2.35 miles). The descent makes for interesting forest walking and lessons in fire ecology because parts were burned and others untouched by the 2013 Rim Fire, creating a mosaic of young trees, tall unburned trees, and, of course, scorched patches. Once along the creek, there are a few camping options, but unfortunately, most of the real estate is far from flat.

Completing the descent, you cross the creek (3.1 miles) and proceed across sandy flats, colorful in good wildflower years, before making a steep descent to Kibbie Creek (4.3 miles). This crossing is a delightful location because the creek, robust in spring and early summer, disperses across broad granite slabs, decorated at the edges with the large-leafed Indian rhubarb and dogwoods. At the highest of flows, you'll have to take care at this crossing. Beyond you enter more severely burned landscape—even some large boulders have fractured from the heat—and must pay more attention to the trail's route; traverse right (southwest) with only moderate elevation loss. Before long you reach a T-junction (5.7 miles), where you turn right, and soon reach the Kibbie Ridge road (5.85 miles). At this point only the car fetcher must continue up the hill.

That person will walk along the road 0.15 mile until she notes a pullout to the right (east). The old Kibbie Ridge Trail begins at the back of this pullout, heading upward approximately parallel to the road. It is all uphill but a quite pleasant walk, with long stretches of intact conifer forest and only brief stretches of brush. It leads up to Shingle Spring and, just beyond, your car (7.8 miles).

hike.) Take FS 17 for 5.3 miles to a junction with paved Hetch Hetchy Road (FS 12), and branch left. Still on FS 17, go a very slow, windy 17.6 miles to reach a T-junction with Cottonwood Road (FS 1N04). If you're

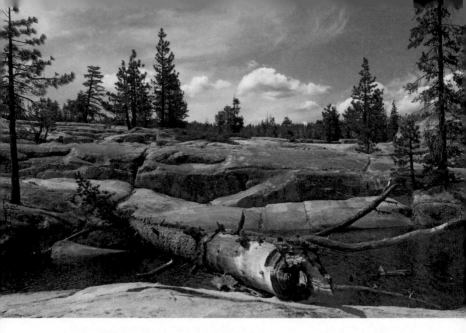

A precarious log *spans a deep outlet of Kibbie Lake.*

in search of a campground, turn left at the T-junction and you'll find the Cherry Valley Campground along a road that traverses over to Cherry Lake's southwest shore. Turning right, you reach the signed Cherry Dam parking area in just 0.3 mile; this is the parking December 15–April 1 when vehicular traffic is prohibited across the Cherry Lake Dam. Note that in the past, the road across the dam was also closed during the fall hunting season, but this restriction is currently lifted.

Starting April 15 (usually), you can drive an additional 5.7 miles in distance, making a 1,200-foot ascent to a newer trailhead. To reach it, drive across Cherry Valley Dam, then continue 0.9 mile (measured from the west end of the dam) to a T-junction with FS 1N45Y, which leads right to Lake Eleanor. Staying on the main road, trend left (north), and continue 2.5 miles (still measured from the dam) to pass a trailhead leading to Lake Eleanor, shortly followed by one to the old Kibbie Ridge Trail. Onward, the road climbs alongside Kibbie Ridge, just a short distance below the old trail. Three switchbacks eventually lead up to the trail at a dead end at 5,880 feet. You'll notice a dirt road descending behind the trailhead; just about a minute's walk down this old road is Shingle Spring, with beautiful dogwoods and, most important, water and some large flat areas perfect for camping the night before you begin your hike. There are not, however, any toilets at this trailhead. There is also no potable water, so fill your water bottles at the ranger station when you pick up your permit.

Note the entire 28.6 miles from CA 120 are slow driving and will take you more than an hour, possibly approaching 1.5–2 hours for drivers less comfortable on steep, windy roads.

Trail Description

The trail heads briefly east from the parking area, ▶1 soon turning north to traverse diagonally up a fire-decimated slope. You are on the Kibbie Ridge Trail, but well above its true start 1.9 miles downhill; you happily drove past this lower starting point in the car, but the lower half of the trail still exists and is in decent condition. It continues to be used by parties completing an 11.9-mile circuit to/from Kibbie Lake; see the Option on page 231 for this hiking alternative. The slope you are crossing was first burned in the 2003 Kibbie Complex Fire and then rescorched in the 2013 Rim Fire, removing the previously used descriptors *cooler, forested* from adjectives that can be accurately applied to the landscape. Instead it is a mostly open slope of rapidly growing, generally thorny brush, with the occasional lollipop tree—my description of those tall trees where all lower branches have been burned and just a small round circle of greenery continues to grow on the top branches, helpful as a seed source for regeneration but hopeless at providing shade. Switchbacks still sporting a handful of trees lead to a broad saddle with dense clusters of young trees—fortunately not touched by the 2013 flames—and a trail junction (1.2 miles). ▶2 Left leads up Kibbie Ridge into Emigrant Wilderness and the incredible slab country in the upper Cherry Creek drainage, while you head right on the Kibbie Lake Trail.

Skirting a small seasonal pond, the trail trends east and soon enters Yosemite National Park and winds down an open slope, working its way around boulders and slabs. Reaching sodden bottomland, the trail trends north (left) and becomes indistinct due to a jumble of downed logs. If you lose the trail, stay on the west (left) side of the marshy area and continue due north. In May and June wildflowers thrive in the moisture, enticing travelers to linger, while mosquitoes will no doubt urge you on! Shortly, the trail trends farther east (right) again, climbing northeast onto granitic slabs mottled by huckleberry oaks to a 6,500-foot saddle (3.0 miles). ▶3

The rocky route next descends to cross a tributary of Kibbie Creek under a south-facing dome; then you closely parallel pools along Kibbie Creek, enjoying some glades of unburned lodgepole pines. You transition into a slab-dominated landscape and enjoy ever more stands of live trees as the patches of bare rock impeded the fire's progress. Just before you descend to cross Kibbie Creek, an unmarked use trail heads to your left, climbing over slabs along the west shore of Kibbie Creek; this is the best spring and early-summer route to take if you plan to camp on the stupendous slabs on the west shore of Kibbie Lake because the crossing options closer to the lake are notably tricky. The most sporting option is a single, long, slightly bouncy log that has been delicately placed high across a deep inlet channel; I wouldn't enjoy crossing it with a full pack. In addition, once close to the lake, Kibbie Creek flows rapidly across slabs and through notches, making it difficult to cross if water levels are high. Instead take this use trail the final 0.4 mile to the lake.

Meanwhile, the main trail angles down to a 20-foot rock hop of Kibbie Creek (3.7 miles); ►4 bouldery underfoot, this requires a shoes-on wade if the water levels are too high. Across the ford, among lodgepoles, is a very good camp. The trail turns upstream, climbing over blasted granitic ledges, the route indicated by rock ducks.

After passing lagoons foreshadowing 106-acre, 6,513-foot-high Kibbie Lake, you see its south shore through trees and leave the trail (4.1 miles), ►5 heading toward camps in a lodgepole–and–Labrador tea fringe on the south shore. Note that no campfires are permitted within 0.25 mile of Kibbie Lake. Kibbie Lake is bounded on the west by gently sloping granite, while the east shore is characterized by steep, broken bluffs and scrub. To find abundant secluded campsites, traverse north along the west shore. The relatively warm lake is mostly shallow, with an algae-coated, sandy bottom, where distinctively orange-colored California newts may take your bait if a rainbow trout doesn't. Especially along its west shore there are many spots for swimming, sunbathing, and fishing. When finished, return the way you came (8.2 miles), ►6 or see the Option on page 231 for an alternative route back.

🚶 MILESTONES		
►1	0.0	Start at Kibbie Ridge Trailhead
►2	1.2	Right at Kibbie Lake–Kibbie Ridge junction
►3	3.0	Saddle
►4	3.7	Kibbie Creek crossing
►5	4.1	Kibbie Lake
►6	8.2	Return to Kibbie Ridge Trailhead

Laurel Lake and Lake Vernon

This relatively low-elevation loop, a good early-summer conditioner, visits two fairly large lakes—Laurel and Vernon—both good rainbow trout fisheries. If you hike only to Laurel Lake, you go only 7.5 miles each way, and your total elevation gain and loss will be about +3,350/-3,350 feet. If you hike only to Lake Vernon, you go only 9.9 miles each way, and the elevation gain and loss will be about +4,080/-4,080 feet. These two lakes are popular weekend destinations spring through fall, and most hikers go no farther, despite a network of trails allowing those with more time to broadly explore the lands of northwestern Yosemite. At 6,490 feet, Laurel Lake is the lowest of any large natural lake in the park that is reached by trail, and it provides relatively warm swimming. This conifer-ringed lake lacks the steep granite backdrop of the park's higher lakes, but in spring the azalea-lined banks, in summer the warm swimming temperature, and at all times the flat camping options around its lengthy—and picturesque—shore make it a desirable destination. Lake Vernon, at 6,564 feet, is just a bit higher but has a wholly different feel because, unlike forest-ringed Laurel Lake, it is mostly encapsulated by slabs, great for sunbathing or warming up after a swim.

Permits

Overnight visitors require a wilderness permit for the Beehive Meadow Trailhead, issued by Yosemite National Park. Pick up your permit at the Hetch Hetchy Entrance Station.

TRAIL USE
Backpack, Horse
LENGTH
21.1 miles, 10–16 hours
(over 2–4 days)
VERTICAL FEET
One-way:
+3,860', –1,100'
Round-trip: ±4,540'
DIFFICULTY
– 1 2 3 **4** 5 +
TRAIL TYPE
Out-and-Back

FEATURES
Lake
Stream
Wildflowers
Great Views
Camping
Swimming
Secluded
Granite Slabs
Geological Interest

FACILITIES
Bear Boxes
Campground
Restrooms
Water

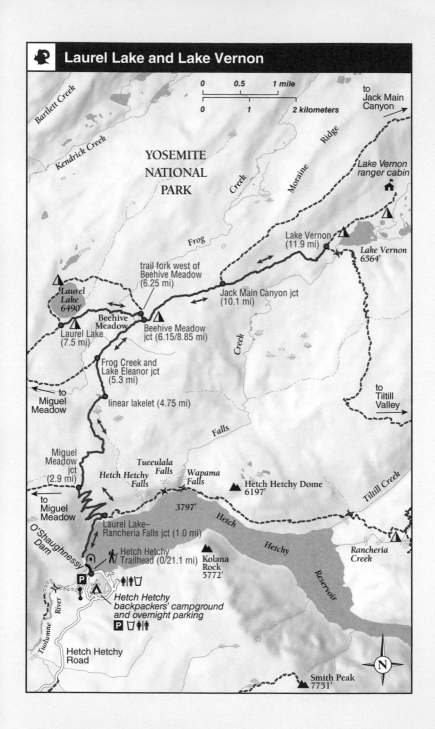

to Jack Main Canyon

Bartlett Creek

Kendrick Creek

YOSEMITE NATIONAL PARK

0   0.5   1 mile

0   1   2 kilometers

Frog

Creek

Moraine

Ridge

Lake Vernon ranger cabin

Lake Vernon 6564'

Lake Vernon (11.9 mi)

trail fork west of Beehive Meadow (6.25 mi)

Jack Main Canyon jct (10.1 mi)

Laurel Lake 6490'

Beehive Meadow

Beehive Meadow jct (6.15/8.85 mi)

Laurel Lake (7.5 mi)

Frog Creek and Lake Eleanor jct (5.3 mi)

to Miguel Meadow

linear lakelet (4.75 mi)

Creek

to Tiltill Valley

Falls

Miguel Meadow jct (2.9 mi)

Tueeulala Falls

Wapama Falls

Hetch Hetchy Dome 6197'

Tiltill Creek

Hetch Hetchy Falls

to Miguel Meadow

3797'

Hetch

Hetchy

O'Shaughnessy Dam

Laurel Lake–Rancheria Falls jct (1.0 mi)

Hetch Hetchy Trailhead (0/21.1 mi)

Kolana Rock 5772'

Reservoir

Rancheria Creek

Tuolumne River

Hetch Hetchy backpackers' campground and overnight parking

Hetch Hetchy Road

Smith Peak 7751'

N

Maps

This trail is covered by the Tom Harrison *Hetch Hetchy* map (1:63,360 scale), the National Geographic Trails Illustrated *#307 Yosemite NW* map (1:40,000 scale), and the USGS 7.5-minute series *Lake Eleanor, Kibbie Lake,* and *Tiltill Mountain* maps (1:24,000 scale).

Best Time

The trails up to both lakes are mostly snow-free by late May, but mosquitoes can linger well into July. Following wetter winters or springs, June and early July yield a plethora of wildflowers, with small annuals densely decorating sandy flats. Mid-July–early August are the best swimming months, when lakes are at their maximum temperatures. A September hike is also rewarding, after most of the hikers have left, and for solitude, the first half of October is even better, though nights and mornings can dip below freezing. An advantage of hiking in these two months is that the long ascent, which can be hot in summer, is a lot more bearable.

Finding the Trail

Driving east along CA 120 (Tioga Road), turn left onto Evergreen Road, located just 0.6 mile west of Yosemite National Park's boundary at the

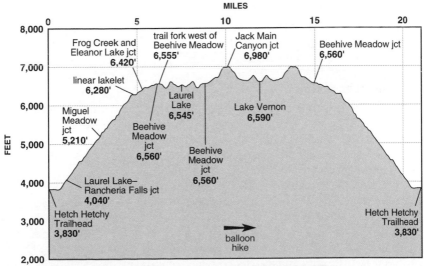

TRAIL 24 Laurel Lake and Lake Vernon Elevation Profile

Big Oak Flat Entrance Station. Drive 7.4 miles north on Evergreen Road to its junction with Hetch Hetchy Road, an intersection located right in the middle of the small community of Mather. Turn right, drive beneath an archway, and continue 1.3 miles to the Hetch Hetchy Entrance Station/Mather Ranger Station.

Road use is restricted near O'Shaughnessy Dam. In midsummer the road is open 7 a.m.–8 p.m., but open hours decrease with dwindling daylight hours. The current hours are posted where you turn onto Evergreen Road or on the Yosemite National Park website; just search for "Hetch Hetchy open hours." At the entrance, your license plate is registered and you are given a placard to display on your dash.

Once past this bottleneck, drive 7.1 miles to a junction branching left for the Hetch Hetchy backpackers' campground. Backpackers turn here, park in the obvious parking area by the road's start, then walk 0.45 mile on the road to O'Shaughnessy Dam. Day hikers continue driving 0.7 mile past the junction to the dam, just beyond which is the trailhead parking. If you are just day hiking and want to stay in a relatively nearby campground, the Dimond O Campground is along Evergreen Road, and Hodgdon Meadow Campground is along CA 120 just inside Yosemite. Backpackers can stay at the trailhead backpackers' campground for a night before and/or after their trip. There are toilets and water faucets at the backpackers' parking area or, for day hikers, in a pullout on the right, just before you reach the reservoir's shore.

Trail Description

Backpackers, starting from their parking area, will add 0.9 mile to their round-trip distance. Summer hikers should start early in the morning because the switchbacking route up from the reservoir is only partly shaded, and temperatures can reach into the 90s by noon. Carry sufficient water; by late summer it's 5.6 miles before you come to water.

You begin by starting across the top of O'Shaughnessy Dam (3,814') at Hetch Hetchy Reservoir. ▶1 On the south wall, the prow of Kolana Rock soars 2,000 feet above the reservoir, while to its north, tiered Hetch Hetchy Dome rises 2,400 feet above the water. In a shaded cleft on the dome's west flank, two-stepped Wapama Falls plunges an aggregate of 1,400 feet. In early summer its gossamer companion, Tueeulala Falls, spills over a near-vertical face slightly farther west. Yet farther west is the informally named Hetch Hetchy Falls, whose water spills down slabs rather than free-falling downward.

Across the 600-foot-long dam, you enter a 500-foot-long tunnel blasted through solid granite when the original dam was raised 85 feet in 1938. Emerging from this bat haven, the formerly paved road traverses just above the rocky west shore of Hetch Hetchy Reservoir. Along much of this length, a pleasant grove of Douglas-fir, gray pine, big-leaf maple, and bay trees shade your progress, though in places the trees were burned in the 2013 Rim Fire. Soon you reach a junction where the Rancheria Falls Trail (Trail 25) branches right (1.0 mile), ▶2 while you continue briefly straight ahead, soon encountering the route's first switchback.

Keeping to the former road, you ascend moderately steep switchbacks and have ever-broader views up the reservoir to Le Conte Point and the Grand Canyon of the Tuolumne River. As you ascend, fairly open, lower slopes give way to live oak–shaded slopes, then near the top to some patches shaded by surviving oaks and conifers. This slope, like much of the route to come, was burned in the 2013 Rim Fire. Most badly burned conifers die, but remarkably many of the live oaks along this slope rapidly resprouted from the trunk and should again provide some shade by the time you read this.

The last of eight switchbacks swings north into a gully and then to a trail junction on a small flat, where left heads to Miguel Meadow along the old road and you trend right, ascending a narrower trail (2.9 miles). ▶3 With one-third of the distance to Laurel Lake covered and half of the elevation gain under your belt, you start up a trail through a partly burned conifer forest. In 0.25 mile you reach a mile-high creeklet, which, though diminutive, usually flows through the summer. This is your first *usually* reliable water, but camping is not permitted here since you are less than 4 trail miles from the trailhead. Up the trail about 600 feet past the creeklet, and about 3.2 miles from the trailhead, you'll see a shallow gully on your right, which is the start of a 1.5-mile-long (each way) cross-country route east to the brink of Wapama Falls, a stunning viewpoint; if you find the brush-free bench, this is an easy route, but otherwise it can be cumbersome.

Unlike the closed road you ascended, which maintains a nearly constant grade, your ascending trail varies, being locally steep, moderate, gentle, or even briefly down. You'll eventually climb 1,000 feet above the creeklet before the serious climbing ends with a curve east to cross the crest

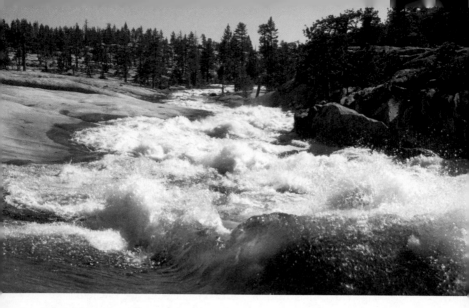

Creek *below Lake Vernon*

of a lateral moraine. On this ascent, look for linear deposits, which are also lateral moraines. Once on top, take a break; you deserve it.

Your hike ahead is now relatively easy. You descend briefly, curving around the eastern tip of a small, seasonal, linear lakelet (4.75 miles) ▶4, as the trail crosses the broad moraine's crest. Shade has been lacking for much of the ascent, the consequence of a sequence of fires that have torn through the area. Near the lakelet the landscape is almost completely devoid of trees, with just a few blackened trunks standing tall as totems. In early spring wildflowers decorate the trail's verges, but with summer heat only the spiny shrubs keep you company as you traipse along. The next junction will be a welcome sight, where you stay straight ahead, while left is signposted for Frog Creek and Lake Eleanor (5.3 miles). ▶5 Laurel Lake, though only 0.75 mile northwest of you, is at least 2.2 trail miles away by either trail you can take, and one wonders why a trail was not built directly to it because the circuitous routes also include excess elevation loss and gain. If you're short on water, take the trail southwest 0.25 mile down to reliable Frog Creek.

If not diverting for water, follow the now shadier trail northeast (right), dip to cross a bracken-bordered creeklet, then soon hike alongside a linear meadow, which in season is profuse with wildflowers. The first meadow pinches off at a low gap, beyond which you quickly find yourself in the southwest corner of a triangular meadow. Staying among white firs and lodgepole pines, you parallel the meadow's edge northeast over to its east corner, called the Beehive, the site of an 1880s cattle-men's camp, where there is a trail junction (6.15 miles). ►6 About 60 feet before it, just within the meadow, is a usually reliable, but well-concealed, spring. Just beyond the junction, among trees, is a spacious campsite.

With most of your ascent behind you, you turn left and walk along the northern edge of Beehive Meadow on the Laurel Lake Trail to reach another trail split within 200 steps (6.25 miles). ►7 Here a path that loops around Laurel Lake's north shore branches north (right), while a shorter trail to the lake's outlet strikes west (left). Not only is the westerly route shorter, but it is also in much better condition—the northerly trail is easy to lose in several locations, due to the regrowth of brush follow-ing fires. Staying left, you drop easily down into a gully and then ford broad Frog Creek, which could be a wet, bouldery ford in late spring and early summer—and indeed impassable at the highest flows. Along its north bank you contour west briefly, then ascend steeply to a heavily forested ridge before gently dropping to good camps near Laurel Lake's outlet. A brief stint brings you to a junction with the north-shore loop trail (7.5 miles) ►8—branching right (northwest) from here leads to more secluded campsites, especially near the northern tip of the lake. At fairly deep 60-acre Laurel Lake, western azalea grows thickly just back of the locally grassy lakeshore, a fragrant accompaniment to huckleberry and thimbleberry. Fishing is fair for rainbow trout, but swimming, especially in July and early August, can be wonderful.

After your stay at the lake, return to the Beehive junction (8.85 miles). ►9 If you want to proceed to Lake Vernon, take the eastbound (left) trail, which winds 1.25 miles easily through burned forest and past moist openings replete with wildflowers—lupines, fireweed, camas lilies, monkeyflowers, and more—up to a moraine-crest junction with the trail branching left to Jack Main Canyon (10.1 miles). ►10 This trail climbs along the crest of Moraine Ridge before dropping into Jack Main Canyon some 4 miles farther north.

From the junction you descend right to an open, granite bench. Now on bedrock, you follow a well-ducked (marked by stones) trail down past excellent examples of smooth glacier-polished rock and glacier-transported boulders, termed glacial erratics. Along this section you can look across the far wall of slab-lined Falls Creek canyon. Just after a small knob obstructs your view, you angle southeast and follow a winding, ducked route up toward the point, soon crossing a low ridge just north of it. Below you lies Lake Vernon, filling a broad, flat-floored canyon, with endless granite slabs spreading to its south, dissected by Falls Creek racing toward the lip of Wapama Falls.

From this inspirational ridge you descend generally northeast to a junction with a spur trail (11.9 miles). ▶11 The distance to Lake Vernon is measured to this point, but depending on your preference, reaching a choice campsite may require up to another mile of walking. Those in search of tent sites nestled among slabs will choose to take the main trail southeast briefly to a bridge across Falls Creek, just below the lake. From here you can explore broadly, even descending a short stretch of Falls Creek to sandy flats with possible campsites southeast of the trail. Parties hunting for tree-sheltered homes will take the spur trail that branches left and follows the western shore of Lake Vernon for 1.3 miles, petering out past a snow-gauge marker and adjacent park cabin. Most lakeside campsites are small and almost all are well hidden from the trail; the largest one is about one-third of the way north along the western shore in a large stand of lodgepole pines. There is also a large camp at the north end of the lake close to where the creek angles from northeast to north and its gradient increases dramatically. The lake, mostly shallow and lying at about 6,564 feet, is one of the warmer park lakes for swimming. After a lovely evening in your chosen locale, return to the Hetch Hetchy Trailhead the way you came (21.1 miles). ▶12

🚶	**MILESTONES**	
▶1	0.0	Start at Hetch Hetchy Trailhead
▶2	1.0	Left at Laurel Lake–Rancheria Falls junction
▶3	2.9	Right at Miguel Meadow junction
▶4	4.75	Linear lakelet
▶5	5.3	Right at Frog Creek and Lake Eleanor junction
▶6	6.15	Left at Beehive Meadow junction
▶7	6.25	Left at trail split west of Beehive Meadow
▶8	7.5	Laurel Lake
▶9	8.85	Left at Beehive Meadow junction
▶10	10.1	Right at Jack Main Canyon junction
▶11	11.9	Lake Vernon
▶12	21.1	Return to Hetch Hetchy Trailhead

Wapama Falls and Rancheria Falls Camp

A stately grove of pines and incense cedars harboring a spacious camping area near Rancheria Falls marks the terminus of this hike. Its cascades and pools are the goals for some, but also rewarding are inspirational vistas of the awesome cliffs and two waterfalls, Tueeulala and Wapama, seen along the undulating path on the north wall of Hetch Hetchy Reservoir. Because you are traversing above a reservoir, you might think that this is an easy hike, but you face gains and losses of hundreds of feet as the trail traverses along ledges in steep granite slabs rising above the water. The route, being quite open and at a relatively low elevation, can be quite sunny and hot, so on a summer's day it is best begun in early morning. On some late-fall and winter days you will share the path with many California newts on their annual migration.

Permits

Overnight visitors require a wilderness permit for the Rancheria Falls Trailhead, issued by Yosemite National Park. Pick up your permit at the Hetch Hetchy Entrance Station.

Maps

This trail is covered by the Tom Harrison *Hetch Hetchy* map (1:63,360 scale), the National Geographic Trails Illustrated *#307 Yosemite NW* map (1:40,000 scale), and the USGS 7.5-minute series *Lake Eleanor* and *Hetch Hetchy Reservoir* maps (1:24,000 scale).

TRAIL USE
Day Hike, Backpack, Horse, Run

LENGTH
12.8 miles, 6–10 hours (over 1–2 days)

VERTICAL FEET
One-way:
+2,040', −1,190'
Round-trip: ±3,230'

DIFFICULTY
− 1 2 **3** 4 5 +

TRAIL TYPE
Out-and-Back

FEATURES
Canyon
Lake
Stream
Waterfall
Wildflowers
Great Views
Camping
Granite Slabs
Geological Interest

FACILITIES
Bear Boxes
Campground
Restrooms
Water

243

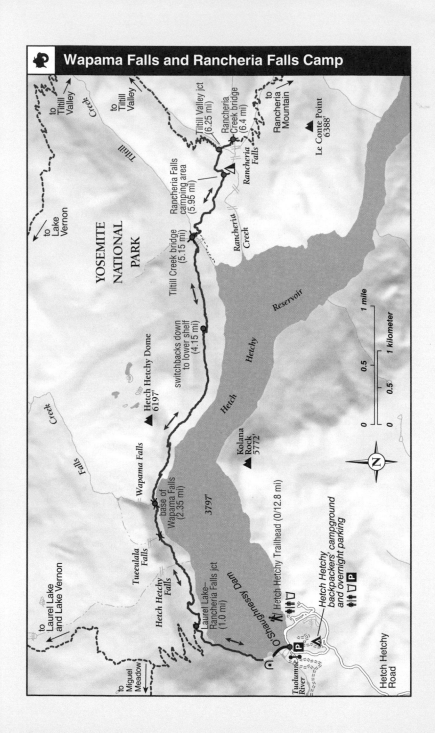

Wapama Falls and Rancheria Falls Camp

Tueeulala Creek

to Tiltill Valley

to Tiltill Valley

Tiltill Valley jct (6.25 mi)

Rancheria Creek bridge (6.4 mi)

to Rancheria Mountain

Tiltill Creek

Le Conte Point 6388'

YOSEMITE NATIONAL PARK

to Lake Vernon

Rancheria Falls

Rancheria Falls camping area (5.95 mi)

Rancheria Creek

Tiltill Creek bridge (5.15 mi)

Reservoir

switchbacks down to lower shelf (4.15 mi)

Hetch Hetchy Dome 6197'

Hetchy

Creek

Hetch

Kolana Rock, 5772'

Wapama Falls

Falls

base of Wapama Falls (2.35 mi)

3797'

Tueeulala Falls

Hetch Hetchy Trailhead (0/12.8 mi)

Hetch Hetchy Falls

Hetch Hetchy backpackers' campground and overnight parking

O'Shaughnessy Dam

Laurel Lake–Rancheria Falls jct (1.0 mi)

to Laurel Lake and Lake Vernon

Laurel Lake and Lake Vernon

to Miguel Meadow

Tuolumne River

Hetch Hetchy Road

1 mile

1 kilometer

0.5

0.5

0

0

N

Best Time

The road to the Hetch Hetchy Trailhead is usually open by April (or earlier), but if you are after the two waterfalls and the wildflowers, May and June are best. After June, Tueeulala Falls quickly fades into oblivion, though Wapama Falls remains impressive through about mid-July, gradually diminishes through the summer months, but persists throughout the hiking season. The Rancheria Falls camping area is well used May–October, with different months deemed perfect based on your preferences: April–June for wildflowers; July–August for swimming, because Rancheria Creek's pools are usually safe to enter by then; and September–November for cooler temperatures, solitude, and the yellow-orange hues of autumn.

> Before the
> O'Shaughnessy
> Dam was completed
> in 1923, the Hetch
> Hetchy Valley was
> said to rival Yosemite
> Valley in beauty.

Finding the Trail

Driving east along CA 120 (Tioga Road), you turn left onto Evergreen Road, located just 0.6 mile west of Yosemite National Park's boundary at the Big Oak Flat Entrance Station. Drive 7.4 miles north on Evergreen Road to its junction with Hetch Hetchy Road, an intersection located right in the middle of the small community of Mather. Turn right,

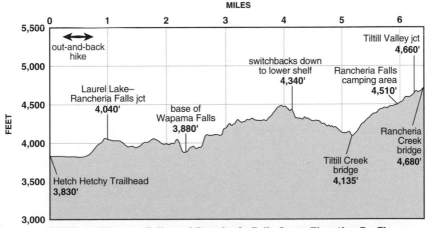

TRAIL 25 Wapama Falls and Rancheria Falls Camp Elevation Profile

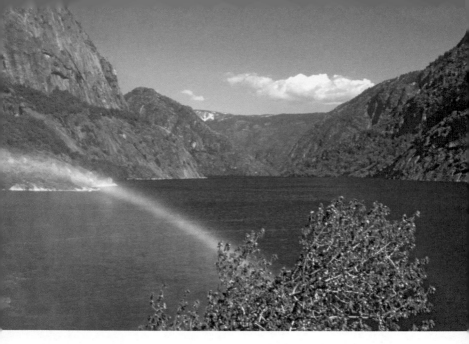

A rainbow *is formed by the spray of Wapama Falls as it tumbles into Hetch Hetchy Reservoir.*

drive beneath an archway, and continue 1.3 miles to the Hetch Hetchy Entrance Station/Mather Ranger Station.

Road use is restricted near O'Shaughnessy Dam. In midsummer the road is open 7 a.m.–8 p.m., but open hours decrease with dwindling daylight hours. The current hours are posted where you turn onto Evergreen Road or on the Yosemite National Park website; just search for "Hetch Hetchy open hours." At the entrance, your license plate is registered and you are given a placard to display on your dash.

Once past this bottleneck, drive 7.1 miles to a junction branching left for the Hetch Hetchy Backpackers' Campground. Backpackers turn here, park in the obvious parking area by the road's start, then walk 0.45 mile on the road to O'Shaughnessy Dam. Day hikers continue driving 0.7 mile past the junction to the dam, just beyond which is the trailhead parking. If you are just day hiking and want to stay in a relatively nearby campground, the Dimond O Campground is along Evergreen Road, and Hodgdon Meadow Campground is along CA 120 just inside Yosemite. Backpackers can stay at the trailhead backpackers' campground for a night before and/or after their trip. There are toilets and water faucets at the backpackers' parking area or, for day hikers, in a pullout on the right, just before you reach the reservoir's shore.

Trail Description

Backpackers, who start from the overnight parking area, will add 0.9 mile to their round-trip distance. Summer hikers should start early in the morning because the walk around the reservoir is in the full sun and temperatures can reach into the 90s by noon. Carry sufficient water; the only reliable—and accessible—water sources are Falls Creek (at Wapama Falls) and then Rancheria Creek. Tiltill Creek flows but is cumbersome to reach because the trail crosses the creek on a bridge above a steep gorge.

You begin by starting across the top of O'Shaughnessy Dam (3,814') at Hetch Hetchy Reservoir. ▶1 On the south wall, the prow of Kolana Rock soars 2,000 feet above the reservoir, while to its north, tiered Hetch Hetchy Dome rises yet 400 feet higher. In a shaded cleft on the dome's west flank, two-stepped Wapama Falls plunges an aggregate of 1,400 feet. In early summer its gossamer companion, Tueeulala Falls, spills 880 feet over the lip slightly farther west.

Across the 600-foot-long dam, you enter a 500-foot-long tunnel blasted through solid granite when the original dam was raised 85 feet in 1938. Emerging from this bat haven, the formerly paved road traverses just above the rocky west shore of Hetch Hetchy Reservoir. Along much of this length a pleasant grove of Douglas-fir, gray pine, big-leaf maple, and bay trees shade your progress, though in places the trees were burned in the 2013 Rim Fire. Soon you reach a junction where the trail to Laurel Lake (Trail 24), following the old road, continues straight ahead (1.0 mile), ▶2 while you turn to the right on a broad granite shelf.

On it you descend gently, first south and then east, across an exfoliating granitic nose, then switchback once down to a broad, sloping ledge, sparingly shaded by the grayish-green foliage of gray pines. From April to June it is often decorated with an assortment of wildflowers in bloom because the granite slabs are quite impervious and the water pools atop them, creating miniature vernal wetlands and moist soils. Species you might see by the hundreds include centaury, clarkias, and monkeyflowers, while other gems like the butterfly mariposa lily and harvest brodiaea occur in smaller clusters. By midsummer it is parched and yellow. You follow this ledge 0.5 mile to a minor stream that descends, until about early summer, as informally named Hetch Hetchy Falls (and incorrectly marked as Tueeulala Falls on many maps). Beyond it you wind down along the north shore of Hetch Hetchy Reservoir to a bridge over a steep, generally dry cleft, where your views east to the lake's head expand impressively. Opposite you towers Kolana Rock, which forces a constriction in the 8-mile-long reservoir's tadpole shape, while the prow of Hetch Hetchy Dome descends to lake level beyond Wapama Falls. Just past the bridge is a seasonally wet, bouldery crossing, the outflow from Tueeulala Falls, lying 0.2 mile east of where it is marked on most maps. It either spills forcefully down a near-vertical wall or is absent because it is created by an overflow channel from Falls Creek. While most of the volume of Falls Creek forms Wapama Falls, at the highest of flows, Falls Creek spills into a subsidiary channel that drops over the lip at Tueeulala Falls. As soon as Falls Creek's volume decreases enough to stop spilling over, Tueeulala Falls instantly vanishes.

A few minutes of easy traverse east from here end at a steep, dynamited descent through a field of huge talus blocks under a tremendous precipice. Soon, if you're passing this way in early summer, flecks of spray dampen your path, as you approach the first of several bridges below the base of Wapama Falls (2.35 miles). ▶3 During some high-runoff years, even these high, sturdy bridges are inundated by seasonally tumultuous Falls Creek and must be crossed very carefully, and on rare occasions the national park will close this route due to dangerous conditions.

Just east of Wapama Falls, the oak trees that have provided shade vanish as you cross a 300-foot-long near-barren field of talus; this was the site of a rockslide in spring 2014, when granite slabs broke loose from nearly 1,000 feet above your head on Hetch Hetchy Dome and pummeled the slope, breaking off nearly every tree. Reentering tree cover, you will now appreciate that the scattered moss-covered boulders on the slope are simply remnants of long-ago rockfalls. Your rocky path leads up around the base of a steep bulge of glacier-polished and striated granite, still under a fly-infested canopy of canyon live oak, bay tree, poison oak, and wild grapevines. After your terrace tapers off, the frequently dynamited trail leaves forest cover and undulates along a steep hillside in open chaparral of yerba santa and mountain mahogany, switchbacking on occasion to circumvent some cliffy spots. The longest descent occurs where the main shelf peters out and you descend to a lower one (4.15 miles). ▶4 Eventually your path descends to the shaded gorge cut by Tiltill Creek, and you cross two bridges, the second one high above the creek (5.15 miles). ▶5 You can get water just above this bridge by making a cautious traverse over to a pool at the brink of the creek's fall. When the current is not too strong, the pool is great to dip in on a hot day; however, at strong flows it is best to wait until Rancheria Creek to refill your water.

Beyond the creek your route climbs the gorge's east slope via a set of tight switchbacks to emerge 250 feet higher on a gentle hillside. Where this ascent eases off, you may see, on your right, the start of an old trail that follows a descending ridge just south of Tiltill Creek, ending just above Hetch Hetchy Reservoir.

Soon you spy Rancheria Creek, and by walking a few paces right, you have an excellent vantage point of it. The creek here slides invitingly over broad rock slabs, its pools superb for skinny-dipping when the creek isn't swift. Every step of your way has been on granite, but just 0.2 mile past this vantage point you may note a tiny remnant of a once much larger volcanic deposit that was transported to this spot in a south-directed eruption of latite tuff about 9.5 million years ago. Just 0.1 mile past the volcanic remnant you reach a junction with a short trail to the spacious Rancheria Falls Camp (5.95 miles). ►6

Once you have dropped your packs—and stored your food securely in your bear canister (this popular camping area is often visited by black bears)—I suggest you walk a stretch along Rancheria Creek. You may choose to simply walk to the river's shore near the camp and head up and down it in pursuit of cascades and pools. One nearby cascade is a small fall, about 25 feet high, which in high volume shoots over a ledge of resistant, dark, intrusive rock. Alternatively you can continue a short distance up the main trail, first turning right at a junction, where left leads to Tiltill Valley and right to Rancheria Mountain (6.25 miles) ►7 and soon thereafter reaching a bridge spanning Rancheria Creek (6.4 miles). ►8 Watching the water plummet past here is mesmerizing and, at low flows, descending below the bridge yields additional swimming holes. Fishing along the creek might yield pan-size rainbow trout. After a lengthy break—or a good night's sleep—return to the Hetch Hetchy Trailhead (12.8 miles). ►9

🚶 MILESTONES

►1	0.0	Start at Hetch Hetchy Trailhead
►2	1.0	Right at Laurel Lake–Rancheria Falls junction
►3	2.35	Wapama Falls
►4	4.15	Switchbacks down to lower shelf
►5	5.15	Tiltill Creek bridge
►6	5.95	Rancheria Falls camping area
►7	6.25	Right at Tiltill Valley junction
►8	6.4	Rancheria Creek bridge
►9	12.8	Return to Hetch Hetchy Trailhead

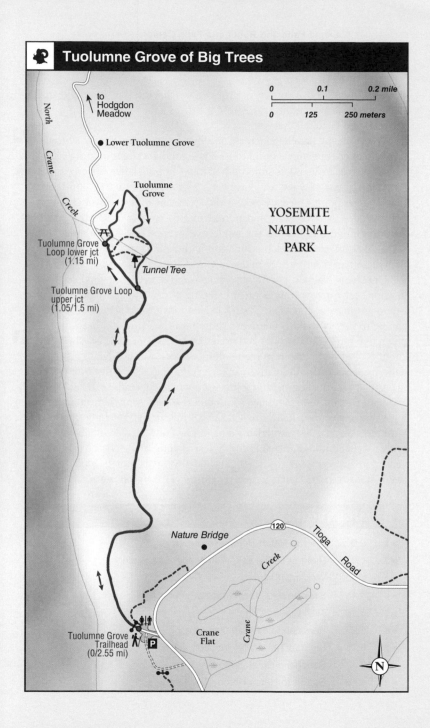

Tuolumne Grove of Big Trees

to Hodgdon Meadow

North Crane Creek

● Lower Tuolumne Grove

Tuolumne Grove

YOSEMITE NATIONAL PARK

Tuolumne Grove Loop lower jct (1.15 mi)

Tunnel Tree

Tuolumne Grove Loop upper jct (1.05/1.5 mi)

Nature Bridge ●

120

Tioga Road

Creek

Crane

Tuolumne Grove Trailhead (0/2.55 mi)

P

Crane Flat

N

0   0.1   0.2 mile

0   125   250 meters

Tuolumne Grove of Big Trees

The Tuolumne Grove has more than a dozen trees at least 10 feet in diameter near the base, and though this pales in comparison with the much larger Mariposa Grove's (Trail 43) approximately 200 trees of similar or larger size, you'll certainly see fewer tourists. Being smaller and less crowded means that you will share the small loop trail through the grove with relatively few people, allowing a more intimate connection with the forest. The small loop trail in the grove takes you through stands of young trees, past fallen logs, and through the Tunnel Tree.

Maps

This trail is covered by the Tom Harrison *Yosemite National Park* map (1:126,720 scale), the National Geographic Trails Illustrated *#306 Yosemite SW* map (1:40,000 scale), and the USGS 7.5-minute series *Ackerson Mountain* map (1:24,000 scale).

Best Time

Any time early April–mid-November, when the closed road usually is snow-free, is fine. It also makes a fine snowshoe trip in winter. There are no prominent wildflower displays in the grove itself, but in spring scattered wildflowers, including orchids and wild roses, dot the roadside.

Finding the Trail

CA 120 turns left (northeast) at Crane Flat, aligning itself with eastbound Tioga Road, while Big Oak Flat Road continues straight ahead toward Yosemite Valley. From this T-junction, drive 0.5 mile east along Tioga Road to a large parking area on your

TRAIL USE
Day Hike, Stroller
Access, Child-Friendly

LENGTH
2.55 miles, 1–3 hours

VERTICAL FEET
One-way: +5', –505'
Round-trip: ±510'

DIFFICULTY
– 1 **2** 3 4 5 +

TRAIL TYPE
Balloon

FEATURES
Wildflowers
Giant Sequoias
Historical Interest

FACILITIES
Bear Boxes
Campground Store
Restrooms

left. There are toilets at the trailhead, but the closest water is at the Crane Flat store—you currently have to use the bathroom sink.

Trail Description

In the area covered by this book's scope, there are three sequoia groves, Merced, Tuolumne, and Mariposa. What they have in common today are similar elevations, between 5,000 and 6,000 feet, and perhaps more important, some underlying metamorphic bedrock. Metamorphic bedrock weathers to produce soils with more nutrients and more groundwater-holding capacity than soils derived from granitic bedrock, and in times of warmer, drier climates, such as a few thousand years ago, metamorphic soils may have enabled our sequoias to survive.

Excepting the short loop at the midpoint of the walk, this route is paved, making it passable to strollers but too steep for comfort for most wheelchair users. However, the gradient is, in places, quite steep, so make sure you have a good grip on the stroller.

The route, an old road closed to vehicles since 1993, is obvious. ▶1 It first curves 0.25 mile over to a gully below the back side of Nature Bridge, an environmental education organization based in Yosemite. This gully is impressively colored by a thicket of yellow coneflowers in early summer. Looking downslope you will notice many dead and charred trees, the result of back burns on this slope that successfully stopped the 2013 Rim

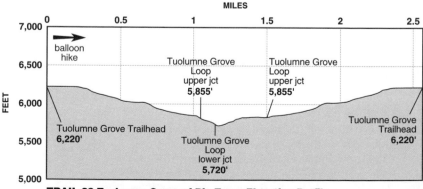

TRAIL 26 Tuolumne Grove of Big Trees Elevation Profile

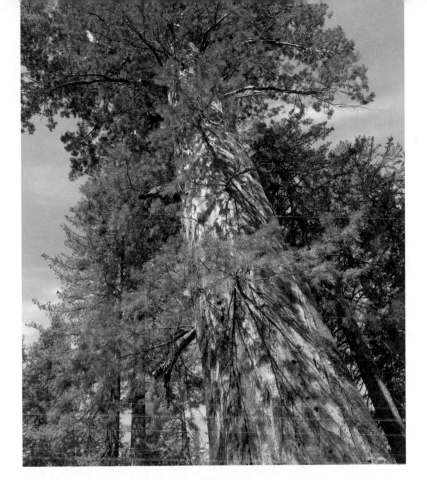

Looking up *the trunk of a massive sequoia*

Fire from damaging the sequoias, but unfortunately killed many beautiful sugar pines. The road soon takes on a steeper gradient as it first descends to a switchback west, then to one north. Just past it, you enter the Tuolumne Grove and spy the first giant trees through the conifer canopy. Seeing the massive red trunks scattered among notably large pines and firs certainly emphasizes the sequoia's girth. Indeed, this is the best of Yosemite's three sequoia groves to admire the trees growing side by side with other species. About 0.2 mile farther down the road, you come to a junction beside an impressive sequoia about 15 feet in diameter (1.05 miles). ▶2 For now continue along the main road, but you will return via the trail to your right. Standing here, you are among some of the largest trees in the grove, looming tall in the forest, but still intermingled with a collection of other conifers including white fir and sugar pine.

Continue 0.1 mile down along the paved road to a picnic table and cluster of small trails (1.15 miles). ►3 Beyond, the road descends about 4.5 miles to Hodgdon Meadow Campground, which lies just east of the Big Oak Flat Entrance Station. Along the trail on the right (north) side of the road, you now take the leftmost option—it is lined with a hewn log fence and follows the banks of a small creek. This self-guiding nature walk winds past several fallen trees, as well as a grove of young individuals, eventually leading to an opening where you can admire the upended roots of a large tree. From this location, your route heads left around the top of these roots, steps across two small creeks on wooden bridges, and shortly reaches the famous Tunnel Tree, a dead, charred hulk with a base diameter of 29.5 feet. In its glory, it must have been one of Yosemite's tallest specimens. A tunnel was carved in it back in 1878, long after a fire shaped its cathedral-like form. The wood is so resistant to decay that it maintains this form centuries after the fire. Walk through the tunnel, enjoying its skylight, and ascend briefly to a reunion with the main road (1.5 miles). ►4 From here, retrace your steps up the road to the trailhead (2.55 miles). ►5

🚶	**MILESTONES**	
►1	0.0	Start at Tuolumne Grove Trailhead
►2	1.05	Left at Tuolumne Grove Loop upper junction
►3	1.15	Right at Tuolumne Grove Loop lower junction
►4	1.5	Left at Tuolumne Grove Loop upper junction
►5	2.55	Return to Tuolumne Grove Trailhead

El Capitan from Tamarack Flat

The 3,000-foot-high vertical walls of El Capitan attract rock climbers from all over the world, and more than five dozen extremely difficult routes ascend it. For nonclimbers this hike provides a more practical means to attain El Capitan's summit. This walk is not particularly distinguished by its terrain or wildflowers and passes no lakes, but reaching the flat-topped El Capitan is sufficient reward for your efforts. Though the round-trip distance is nearly 17 miles, I nevertheless recommend this trail as a day hike in mid- to late summer and fall because the main source of water along this trail is Ribbon Creek, which dries up around midsummer.

Permits

Overnight visitors require a wilderness permit for the Tamarack Creek Trailhead (route as described) or Old Big Oak Flat Road Trailhead (alternative start), issued by Yosemite National Park. Pick up your wilderness permit at the Big Oak Flat Information Station or the Yosemite Valley Wilderness Center.

Maps

This trail is covered by the Tom Harrison *Yosemite National Park* map (1:126,720 scale), the National Geographic Trails Illustrated *#306 Yosemite SW* map (1:40,000 scale), and the USGS 7.5-minute series *Tamarack Flat* and *El Capitan* maps (1:24,000 scale).

Best Time

Despite being mostly snow-free by mid-June and staying that way usually until late October, this trail has a shorter hiking season. The reason for

TRAIL USE
Day Hike, Backpack, Horse, Run

LENGTH
16.8 miles, 7–12 hours (over 1–2 days)

VERTICAL FEET
One-way:
+2,470', −1,245'
Round-trip: ±3,715'

DIFFICULTY
− 1 2 3 **4** 5 +

TRAIL TYPE
Out-and-Back

FEATURES
Summit
Wildflowers
Great Views
Camping
Secluded

FACILITIES
Bear Boxes
Campground
Horse Staging
Restrooms

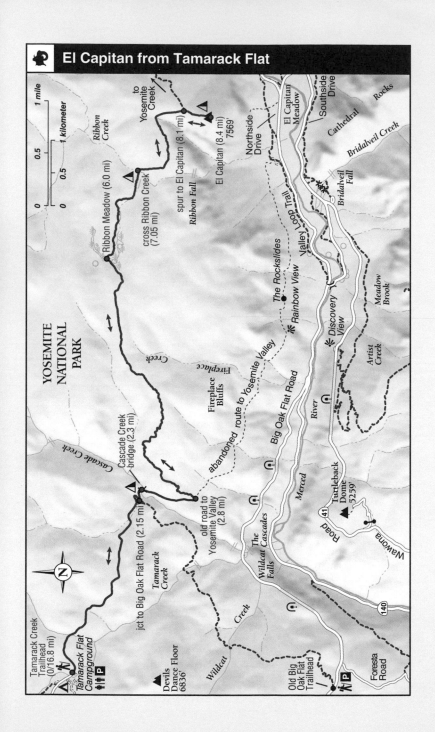

El Capitan from Tamarack Flat

1 mile
0.5
0

1 kilometer
1
0.5
0

YOSEMITE NATIONAL PARK

Ribbon Creek

to Yosemite Creek

spur to El Capitan (8.1 mi)

Ribbon Fall

El Capitan (8.4 mi) 7569

Ribbon Meadow (6.0 mi)

cross Ribbon Creek (7.05 mi)

Northside Drive

El Capitan Meadow

Southside Drive

Cathedral Rocks

Bridalveil Creek

Bridalveil Fall

Creek

Fireplace Creek

Fireplace Bluffs

The Rockslides

Rainbow View

Valley Loop Trail

Discovery View

Meadow Brook

Artist Creek

abandoned route to Yosemite Valley

Big Oak Flat Road

Cascade Creek

Cascade Creek bridge (2.3 mi)

old road to Yosemite Valley (2.8 mi)

Merced River

jct to Big Oak Flat Road (2.15 mi)

Tamarack Creek

Devils Dance Floor 6836'

The Wildcat Cascades Falls

Turtleback Dome 5259'

41

Wawona Road

Tamarack Creek Trailhead (0/16.8 mi)

Tamarack Flat Campground

Wildcat Creek

Old Big Oak Flat Trailhead

Foresta Road

140

N

this is that the road down to Tamarack Flat Campground is open only from about early July (or mid-June) to early October, and when the road is closed, the hike is too long to be rewarding for most people. It then involves an additional 1.2 miles (round-trip) and 1,100 feet of ascent (and of course 1,100 feet of descent), as you would start the walk from the little-used Old Big Oak Flat Road Trailhead along Big Oak Flat Road near the Foresta turnoff.

Finding the Trail

CA 120 turns left (northeast) at Crane Flat, aligning itself with eastbound Tioga Road, while Big Oak Flat Road continues straight ahead toward Yosemite Valley. From this T-junction, drive northeast 3.75 miles up Tioga Road (CA 120 eastbound) to the Tamarack Flat Campground turnoff, immediately before the Gin Flat scenic turnout. Drive southeast down to the east end of Tamarack Flat Campground (along Old Big Oak Flat Road), 3.05 miles from Tioga Road. There are toilets in the campground, but the closest water is at the Crane Flat store—you currently have to use the bathroom sink.

To reach the alternative trailhead, instead of turning onto CA 120 eastbound, drive 5.9 miles along Big Oak Flat Road toward Yosemite Valley to a small parking area on the right. The trail is just across the road. There are no facilities at this trailhead—the closest water is at the Crane Flat store.

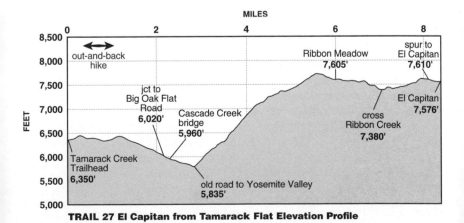

TRAIL 27 El Capitan from Tamarack Flat Elevation Profile

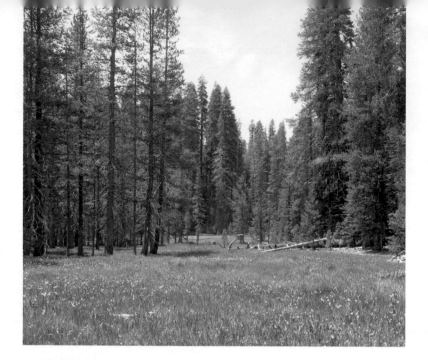

Ribbon Meadow

Trail Description

From Tamarack Creek Trailhead in Tamarack Flat Campground, ►1 you ascend slopes on the old (original) Big Oak Flat Road for a 100-foot elevation gain. Here, white firs are the dominant trees, and along both sides of the road, you'll see large, partly buried granitic boulders. Just before you reach a prominent cluster of rocks, your road begins a steady descent to Cascade Creek. At a road switchback you'll see a junction with a trail to the new Big Oak Flat Road, where you continue left (2.15 miles). ►2 This is the direction from which you would come if the road to Tamarack Flat Campground is closed, necessitating a start along the new Big Oak Flat Road. Down at this lower, warmer, drier elevation, you'll find ponderosa and sugar pines intermingled with the firs, though with each year, more and more of the park's majestic sugar pines are dying, the species hardest hit by the 2012–2016 drought and ongoing bark beetle attacks. Continuing along the old road, you soon reach a sturdy bridge spanning Cascade Creek (2.3 miles). ►3 It is unlikely that you will choose to camp this close to your starting point, but there are small campsites just before the bridge, and in late summer small pools along Cascade Creek make nice swimming holes. Before then the creek is likely to be too swift for safe frolicking, particularly because the water-polished

rock can be quite slippery. The large-leaved Indian rhubarb, dogwoods, ✽
willows, western azaleas, and serviceberries make fine creekside companions. If you are hiking later than about early August, this may be your
last reliable water, so carry enough to last.

Bound for El Capitan, you continue 0.5 mile down
Old Big Oak Flat Road—now more like a trail—to a
junction where you turn left, toward El Capitan, part-
ing ways with the old road (2.8 miles). ►4 The old
road now continues its descent to Yosemite Valley via
a route that is in part completely obliterated by massive rockslides (also known as The Rockslides). To
think, this was once the only way into the valley and
is now even walked only rarely—and with difficulty.
But returning our thoughts to our route to El Capitan,
you now begin a major climb of almost 2,000 feet.

> **World-class climbers
> can climb the face of
> El Capitan in about
> the same time that the
> average hiker takes
> to reach the summit
> by trail.**

Starting in a forest of incense cedar, ponderosa
and sugar pines, and white fir, you climb hundreds of feet—steeply at
times—up to drier slopes dotted with clusters of greenleaf manzanita and
huckleberry oak. Occasionally you see black oaks, but these diminish to
shrub height as you climb higher, disappearing altogether by the time you
reach a small drop on a ridge. Eventually you emerge onto a sandy ridge
speckled with beautiful Jeffrey pines and, in spring, a thin veneer of wildflowers. Granite slabs lie just below the surface of the shallow soils, and ✽
the slope is parched as the summer progresses.

From the top you make a short descent to a sedge-filled damp
meadow, the western outskirts of Ribbon Meadow (6.0 miles), ►5 which
sprouts water-loving wildflowers, especially dense tracts of shooting stars
and corn lilies. The meadow guides you to a crossing of a Ribbon Creek ✽
tributary—a wide bog in early summer, but later dry—and back into forest, still designated part of Ribbon Meadow, but now more a dense lodgepole forest. On the trees' bark you'll see blazes to guide you where the
route becomes a little vague. Paralleling the tributary that flows through
Ribbon Meadow, the trail heads east down to Ribbon Creek (7.05 miles).
►6 Along the banks of Ribbon Creek are the trail's most used campsites— ⚠
pleasant in spring and early summer but waterless when the creek dries
up about midsummer.

No longer far from your goal, you make a brief climb, an equally
brief descent, and then an ascending traverse east to the top of El Capitan
Gully. Your first views of El Capitan and the south wall of Yosemite Valley

appear on this traverse and continue to expand as you climb south from the gully to a junction with the El Capitan spur trail (8.1 miles). ▶7 At this junction, you head right (south) toward El Capitan, but if you are hiking this trail after Ribbon Creek has dried up and are short on water, you may want to continue on the main trail (left branch) 0.5 mile northeast to two trickling springs.

Along the short spur trail south to El Capitan's broad, rounded summit (8.4 miles), ▶8 you can gaze upcanyon and identify unmistakable Half Dome, at the valley's end; barely protruding Sentinel Dome, above the valley's south wall; and fin-shaped Mount Clark, on the skyline above the dome. Take your time exploring El Capitan's large, domed summit area, but don't stray too far from it. The first 0.1 mile below it is safe, but then the summit's slopes gradually get steeper and you could slip on loose, weathered crystals, giving yourself a one-way trip to the bottom. If you have carried enough water with you, there are some fine sandy flats on the summit that would make stunning campsites. When you are done imbibing the view, retrace your steps to the Tamarack Flat Campground (16.8 miles). ▶9

🚶	**MILESTONES**	
▶1	0.0	Start at Tamarack Creek Trailhead (in Tamarack Flat Campground)
▶2	2.15	Left at junction to Big Oak Flat Road
▶3	2.3	Cascade Creek bridge
▶4	2.8	Left to leave old road
▶5	6.0	Ribbon Meadow
▶6	7.05	Cross Ribbon Creek
▶7	8.1	Right at El Capitan spur trail
▶8	8.4	El Capitan's summit
▶9	16.8	Return to Tamarack Creek Trailhead

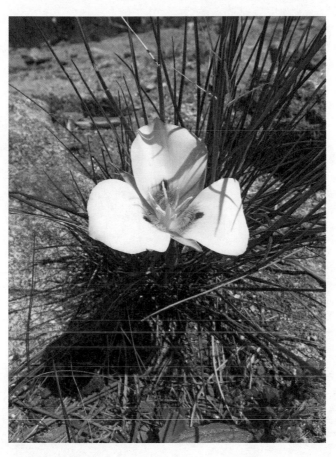

Mariposa lily *on the summit of El Capitan*

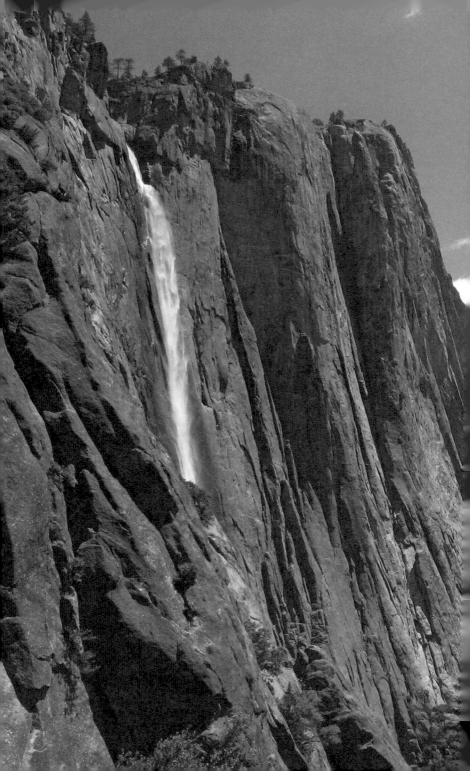

CHAPTER 5

Yosemite Valley

Rightly called The Incomparable Valley, Yosemite Valley is a magnet that attracts visitors from all over the world. As John Muir noted long ago, the Sierra Nevada has several "Yosemites," including Hetch Hetchy to the north, though none of them matches Yosemite Valley in grandeur. Though some of these Yosemites rival or exceed Yosemite Valley in the depth of their canyons and the steepness of their walls, none has the prize-winning combination of its wide, spacious floor; its world-famous waterfalls; and its unforgettable monoliths—El Capitan and Half Dome.

This hiking section is composed of two groups. Trails 28, 29, and 31 are relatively flat, taking you to three tourist destinations: respectively, Bridalveil Fall, Lower Yosemite Fall, and Mirror Lake. The other trails involve climbing, of which Trail 32, to the Vernal Fall Bridge, is the shortest and most popular but, nevertheless, steep. The four others involve strenuous, protracted climbing, and only those in good shape will enjoy them. The first three, to the brink of Upper Yosemite Fall, the top of Nevada Fall, and the summit of Half Dome, can have hundreds of hikers on many summer days. Only along the last, to Merced Lake, do the numbers dwindle to dozens. The plentiful numbers of hikers on all of this chapter's trails attest to the grand views encountered on each. While most hikers ascending the 100-plus switchbacks up the Yosemite Falls Trail go only as far as the upper fall's brink, a few are rewarded with a push to the small summit of Eagle Peak, the highest of the Three Brothers. An even smaller number backpack up to just below Eagle Peak's summit to view the sunset and sunrise over Yosemite Valley.

Opposite: *Upper Yosemite Fall (see Trail 30, page 280)*

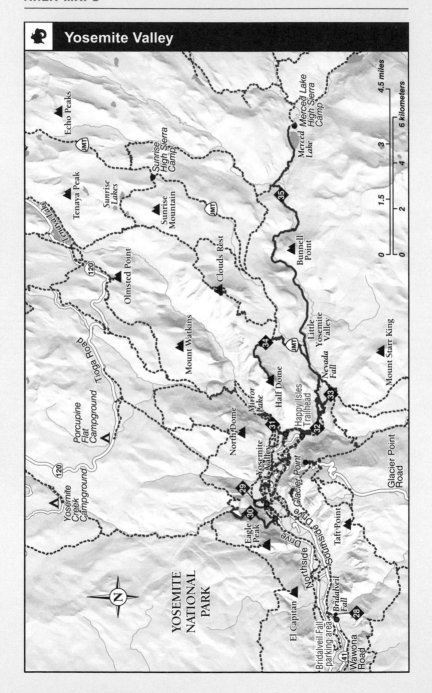

Yosemite Valley

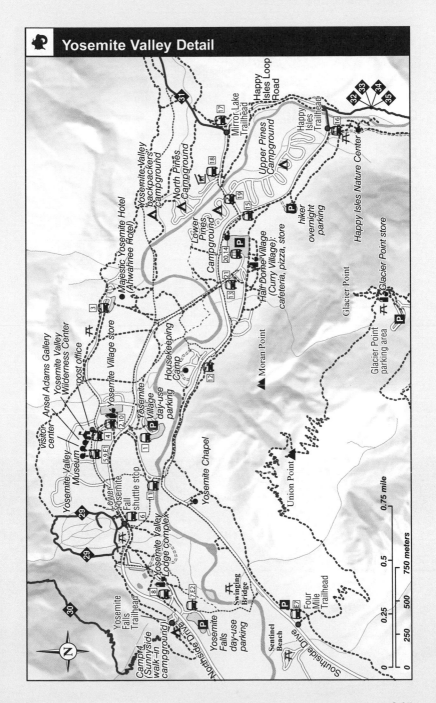

Yosemite Valley Detail

TRAIL FEATURES TABLE

Yosemite Valley

Trail	Difficulty	Length	Type	USES & ACCESS	TERRAIN	NATURE	OTHER
28	1	0.4	Out-and-Back	Day Hiking, Wheelchair Access, Stroller Access, Child-Friendly	Stream, Waterfall		Great Views
29	1	1.2	Loop	Day Hiking, Wheelchair Access, Stroller Access, Child-Friendly	Canyon, Stream, Waterfall		Great Views
30	3	6.3	Point-to-Point	Day Hiking, Backpacking	Canyon, Summit, Stream, Waterfall	Wildflowers	Great Views, Camping, Steep, Geological Interest
31	1	1.9	Balloon	Day Hiking, Running, Wheelchair Access, Stroller Access, Child-Friendly	Canyon, Lake, Stream		Great Views, Geological Interest
32	2	2.0	Point-to-Point	Day Hiking, Stroller Access, Child-Friendly	Canyon, Stream, Waterfall		Great Views, Steep
33	3	6.4	Loop	Day Hiking	Canyon, Stream, Waterfall	Wildflowers	Great Views, Steep, Geological Interest
34	4	14.7	Point-to-Point	Day Hiking, Backpacking	Canyon, Summit, Stream, Waterfall	Wildflowers	Great Views, Camping, Steep, Granite Slabs, Geological Interest
35	5	26.6	Point-to-Point	Backpacking, Horses	Canyon, Lake, Stream, Waterfall	Wildflowers	Great Views, Camping, Swimming, Steep, Granite Slabs, Geological Interest

Legend

TYPE
- Point-to-Point
- Loop
- Out-and-Back
- Balloon

DIFFICULTY
- 1 2 3 4 5 +
- less ——— more

USES & ACCESS
- Day Hiking
- Backpacking
- Horses
- Running
- Wheelchair Access
- Stroller Access
- Child-Friendly
- Caution

TERRAIN
- Canyon
- Summit
- Lake
- Stream
- Waterfall

NATURE
- Autumn Colors
- Wildflowers
- Giant Sequoias

FEATURES
- Great Views
- Camping
- Swimming
- Secluded
- Steep
- Granite Slabs
- Historical Interest
- Geological Interest

Cascades *beneath Bunnell Point (see Trail 35, page 315)*

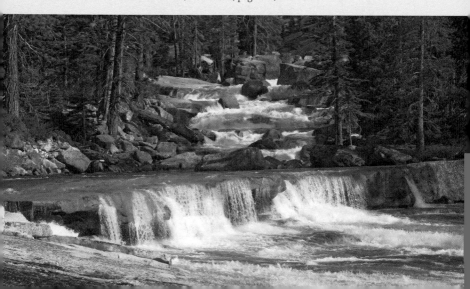

Yosemite Valley

Bridalveil Fall 270

TRAIL 28

Day Hike, Wheelchair
Access, Stroller Access,
Child-Friendly
0.4 mile, Out-and-Back
Difficulty: **1** 2 3 4 5

The hike to a view of Bridalveil Fall is one of four extremely popular, wheelchair-accessible trails in the park, the other three being to the base of Lower Yosemite Fall, out to Glacier Point, and to the lower reaches of the Mariposa Grove. In May and June, when Bridalveil Fall is at its greatest flow, not only do you have a dramatic view of the falls, but you may also be moistened (or even soaked) by its spray. Unlike Yosemite Fall, Bridalveil Fall never completely dries out, making it a good destination for late summer visitors.

Lower Yosemite Fall 274

TRAIL 29

Day Hike, Wheelchair
Access, Stroller Access,
Child-Friendly
1.2 miles, Balloon
Difficulty: **1** 2 3 4 5

From Memorial Day to the Labor Day weekend thousands of visitors daily make a short pilgrimage north to the base of Lower Yosemite Fall, many (if not most) arriving by tour buses and from out of state. And why not? Yosemite National Park is one of the most famous UNESCO World Heritage Sites; Yosemite Valley is its star attraction, and Lower Yosemite Fall is its most accessible fall. On your hike the vast majority of hikers only go to the bridge view of Lower Yosemite Fall and return the way they came, whereas I describe a slightly longer route, a 1.2-mile loop.

Vernal Fall–Nevada Fall Loop 297

Mile for mile, the very popular balloon hike up to the brink of Nevada Fall and back may be the most scenic one in the park. The first part of this loop goes up the famous (or infamous) Mist Trail—a steep, strenuous trail that sprays you with Vernal Fall's mist, cooling you on hot afternoons. Above you enjoy plummeting Nevada Fall and beautiful views of the domes in the lower Merced River canyon.

TRAIL 33

Day Hike
6.4 miles, Balloon
Difficulty: 1 2 **3** 4 5

Half Dome 305

If I as a first-time visitor were allowed to do only one day hike in the park, I would unquestionably choose this hike—the one that I most associate with Yosemite and on whose summit I've sat countless times admiring the surrounding landscape. On a good summer day, 300 hikers attempt this summit—the number set by the number of permits issued by the park—but many turn back, either from exhaustion or from fear. If the summit of Half Dome is also your dream, you will need to plan months ahead to have a good chance at scoring a permit.

TRAIL 34

Day Hike, Backpack
14.7 miles,
Out-and-Back
Difficulty: 1 2 3 **4** 5

Merced Lake 315

Best done in three days with overnight stops at Little Yosemite Valley (on the way up) and Merced Lake, this hike is often done in two by energetic weekend hikers. Its route, up a fantastic river canyon, is one of the Sierra's best. Located at an elevation of about 7,200 feet, relatively large Merced Lake is about 2,000-plus feet lower than the popular ones reached from Tuolumne Meadows' trailheads, and therefore it—and the route to reach it—is snowfree sooner and still pleasantly warm during the autumn months.

TRAIL 35

Backpack, Horse
26.6 miles,
Out-and-Back
Difficulty: 1 2 3 4 **5**

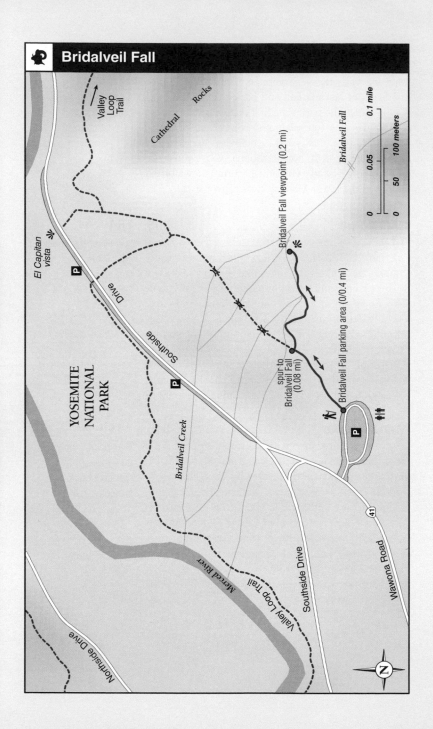

Bridalveil Fall

Valley Loop Trail

Cathedral Rocks

Bridalveil Fall viewpoint (0.2 mi)

Bridalveil Fall

El Capitan vista

P

Southside Drive

YOSEMITE NATIONAL PARK

Bridalveil Creek

P

Merced River

spur to Bridalveil Fall (0.08 mi)

Bridalveil Fall parking area (0/0.4 mi)

Valley Loop Trail

Southside Drive

Northside Drive

P

41

Wawona Road

0   0.05   0.1 mile
0   50   100 meters

N

270   **Top Trails Yosemite**

Bridalveil Fall

The hike to a view of Bridalveil Fall is one of four extremely popular, wheelchair-accessible trails in the park, the other three being to the base of Lower Yosemite Fall (Trail 29), out to Glacier Point (Trail 39), and to the lower reaches of the Mariposa Grove (part of Trail 43). In May and June, when Bridalveil Fall is at its greatest flow, not only do you have a dramatic view of the fall, but you may also be moistened (or even soaked) by its spray. Unlike Yosemite Fall, Bridalveil Fall never completely dries out, making it a good destination for late summer visitors.

Maps

This trail is covered by the Tom Harrison *Yosemite Valley* map (1:24,000 scale), the National Geographic Trails Illustrated *#306 Yosemite SW* map (1:40,000 scale), and the USGS *Yosemite Valley* map (1:24,000 scale).

Best Time

Snowmelt feeding Bridalveil Creek and other Yosemite Valley falls is greatest in May and June, which are the best months to visit all of these falls. If you don't mind visiting a diminished Bridalveil Fall, then you can take the trail April–November. December–March the trail can be snowbound and/or icy, making it slippery, but it is possible to visit it year-round.

Finding the Trail

The trail starts at Bridalveil Fall parking lot, less than 0.1 mile before the descending Wawona Road (CA 41) reaches a junction on the floor of Yosemite Valley. If you are driving east on the main

TRAIL USE
Day Hike, Wheelchair Access, Stroller Access, Child-Friendly
LENGTH
0.4 mile, 10–30 minutes
VERTICAL FEET
One-way: +50', –0'
Round-trip: ±50'
DIFFICULTY
– **1** 2 3 4 5 +
TRAIL TYPE
Out-and-Back

FEATURES
Stream
Waterfall
Great Views

FACILITIES
Bear Boxes
Campgrounds
Lodging
Restrooms
Store
Visitor Center
Water

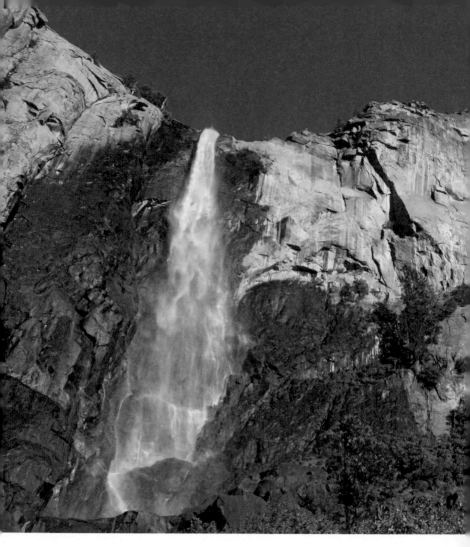

Bridalveil Fall

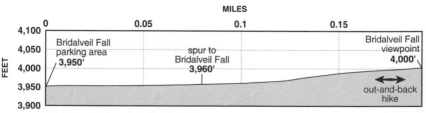

TRAIL 28 Bridalveil Fall Elevation Profile

MILES

FEET

Bridalveil Fall
parking area
3,950'

spur to
Bridalveil Fall
3,960'

Bridalveil Fall
viewpoint
4,000'

out-and-back
hike

Yosemite Valley loop (Southside Drive), turn right onto the road signed for Wawona (CA 41) and almost immediately turn into the Bridalveil Fall parking lot. There are toilets at the trailhead, but to fill water bottles you will need to visit one of the more easterly Yosemite Valley destinations, such as Yosemite Village or Yosemite Valley Lodge.

The valley's Miwok Indians named the fall Pohono, "fall of the puffing winds," for at low volume its water is pushed around by gusts of wind.

Trail Description

Starting from the northeast end of the Bridalveil Fall parking lot, ►1 you hike just 2 or 3 minutes on a paved trail to a junction with a spur trail (0.08 mile). ►2 Veer right onto it and parallel a Bridalveil Creek tributary as you climb an equally short trail to its end at the Bridalveil Fall viewpoint (0.2 mile). ►3 During May and June, when Bridalveil Fall is at its best, your viewpoint will be drenched in spray, making the last part of the trail very slippery and making photography from this vantage point nearly impossible. If you are dressed for the spray, it is exhilarating, not annoying, and of course, kids love the spray. Bridalveil Fall dances with the wind, especially once its flow has started to taper. Of Yosemite's other falls, only Vernal Fall leaps free over a dead-vertical cliff, but its flow—the Merced River—is too strong to be greatly affected by the wind. The other major falls drop over cliffs that are less than vertical, and hence the falls partly glide down them. Eventually pulling yourself free from the mesmerizing falls, retrace your steps to the car (0.4 mile). ►4

☆ MILESTONES

►1	0.0	Start at Bridalveil Fall parking lot
►2	0.08	Right onto Bridalveil Fall spur trail
►3	0.2	Bridalveil Fall viewpoint
►4	0.4	Return to Bridalveil Fall parking lot

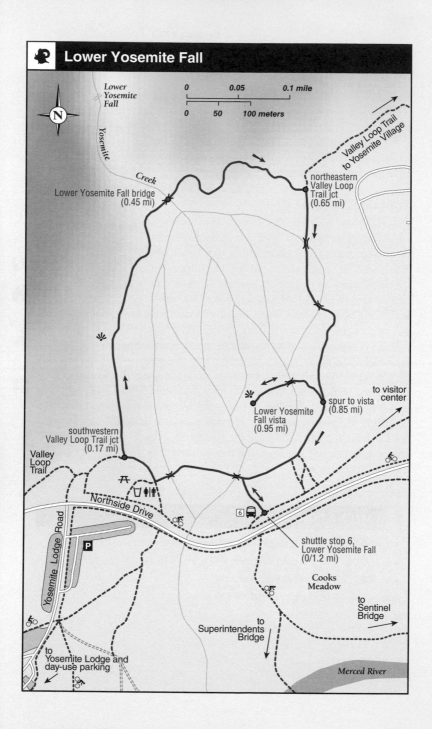

Lower Yosemite Fall

Lower
Yosemite
Fall

0   0.05   0.1 mile

0   50   100 meters

N

Yosemite

Creek

Valley Loop Trail
to Yosemite Village

Lower Yosemite Fall bridge
(0.45 mi)

northeastern
Valley Loop
Trail jct
(0.65 mi)

to visitor
center

Lower Yosemite
Fall vista
(0.95 mi)

spur to vista
(0.85 mi)

southwestern
Valley Loop Trail jct
(0.17 mi)

Valley
Loop
Trail

Northside Drive

Yosemite Lodge Road

P

6

shuttle stop 6,
Lower Yosemite Fall
(0/1.2 mi)

Cooks
Meadow

to
Sentinel
Bridge

to
Superintendents
Bridge

to
Yosemite Lodge and
day-use parking

Merced River

Lower Yosemite Fall

From Memorial Day to the Labor Day weekend, more than a thousand visitors daily make a short pilgrimage north to the base of Lower Yosemite Fall, many (if not most) arriving by tour buses and from out of state. And why not? Yosemite National Park is one of the most famous UNESCO World Heritage Sites; Yosemite Valley is its star attraction, and Lower Yosemite Fall is its most accessible fall. On your hike the vast majority of hikers only go to the bridge view of Lower Yosemite Fall and return the way they came, whereas I describe a slightly longer route, a 1.2-mile loop. The route is elegantly designed, with information placards and statues further enriching your walk.

Maps

This trail is covered by the Tom Harrison *Yosemite Valley* map (1:24,000 scale), the National Geographic Trails Illustrated *#306 Yosemite SW* map (1:40,000 scale), and the USGS *Yosemite Valley* map (1:24,000 scale).

Best Time

Snowmelt feeding Yosemite Creek and other Yosemite Valley falls is greatest in May and June, which are undeniably the best months to visit all of these falls. By mid-August there may be very little water plunging over Lower Yosemite Fall's brink, and in September and into October, the fall can be completely dry. Once the rains return, followed by snow, the fall is resurrected, and though not nearly at full volume, it can be inspirational November–April.

TRAIL USE
Day Hike, Wheelchair Access, Stroller Access, Child-Friendly
LENGTH
1.2 miles, 30 minutes–1 hour
VERTICAL FEET
Round-trip: ±160'
DIFFICULTY
– **1** 2 3 4 5 +
TRAIL TYPE
Balloon

FEATURES
Canyon
Stream
Waterfall
Great Views

FACILITIES
Campgrounds
Lodging
Picnic Tables
Restrooms
Shuttle Stop
Store
Visitor Center
Water

In the 1890s it was suggested to build a dam above the brink of Yosemite Falls so that visitors could enjoy the falls throughout the summer.

Midwinter the rock walls are often ice-glazed behind the thin shield of water.

For any popular Yosemite Valley hike, but especially this one, also consider the best time of day to visit. In the early morning you can surprisingly enjoy the alcove holding Lower Yosemite Fall nearly to yourself, as the tour buses do not arrive until late morning. However, the best lighting on the falls is at midday when the sun shines past the steep walls guarding the fall and illuminates it.

Finding the Trail

If you are staying at a campground or lodge in Yosemite Valley, leave your car there, head to the shuttle, and take the free Yosemite Valley shuttle bus to stop 6. If you are a day-use visitor, park your car in Yosemite Falls day-use lot, located just west of the Yosemite Valley Lodge complex, and walk east along use trails on either side of Northside Drive to a junction with the Valley Loop Trail at the southwestern corner of this hike, beginning (and ending) your loop here. This adds 0.5 mile to the walk each direction but is faster than taking the shuttle. There is also a large day-use lot near Yosemite Village, from which you could take the Yosemite Valley shuttle bus to stop 6. Alternatively, if you are driving, you might find parking on both sides of Northside Drive just east of stop 6, but don't count on it. There are water faucets just beyond the toilets a short distance into this hike.

Trail Description

As described here, the Lower Yosemite Fall loop trail begins along Northside Drive from shuttle stop 6, which is just east of the Lower Yosemite

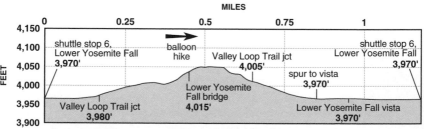

TRAIL 29 Lower Yosemite Fall Elevation Profile

Fall complex. ▶1 But because the loop begins by paralleling Northside Drive west, you can begin (and end) wherever along Northside Drive is most convenient to your parking spot. From the shuttle stop you can take the slightly shorter paved path directly adjacent to Northside Drive or—my recommendation—take a path 200 feet north to a junction and then turn right to follow a quieter route. You'll be finishing your loop on this same path, coming from the northeast. You head left (west), bridging two branches of Yosemite Creek on your way to a building with restrooms and, immediately west of it, a drinking fountain and tables. In front of the building is a display that introduces you to this area. More displays lie ahead along your loop.

You are at the southwest edge of the Lower Yosemite Fall complex, and where you reach a T-junction, turn right onto an arrow-straight path north (0.17 mile). ▶2 Ahead, your broad path aims directly toward Lower Yosemite Fall and Upper Yosemite Fall behind it, this view courtesy of many trees felled long ago to present visitors with this Kodak moment. It seems that virtually all visitors try to take a photo of the falls and their family/friends, trying not to include all the others attempting the same task. Selfie sticks have not made this quest any easier.

The path north to the lower fall is obvious, and your photogenic path soon reaches an alcove marked with engaging displays. On the continued path north, you quickly encounter rocks on your left, many the size of cabins and several the size of houses. These broke loose from the cliffs above, and indeed rockfalls occur in Yosemite Valley nearly annually. The walks beyond Mirror Lake and to the Happy Isles Nature Center both provide glimpses of recent impressive rockslides. Soon the paved path begins to climb and curve gently, then moderately (the only part tough in a wheelchair), and after several minutes you arrive at a wide bridge across Yosemite Creek (0.45 mile), ▶3 which offers an impressive view of Lower Yosemite Fall. In late spring and early summer, visitors are treated to the thunderous roar of the fall, a sound that reverberates in the alcove cut in this rock. During this time visitors are further treated to the fall's spray. But by mid-July Yosemite Falls are somewhat diminished, and by August the lower fall is usually reduced to a mist, and even this can be gone by the Labor Day weekend. Dry or not, the rounded rocks in boulder-choked Yosemite Creek are water polished to an icelike finish, making them extremely slippery. Only explore the boulder field at the base of the fall if water levels are very low. In winter, the minuscule ledges on the rock face usually hold patches of ice, providing yet another

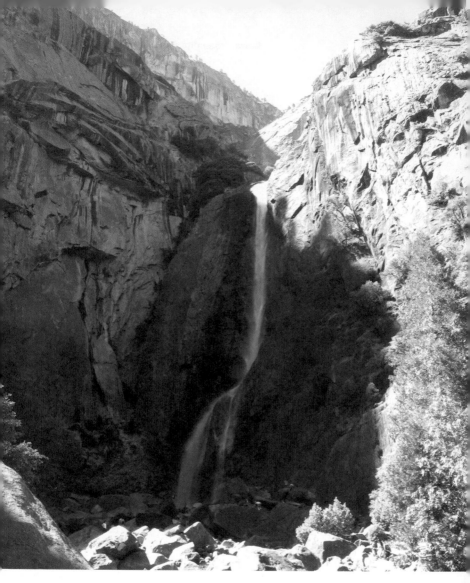

Lower Yosemite Fall

seasonal variant. My favorite might just be the moonbow—on full moon nights in February and March, the evening moon shines onto the falls, creating a surreal, faint, silvery rainbow.

From the bridge, most folks return the way they came, and those with wheelchairs or strollers must retreat here. But keeping to the clockwise loop, you take the paved path briefly northeast toward a cliff, then wind along boardwalks between boulders and trees as you traverse around talus piles and boulders. In this vicinity you may hear or see climbers on one of about a dozen difficult routes up the cliff just north of you. While some routes are short, others ascend to a long, linear ledge known as Sunnyside Bench, about 400 feet above you. After a couple of minutes walking eastward, you reach a junction (0.65 mile). ►4 The Valley Loop Trail continues straight ahead, while you turn right, taking a gently winding, forested path south and slightly down between two branches of Yosemite Creek. In early summer, keep your eyes peeled for delicious black raspberries along this stretch—you are permitted to sample a few of them.

Soon you reach a small junction (0.85 mile). ►5 Turning right takes you down a short spur trail to another view of the fall from a dead end above a branch of Yosemite Creek, where you'll find a James Hutchings bench and a John Muir plaque (0.95 mile). ►6 Most important, there is another convenient gap in the trees here, allowing you to photograph the fall. An added advantage of this brief detour is that it attracts fewer people, and you can quite likely take a picture of your family without other people in the foreground.

Retracing your steps to the main trail, turn right (south) and continue past an informative exhibit, complete with benches and a fine view of Upper Yosemite Fall, back to Northside Drive. You arrive at a spot about 300 feet east of the start of your loop. Once again avoiding the paved variant, branch right at the north edge of the area and take a path that parallels a creek branch west, an especially scenic alternative when Yosemite Creek is flowing briskly. Soon you reach a junction that you will recognize from the start of your walk and turn left, retracing your steps south to the shuttle stop (1.2 miles). ►7

---

† MILESTONES

►1	0.0	Start at shuttle stop 6, Lower Yosemite Fall
►2	0.17	Right at southwestern junction with Valley Loop Trail
►3	0.45	Lower Yosemite Fall bridge
►4	0.65	Right at northeastern junction with Valley Loop Trail
►5	0.85	Right at junction with spur trail to vista
►6	0.95	Lower Yosemite Fall vista
►7	1.2	Return to shuttle stop 6, Lower Yosemite Fall

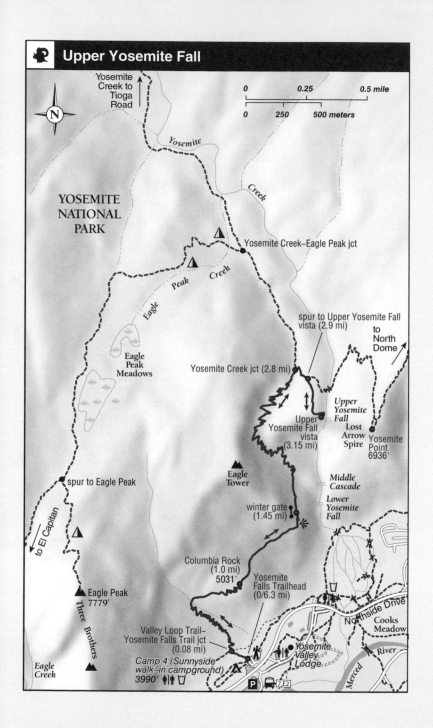

Upper Yosemite Fall

Yosemite Creek to Tioga Road

N

0   0.25   0.5 mile

0   250   500 meters

Yosemite

YOSEMITE
NATIONAL
PARK

Creek

⚠ Yosemite Creek–Eagle Peak jct

⚠ *Eagle* *Peak* *Creek*

Eagle

spur to Upper Yosemite Fall
vista (2.9 mi)

to
North
Dome

Eagle
Peak
Meadows

Yosemite Creek jct (2.8 mi)

*Upper
Yosemite
Fall*

Upper
Yosemite Fall
vista
(3.15 mi)

Lost
Arrow
Spire

Yosemite
Point
6936'

▲ Eagle
Tower

*Middle
Cascade*

spur to Eagle Peak

*Lower
Yosemite
Fall*

winter gate
(1.45 mi)

⚠

to El Capitan

Columbia Rock
(1.0 mi)
5031'

Yosemite
Falls Trailhead
(0/6.3 mi)

Northside Drive

▲ Eagle Peak
7779'

Cooks
Meadow

Three Brothers

Merced

River

Valley Loop Trail–
Yosemite Falls Trail jct
(0.08 mi)

Yosemite
Valley
Lodge

*Eagle
Creek*

⛺ *Camp 4 (Sunnyside
walk–in campground)
3990'*

P 🚌 7, E2

Upper Yosemite Fall

Far above the crowds concentrated at the base of Lower Yosemite Fall (Trail 29), this popular trail gets you to the brink of Upper Yosemite Fall. The hike to this falcon's aerie leads you up switchbacks beside the plunging falls, providing an ongoing view of your destination. For some, the hike is quite strenuous, and many ascend only to Columbia Rock, which is a worthy goal in itself.

An optional extension of Trail 30, to strategically located Eagle Peak, highest of the Three Brothers, provides commanding views both up and down Yosemite Valley. Doing it will increase your round-trip distance from 6.3 to 12.0 miles and your total elevation gain by about 1,500 feet, to 4,900 feet—and of course, you will have to descend the same amount. A somewhat shorter but also rewarding alternative is the 1.9-mile round-trip journey to Yosemite Point. Both trails are shown on the map for the hike.

Permits

Overnight visitors require a wilderness permit for the Yosemite Falls Trailhead, issued by Yosemite National Park. Pick up your wilderness permit at the Yosemite Valley Wilderness Center.

Maps

This trail is covered by the Tom Harrison *Yosemite Valley* map (1:24,000 scale), the National Geographic Trails Illustrated *#306 Yosemite SW* map (1:40,000 scale), and the USGS *Yosemite Valley* map (1:24,000 scale).

TRAIL USE
Day Hike, Backpack
LENGTH
6.3 miles, 3–7 hours
(over 1–2 days)
VERTICAL FEET
One-way: +2,910', −380'
Round-trip: ±3,290'
DIFFICULTY
− 1 2 **3** 4 5 +
TRAIL TYPE
Out-and-Back

FEATURES
Canyon
Summit
Stream
Waterfall
Wildflowers
Great Views
Camping
Steep
Geological Interest

FACILITIES
Bear Boxes
Campgrounds
Lodging
Restrooms
Shuttle Stop
Store
Visitor Center
Water

281

Best Time

Snowmelt feeding Yosemite Creek and other Yosemite Valley falls is greatest in May and June, which are the best months to visit all of Yosemite's falls. If you are backpacking to sites above the falls, then the first half of July may be better because Upper Yosemite Fall is still impressive, but the upland's mosquito population is greatly diminished and Yosemite Creek has some lovely swimming pools *far* upstream of the falls. In August not much water plunges over the brink of Upper Yosemite Fall, and in September—or sometimes earlier—and into October, the fall can be completely dry. Between approximately December and late March, the trail is usually gated at about the midpoint, right before the trail traverses a ledge that can be filled with an icy, sloping snowfield. During these months there is some chance that you will be unable to complete this hike, but the hike to Columbia Rock is possible anytime deep snow on the valley floor doesn't impede your progress.

> The last glacier advanced to the fall's brink and was about 600 feet thick where it calved icefalls over the cliff onto the valley's glacier, more than 1,000 feet below.

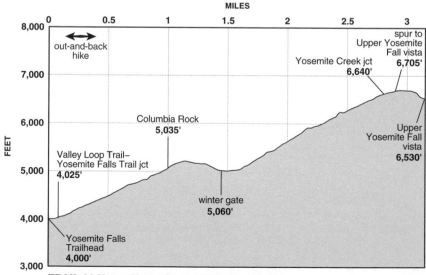

TRAIL 30 Upper Yosemite Fall Elevation Profile

Finding the Trail

The trailhead is located at the back of the Camp 4 (Sunnyside walk-in campground) parking lot. This lies on the north side of the Yosemite Valley loop road (Northside Drive), just west of Yosemite Lodge. Day hikers can park in the Yosemite Falls day-use lot located almost exactly across Northside Drive from Camp 4, at the west end of the Yosemite Valley Lodge complex. Day hikers staying in Yosemite Valley overnight are encouraged to leave their vehicles at their campsite or lodging and use the free shuttle buses to reach the trailhead, located near stop 7. Overnight hikers must park in the backpackers' parking lot, located along the road to Happy Isles; you continue briefly past the NO ACCESS signs and then turn to your right at the trailhead parking signs. From here, you must retrace your steps to Half Dome Village (Curry Village) to catch the shuttle bus. Take the bus to stop 7, Camp 4. (Note that mileages are measured from the trailhead; starting at the shuttle stop adds 0.35 mile *each direction* to your walk.) There are toilets and water faucets in the adjacent campground.

Trail Description

From the back of the Camp 4 parking area, ▶1 you begin on a north-heading trail. Passing an old unmarked trail junction on your right, you soon reach a junction where you turn right up the Yosemite Falls Trail, while the Valley Loop Trail continues to the left (west) (0.08 mile). ▶2 Starting up nearly four dozen short switchbacks, you quickly leave the tall conifers of the valley floor behind and are instead under the shade of canyon live oaks and often pestered by endless gnats that shelter among these trees. The canyon live oaks are the dominant trees on the south-facing walls throughout Yosemite Valley, growing among large boulders and blocking all prospects of a view. The rocks attest to giant rockfalls that shatter Yosemite Valley's peace on a regular basis. Lacking distracting views, you just march upward until you reach a usually dry wash, beyond which you obtain framed views of Leidig Meadow and the valley's central features.

With more than one-fourth of the elevation gain below you, you pass more oaks and an occasional bay tree as you now switchback east to a panoramic viewpoint, Columbia Rock (1.0 miles), ▶3 which at 5,031 feet is just over 1,000 feet above the valley floor. At its safety railing you can study the valley's geometry from the Quarter Domes east of Half Dome west to the Cathedral Spires. Several steep, gravelly switchbacks climb from the viewpoint, and then the trail traverses northeast, drops slightly,

OPTION: Eagle Peak

▲ Should you wish to climb to the very rewarding summit of Eagle Peak, first return to the junction in the gully west of the fall, the Yosemite Creek junction, ►5 from which most people descend 2.8 miles back down to the valley floor. Bound for Eagle Peak, 2.85 miles distant and about 1,160 feet above your junction, you now commence a shady trek 0.6 mile north paralleling Yosemite Creek, climbing out of the gully, descending into a second one, and climbing out of a third to a junction, where you turn left, away from Yosemite Creek.

▲ You soon cross seasonal Eagle Peak Creek, pass a few nice campsites if there is water in the creek, and then climb more than 300 feet, at first steeply, before leveling off in a bouldery area—part of a moraine that was left by a glacier that descended from the west slopes of Mount Hoffmann. Now you turn south, generally leaving Jeffrey pines and white firs for lodgepole pines and red firs as you climb to Eagle Peak Meadows, whose north edge is blocked by another moraine.

Beyond the sometimes boggy meadow, you cross the headwaters of Eagle Peak Creek and in a few minutes reach a hillside junction, signposted for Eagle Peak and located 1.65 miles from the junction where you diverged away from Yosemite Creek. From it, the trail, continuing along the north rim of Yosemite Valley, climbs and drops along a 1.75-mile course to the El Capitan spur trail, an alternative way to this peak's summit (those with access to a car shuttle can hike one-way from here to Tamarack Flat Campground; see Trail 27). From the junction you branch left for a moderate 0.6-mile ascent to the steep-sided summit of Eagle Peak. Note that as you cross a small saddle en route to the summit, you can locate a few small campsites; you'll

▲ have to carry your water from either Eagle Peak Creek or Yosemite Creek, but these sites make a fine perch for those wishing to enjoy a sunset and a sunrise from the summit of Eagle Peak. Indeed, this peak

🅷 boasts far-ranging, near-aerial views, which extend all the way to the Sierra Crest along the park's east boundary. Below, central Yosemite Valley spreads out like a map, and if you've brought along a detailed map of this valley, you should be able to identify most of its major landmarks plus dozens of minor features. After your stay atop Eagle Peak, return directly to your trailhead, a distance of 5.7 miles.

OPTION: View All of the Fall

From the cryptic junction just before ►4, a 150-foot-long trail descends to a railing with an incredible view. Here you look almost directly down on Lower Yosemite Fall and can trace Yosemite Creek up past its cascades to Upper Yosemite Fall. There is no other trail spot on the north side of the valley where you can see the entire falls' sequence. Be forewarned, however: The trail is quite exposed, and a careless step could result in a fatal slip over the brink of a cliff. Only descend what you are confident you can climb back up, and do not deviate from the traveled path.

passes an enormous Douglas-fir, and then drops some more before it bends north for a sudden dramatic view of Upper Yosemite Fall. Here, at a minor low spot in the trail, is a cryptic junction, leading to a no-longer-signposted aerial vista sure to awe sure-footed individuals.

Next, the main trail quickly switchbacks to take you down to a gate (1.45 miles), ►4 which is closed in times of potential danger, such as when the next stretch of trail is covered with snow or when rockfall may be imminent. Traversing a broad ledge beyond the gate, you are now staring straight at Upper Yosemite Fall. In winter, a giant cone of snow can form at the base of the fall, as waterdrops freeze in their descent and pile up at the base. Passing colorful wildflower gardens and reentering forest cover, you may note use trails descending toward the river course; if—and only if—water flows over Lower Yosemite Fall are low, you can indeed descend along the base of the cliff to the edge of the pool at the base of the falls and stare straight up at the surge of descending water.

Soon above this forest patch, you start a long, tough, steep switch-backing ascent of a rocky gully to the west of the fall. The fall itself soon disappears from view as you work your way up this convenient passageway recessed between steep walls. This ravine was likely the route Yosemite Creek took until a glacier pushed it to its current course, probably more than 100,000 years ago. Your climb ends among white firs and Jeffery pines, about 135 switchbacks above the valley floor. Here, in a gully beside a seasonal creeklet, you come to a junction where your route turns right, while the trail up Yosemite Creek and to Eagle Peak continues straight ahead (2.8 miles). ►5 Your trail makes a brief climb east out of the gully and reaches a broad crest. If you are on an overnight trip, as enticing as the ridge to the north appears, you must continue another mile away from the trailhead, either along Yosemite Creek or toward Yosemite Point, before you may legally camp, as you must be 4 trail miles from any Yosemite Valley trailhead before camping. (If you continue up the trail paralleling Yosemite Creek beyond the previously described junction, there are plenty of camping options a mile up.)

Soon you will spy a right-trending spur trail on the ridge (2.9 miles) ▶6; turn south, bound for the brink of Upper Yosemite Fall. Keep to the crest as you follow the spur trail south almost to the valley's rim; then at a juniper you veer east (left) and descend more steps to a fenced-in viewpoint. If you're acrophobic, you should not attempt the last part of this descent, even though it has a handrail, because it is possible, though unlikely, that you could slip on loose gravel or smooth bedrock and tumble beneath the railing. Beside the lip of Upper Yosemite Fall, you see and hear it plunge all the way down its 1,430-foot drop to the rocks below (3.15 miles). ▶7

After returning up the crest, you can briefly take a trail east down to a bridge over Yosemite Creek and obtain water. However, be careful! Occasionally people wading in the creek's icy water slip on the glass-smooth creek bottom and are swiftly carried over the fall's brink—this has even occurred at low-water flows. From the creek's bridge you could continue eastward 0.95 mile up a trail to Yosemite Point, a highly scenic goal, or to Eagle Peak (see the Option on page 284). Afterward, retrace your steps to the trailhead (6.3 miles). ▶8

🚶	**MILESTONES**	
▶1	0.0	Start at Yosemite Falls Trailhead (near Camp 4 kiosk)
▶2	0.08	Right at Valley Loop Trail–Yosemite Falls Trail junction
▶3	1.0	Columbia Rock
▶4	1.45	Winter gate
▶5	2.8	Right at Yosemite Creek junction
▶6	2.9	Right at Upper Yosemite Fall vista spur trail
▶7	3.15	Upper Yosemite Fall vista
▶8	6.3	Return to Yosemite Falls Trailhead

Mirror Lake

First cars and later shuttle buses went to Mirror Lake, but now the paved road is used only by cyclists, pedestrians, and a few cars with special permission. Hikers can also use quieter, parallel paths that are only open to foot traffic. Be forewarned that Mirror Lake is just a broad stretch of Tenaya Creek, not a true lake. In times of high water, it is quite impressive and reflective, but in July the flow diminishes and the width of the "lake" greatly decreases—indeed Tenaya Creek usually stops flowing late summer.

Maps

This trail is covered by the Tom Harrison *Yosemite Valley* map (1:24,000 scale), the National Geographic Trails Illustrated *#306 Yosemite SW* map (1:40,000 scale), and the USGS *Yosemite Valley* map (1:24,000 scale).

Best Time

To see the reflections in Mirror Lake, you need to visit during the time of maximum runoff, which is about early May–late June. Visitors arrive in Yosemite year-round, however, and most visit it later, when the "lake" is merely a wide stretch of Tenaya Creek—Bridalveil Fall (Trail 28) or Vernal Fall (Trail 32) are better choices late in the summer. As water levels drop, pools along Tenaya Creek, just before the end of the trail, become well-used family swimming holes.

Finding the Trail

The trailhead is located at Yosemite Valley shuttle stop 17, along Happy Isles Loop Road a little to the

TRAIL USE
Day Hike, Bike, Run,
Wheelchair Access,
Stroller Access,
Child-Friendly

LENGTH
1.9 miles, 45 minutes–
2 hours

VERTICAL FEET
One-way: +115', –5'
Round-trip: ±120'

DIFFICULTY
– 1 2 3 4 5 +

TRAIL TYPE
Balloon

FEATURES
Canyon
Lake
Stream
Great Views
Geological Interest

FACILITIES
Bear Boxes
Campgrounds
Horse Staging
Lodging
Restrooms
Shuttle Stop
Store
Visitor Center

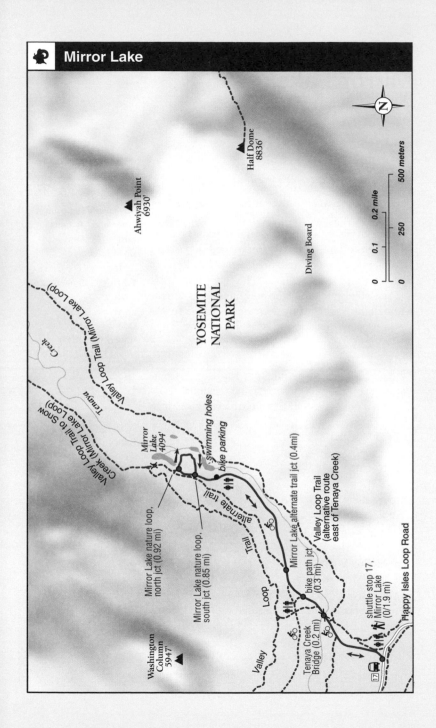

N

Half Dome
8836'

Ahwiyah Point
6930'

Diving Board

500 meters

0.2 mile

0.1

0 250

0

YOSEMITE
NATIONAL
PARK

(Mirror Lake Loop)

Valley Loop Trail

Creek

Tenaya

Valley Loop Trail to Snow
Creek (Mirror Lake Loop)

Mirror
Lake
4094'

swimming holes

bike parking

Mirror Lake nature loop,
north jct (0.92 mi)

Mirror Lake nature loop,
south jct (0.85 mi)

alternate trail

Mirror Lake alternate trail jct (0.4mi)

Valley Loop Trail
(alternative route
east of Tenaya Creek)

Trail

Loop

Valley

bike path jct
(0.3 mi)

Tenaya Creek
Bridge (0.2 mi)

shuttle stop 17,
Mirror Lake
(0/1.9 mi)

Washington
Column
5947'

Happy Isles Loop Road

east of the stables and North Pines Campground. Because this road is closed to vehicular traffic, except the shuttle buses, take the shuttle bus to stop 17. Note that for those staying in one of the three nearby campgrounds, North, Upper, and Lower Pines, it is more efficient to walk east along Happy Isles Loop Road to this trailhead than to take the shuttle. Shuttle users can park their cars in either the Half Dome Village (Curry Village) parking area or the large day-use parking areas near Yosemite Village or the Yosemite Valley Lodge. There are water faucets in the nearby campgrounds or at Half Dome Village but not at the trailhead or along the walk.

Trail Description

The shortest route to Mirror Lake is along the paved bike path from shuttle stop 17 north to the lake. At shuttle stop 17, the low ridge you see just south of Happy Isles Loop Road is the valley's Medial Moraine. Not formed by the converging Tenaya Canyon and Merced Canyon glaciers, as implied by its name, this is actually a recessional moraine left by the retreating Merced Canyon glacier.

The bike path starts north from stop 17, ▶1 from which you'll see an adjacent outhouse plus a path immediately branching right. This spur momentarily reaches a trail that parallels the road and connects the Happy Isles environs to the Mirror Lake environs. It is slightly longer but quieter, more for the nature lovers, and it skirts an area of giant rockfall boulders that testify to the instability of Half Dome. This trail stays on the east side of Tenaya Creek, while the road soon crosses to its west, and at the highest water flows, it can be difficult to cross Tenaya Creek at Mirror Lake, so once you start up this trail, you may have to be content to stay on this side of the creek for your entire walk.

On the virtually level bike path, you walk, bike, or jog, first north then northeast, to Tenaya Creek Bridge (0.2 mile). ▶2 Standing on the Tenaya

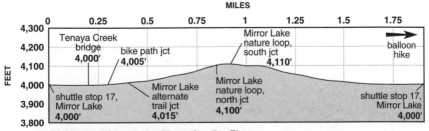

TRAIL 31 Mirror Lake Elevation Profile

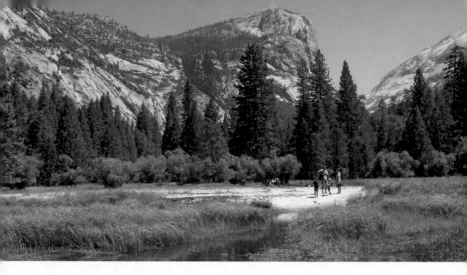

Mirror Lake *and Mount Watkins*

Creek Bridge, you can get a good idea of the status of Mirror Lake. If Tenaya Creek is a raging torrent descending toward you, Mirror Lake will be worth the visit, but if there is only slow water or no water at all, you will have to enjoy the view of Half Dome and Mount Watkins without their reflections.

Immediately before the bridge, a trail heads east to reconnect with the previously described parallel path to the east. Just a couple of minutes past the bridge, you reach a bike path junction on the left toward the Majestic Yosemite Hotel (formerly the Ahwahnee) and on to Yosemite Village (0.3 mile). ▶3

Those bound for Mirror Lake curve right, pass another toilet, and make an easy traverse east over toward Tenaya Creek. Within minutes you will note a little-used junction on your left (0.4 mile). ▶4 This trail is another alternative to the paved route you are following, if you'd like to walk among the trees and boulders; you will reconnect with the paved road close to Mirror Lake. The last part of the path up to the seasonal lake is a moderate ascent alongside the creek, and those on rental bikes have to park them at the start of this ascent. After about 0.25 mile you reach a shallow pond—it was once deeper and until the mid-1990s was a popular summertime swimming hole, but it is paralleling the evolution of adjacent Mirror Lake, reverting to just a broad stretch of Tenaya Creek. Nonetheless, on an early summer visit, it is still crowded with children splashing and playing in the sand.

Passing yet another toilet, the paved road becomes a trail and you soon reach a right-bearing junction, the end of a nature loop taking you to the southwest edge of Mirror Lake (0.85 mile). ▶5 Continue straight ahead for now—you will return along this route. Indeed, in just minutes you reach a second junction (0.92 mile), ►6 and this time bend right toward the lake-shore. Information placards tell you about the human and natural history of Mirror Lake, and of course, you are treated to beautiful views of the face of Half Dome. Here photographers gather to take seasonally reflective photos. Take a minute to look for the light-colored scar to the left of Half Dome, where a large rockslide occurred on Ahwiyah Point in March 2009. The nature loop takes you back to the trail on which you ascended, and you will return to the shuttle stop via this route (1.9 miles). ►7

If you have time to explore further, there are a number of add-ons in the area. To get the mirrored reflection of Mount Watkins (in times of high water), continue straight ahead at the northern junction with the Mirror Lake nature loop and walk out to the lakeshore a little far-ther north on any of the well-used use trails. Farther north again, if you continue onto the Valley Loop Trail, westbound, you can visit the Indian Caves, with several caves located among dozens of house-size boulders, wonderfully enticing to children. To reach these, continue straight ahead at the northern junction with the Mirror Lake nature loop, cross a small bridge, and turn left at the T-junction with the Valley Loop Trail in 0.1 mile. Last, from this same T-junction, if you turn right, you can take a 2.7-mile loop trail that continues northeast along Tenaya Creek, officially the easternmost extent of the Valley Loop Trail. This trail has limited views but is a superb forest-floor walk with abundant birdlife, forest flowers, and towering trees. Along the south side of the loop, you walk through the base of the Ahwiyah Point rockslide, admiring how plants are once again emerging among the rubble. If you take this loop, you will return to the Mirror Lake environs on the far side of Tenaya Creek and must either cross the creek to reach the road or continue along the afore-mentioned parallel trail that also leads to the shuttle stop.

🏃 MILESTONES

►1	0.0	Start at shuttle stop 17, Mirror Lake
►2	0.2	Tenaya Creek Bridge
►3	0.3	Right at bike path junction
►4	0.4	Straight where alternate trail diverges left
►5	0.85	Straight ahead at southern Mirror Lake nature loop junction
►6	0.92	Right onto Mirror Lake nature loop (north end)
►7	1.9	Return to shuttle stop 17, Mirror Lake

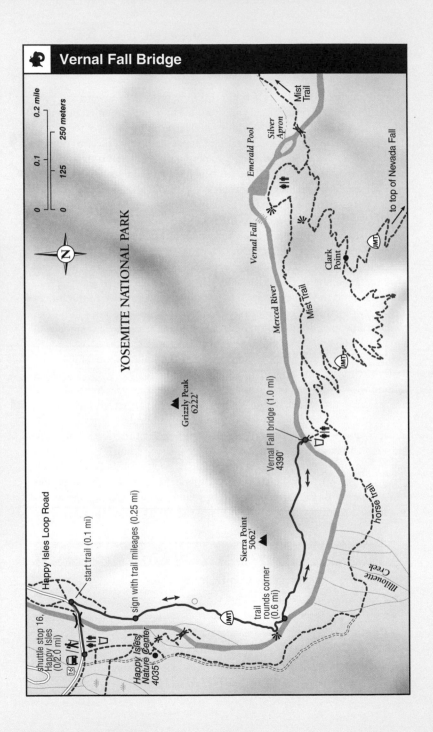

Vernal Fall Bridge

Mist Trail

Silver Apron

Emerald Pool

Vernal Fall

to top of Nevada Fall

JMT

Clark Point

Merced River

Mist Trail

JMT

Grizzly Peak 6222'

YOSEMITE NATIONAL PARK

Vernal Fall bridge 4390' (1.0 mi)

horse trail

Sierra Point 5062'

Illilouette Creek

N

Happy Isles Loop Road

start trail (0.1 mi)

sign with trail mileages (0.25 mi)

JMT

trail rounds corner (0.6 mi)

shuttle stop 16, Happy Isles (0/2.0 mi)

16

Happy Isles Nature Center 4035'

0   0.1   0.2 mile

0   125   250 meters

Vernal Fall Bridge

Like the base of Yosemite and Bridalveil Falls, a popular, paved path leads to the base of Vernal Fall—if you have a full day here, take all three walks because each is unique. However, unlike the other two destinations, the 1.0 mile to the Vernal Fall bridge gains significant elevation. Flatlanders will need to take it at a slow pace, and the grade is too steep for wheelchairs and just doable with a jogging stroller—but the effort is well worth it, as you hike past steep granite flanks to view the pounding falls. Perhaps several thousand hikers make this ascent on any sunny summer day.

TRAIL USE
Day Hike, Stroller
Access, Child-Friendly
LENGTH
2.0 miles, 1–2 hours
VERTICAL FEET
One-way: +475', –115'
Round-trip: ±590'
DIFFICULTY
– 1 **2** 3 4 5 +
TRAIL TYPE
Out-and-Back

FEATURES
Canyon
Stream
Waterfall
Great Views
Geological Interest

FACILITIES
Bear Boxes
Campgrounds
Lodging
Restrooms
Shuttle Stop
Store
Visitor Center
Water

Maps

This trail is covered by the Tom Harrison *Yosemite Valley* map (1:24,000 scale), the National Geographic Trails Illustrated *#306 Yosemite SW* map (1:40,000 scale), and the USGS *Yosemite Valley* map (1:24,000 scale).

Best Time

Because the Merced River flows year-round, you could take the trail to the base of Vernal Fall at almost any time of year, including for much of the winter. Ideally, May–July is best because so much water then leaps over the brink of the fall. However, the walk is also worth embarking on at lower flows because it is still photogenic as a thin film of water framed by the vertical cliffs in the alcove.

Finding the Trail

The trailhead is located at Happy Isles, Yosemite Valley shuttle stop 16, along Happy Isles Loop

A few feet before the spring-fed cistern, a treacherous trail once climbed to Sierra Point but was closed in 1977 following several accidents.

Road. Because this road is closed to vehicular traffic, except the shuttle buses, take the shuttle bus to reach the trailhead. Note that for those staying in Upper Pines Campground, it is more efficient to walk to this trailhead than to take the shuttle—just cut through the campground to Happy Isles Loop Road. Those staying at Lower Pines and North Pines Campgrounds should walk the short distance to shuttle stop 15 to avoid a long shuttle ride back via Half Dome Village (Curry Village) or beyond. Other hikers can park their cars in either the Half Dome Village parking area or the large day-use parking area near Yosemite Village. Water faucets and toilets are at the shuttle stop and just beyond the Vernal Fall bridge, your destination.

Trail Description

From the shuttle stop ►1 you walk briefly east along the road, across a bridge, and then turn right, off the road (0.1 mile). ►2 Now head south along a broad sandy path, soon reaching a sign noting the water level during the destructive floods in January 1997. Just imagine the volume and force of water on that occasion, which washed out the bridge that used to cross the river here. Beyond is the start of the famous John Muir Trail (0.25 mile), ►3 marked by a large wood placard indicating the distances to faraway locations.

Walking along a paved track, up which a determined parent can just push a stroller, you pass through a forest of Douglas-fir, California bay

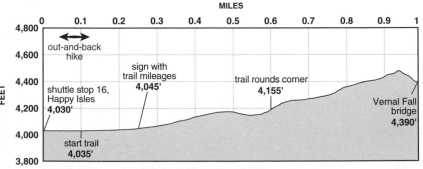

TRAIL 32 Vernal Fall Bridge Elevation Profile

laurel, and incense cedar. After a few minutes you reach a small spring-fed cistern with questionably pure water. Beyond it the climb south steepens, and before bending east you get a glance back at Upper Yosem-ite Fall, partly blocked by the Glacier Point Apron. From a lookout at a distinct left curve in the trail (0.6 mile), ▶4 look west to vertical cliffs rising to the Glacier Point vista. Note the decimated forest at the base of Glacier Point Apron, the aftermath of a massive rockslide in July 1996. The deposit of boulders lies close to the cliff wall, and beyond is a ring of trees, toppled by the air blast that accompanied the slide—the giant,

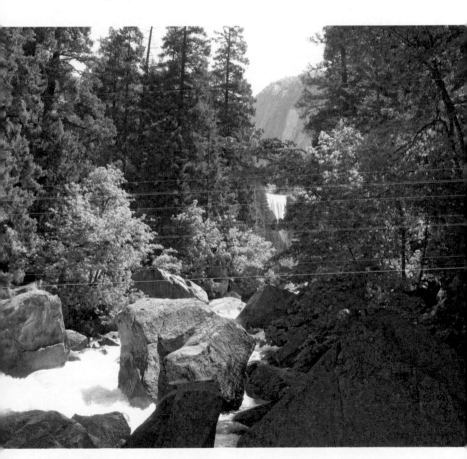

Vernal Fall

largely intact rock slabs were tumbling at an astonishing 270 miles per hour by the time they reached the valley floor. If you look at the apron, you see a series of oblique-angle cliffs—all of them remarkably similar in orientation because they've fractured along the same series of joint planes time and again across geologic history. At the canyon's south end, Illilouette Fall plunges 370 feet over a vertical, joint-controlled cliff. Just east of the fall is a large scar that marks the site of another major rockfall from the winter of 1968–69.

Climbing east now, you head up a canyon whose floor in times past was buried by as much as 1,800 feet of glacier ice. Hiking beneath the unstable, highly fractured south wall of Sierra Point, you soon exit live oak cover and cross a talus slope—an accumulation of rockfall boulders. Entering forest shade once more, you ascend a steep stretch of trail before making a quick drop to the Vernal Fall bridge (1.0 mile). ▶5 From it you see Vernal Fall, a broad curtain of water plunging 320 feet over a vertical cliff before cascading toward you. Looming above the fall are two glacier-resistant masses, Mount Broderick (left) and Liberty Cap (right). Just beyond the bridge are restrooms, a drinking fountain, and an emergency telephone. There are additional views of the falls to be had by continuing up alongside the river for approximately 0.2 mile—or beyond, but then turn to Trails 33 or 34. Return to the Happy Isles shuttle stop by the same route (2.0 miles). ▶6

🚶	MILESTONES	
▶1	0.0	Start at shuttle stop 16, Happy Isles
▶2	0.1	Turn right onto trail
▶3	0.25	Sign with trail mileages at start of official trail
▶4	0.6	Trail rounds corner
▶5	1.0	Vernal Fall bridge
▶6	2.0	Return to shuttle stop 16, Happy Isles

Vernal Fall–Nevada Fall Loop

Mile for mile, the very popular balloon hike up to the brink of Nevada Fall and back may be the most scenic one in the park. The first part of this loop goes up the famous (or infamous) Mist Trail—a steep, strenuous trail that sprays you with Vernal Fall's mist, which cools you on hot afternoons. You next ascend past equally picturesque Nevada Fall. The descent along the John Muir Trail (JMT) and past Clark Point gives you aerial views of the landscape you walked through on your climb. Barely a step of the hike is not worth celebrating, even though your knees may be begging for a rest. The best photos of the falls are taken from late morning through late afternoon, when they are illuminated by the sun.

Maps

This trail is covered by the Tom Harrison *Yosemite Valley* map (1:24,000 scale), the National Geographic Trails Illustrated *#306 Yosemite SW* map (1:40,000 scale), and the USGS *Yosemite Valley* map (1:24,000 scale).

Best Time

To visit Vernal and Nevada Falls in all their glory, it is best to go during the time of the Merced River's maximum runoff, which usually is in May and June. During July there still is plenty of water coming over the falls, but they diminish considerably by August and continue to diminish until sufficient precipitation comes, usually in November. Note that the segment of the Mist Trail alongside Vernal Fall and the JMT alongside Nevada Fall are closed during winter

TRAIL USE
Day Hike
LENGTH
6.4 miles, 3–6 hours
VERTICAL FEET
One-way: +2,125', –220'
Round-trip: ±2,345'
DIFFICULTY
– 1 2 **3** 4 5 +
TRAIL TYPE
Balloon

FEATURES
Canyon
Stream
Waterfall
Wildflowers
Great Views
Steep
Geological Interest

FACILITIES
Bear Boxes
Campgrounds
Lodging
Restrooms
Shuttle Stop
Store
Visitor Center
Water

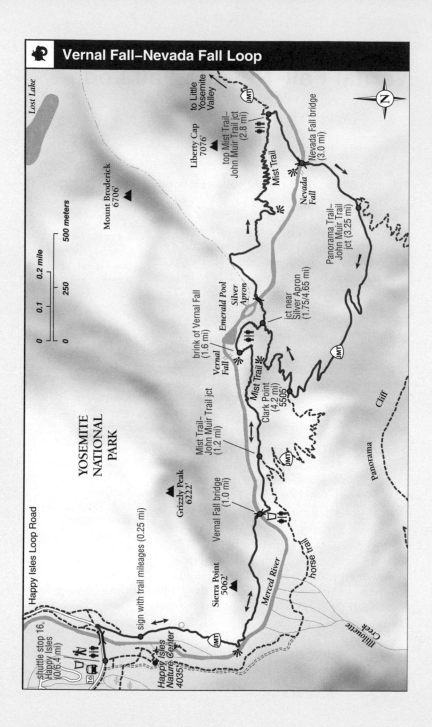

Vernal Fall–Nevada Fall Loop

Lost Lake

to Little Yosemite Valley

JMT

Liberty Cap 7076'

top Mist Trail–John Muir Trail jct (2.8 mi)

Mist Trail

Nevada Fall bridge (3.0 mi)

Mount Broderick 6706'

Nevada Fall

500 meters

250

0.2 mile

0.1

Panorama Trail–John Muir Trail jct (3.25 mi)

250

0

0

Emerald Pool

Silver Apron

brink of Vernal Fall (1.6 mi)

jct near Silver Apron (1.75/4.65 mi)

Vernal Fall

Mist Trail

JMT

YOSEMITE NATIONAL PARK

Clark Point 5505'

Mist Trail–John Muir Trail jct (1.2 mi)

JMT

Happy Isles Loop Road

Grizzly Peak 6222'

Vernal Fall bridge (1.0 mi)

sign with trail mileages (0.25 mi)

Sierra Point 5062'

Merced River

Panorama Cliff

horse trail

shuttle stop 16, Happy Isles (0/6.4 mi)

JMT

Happy Isles Nature Center 4035'

Illilouette Creek

due to icy conditions. You can still piece together a route to the top of Nevada Fall during the winter months (usually late November–March but longer in high-snowfall years), by ascending the JMT to Clark Point, descending the connector trail to the Mist Trail near the Silver Apron bridge, and then climbing the Mist Trail to the top of Nevada Fall, but it is a much longer route.

La Casa Nevada, opened in 1870 and managed by Albert Snow until a fire destroyed it in 1891, once stood on a broad bench above the Silver Apron bridge.

Finding the Trail

The trailhead is located at Happy Isles, Yosemite Valley shuttle stop 16, along Happy Isles Loop Road. Because this road is closed to vehicular traffic, except the shuttle buses, take the shuttle bus to reach the trailhead. Note that for those staying in Upper Pines Campground, it is more efficient to walk to this trailhead than to take the shuttle—just cut through the campground to the loop road. Those staying at Lower Pines and North Pines Campgrounds should walk the short distance to shuttle stop 15 to avoid a long shuttle ride back via Half Dome Village (Curry Village) or beyond. Other hikers can park their cars in either the Half Dome Village parking

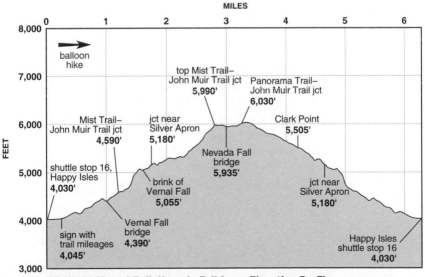

TRAIL 33 Vernal Fall–Nevada Fall Loop Elevation Profile

area or the large day-use parking area near Yosemite Village. There are water faucets and toilets at the shuttle stop and just beyond the Vernal Fall bridge, 1 mile into your hike.

Trail Description

From the shuttle stop ▶1 you walk briefly east across a bridge and then leave the road and head south (right), soon reaching the start of the famous John Muir Trail (JMT) (0.25 mile), ▶2 which heads about 210 miles southward to the summit of Mount Whitney. After a few minutes you reach a small spring-fed cistern with questionably pure water.

Beyond it the climb south steepens, and before bending east you get a glance back at Upper Yosemite Fall, partly blocked by Glacier Point Apron. Note the decimated forest at the base of Glacier Point Apron, the aftermath of a massive rockslide in July 1996. The deposit of boulders lies close to the cliff wall, and beyond is a ring of trees, toppled by the air blast that accompanied the slide—the giant, largely intact rock slabs were tumbling at an astonishing 270 miles per hour by the time they reached the valley floor. If you look at the apron, you see a series of oblique-angle cliffs—all of them remarkably similar in orientation because they've fractured along the same series of joint planes time and again across geologic history. At the canyon's south end, Illilouette Fall plunges 370 feet over a vertical, also joint-controlled cliff.

Climbing east, you head up a canyon whose floor in times past was buried by as much as 1,800 feet of glacier ice. Hiking beneath the unstable, highly fractured south wall of Sierra Point, you are first shaded by live oaks and then cross a talus slope—an accumulation of rockfall boulders that is likely to continue growing over time. Entering forest shade once more, you ascend a steep stretch of trail before making a quick drop to the Vernal Fall bridge (1.0 mile). ▶3 From it you see Vernal Fall, a broad curtain of water plunging 320 feet over a vertical cliff before cascading toward you. Looming above the fall are two glacier-resistant masses, Mount Broderick (left) and Liberty Cap (right). Just beyond the bridge are restrooms, a drinking fountain (including a tap for water bottles), and an emergency telephone.

Climbing under forest cover alongside the river, you soon reach a junction where the Mist Trail continues upriver (left), your route, while the JMT starts a switchbacking ascent to the right (1.2 miles). ▶4 The latter is the route taken by hikers not keen on the steep steps that comprise the Mist Trail as well as those with horses or other pack stock.

Dressed for the upcoming mist, which can really soak you in May or June, start up the Mist Trail and soon, rounding a bend, you receive your first spray as you're crossing steep rocky slabs; be courteous and safe as you pass people here. Relentless, tall rock steps lead you up a verdant slope right of the river. If you're climbing this trail on a sunny day, you may see one, if not two, rainbows come alive in the fall's spray. The spray increases as you advance toward the fall, with just a brief respite as the trail ducks beneath a large boulder.

Beyond the boulder, complete your 300-plus steps, most of them wet, which guide you up the spray-drenched garden into a forested gully. The stairs through this passage have been recently reengineered, but they are still steep and tall—work your way up slowly. Then, reaching an alcove beneath an ominous overhang, you scurry left up a last set of stairs. These, protected by a railing, guide one to the top of a vertical cliff. Pausing here you can study your route, the nearby fall, and the river gorge. The railing leads to the brink of Vernal Fall (1.6 miles), ►5 where peering over you stare down at the pulsing mass of water. Unfortunately, people venture beyond it, and sometimes are swept over the fall; I am fond of the analogies, comparing the river's edge to a cliff face, because both are equally dangerous boundaries. At high flow the risk is more obvious, but even when dry the rock is so smooth that people have lost their footing and fallen into the current. Just above it is Emerald Pool, and due to its treacherous current, wading and swimming are forbidden.

Plunging into the upper end of chilly Emerald Pool is churning Silver Apron, and a bridge spanning its narrow gorge is your immediate goal. The trail is a little vague in this area, due to use paths, but the correct route leaves the river near the pool's far (east) end, and climbs south (right); outhouses are visible in the forest to the right. Ascending a few tight switchbacks, the trail soon angles east across slabs to a somewhat indistinct junction (1.75 miles). ►6 From it a view-blessed trail climbs to Clark Point, where it meets the JMT; this is the route along which you will return. For now, trend left and traverse across slabs decorated by succulent, yellow stonecrops in spring, and then curve left over to the Silver Apron bridge. Beyond it you have a short, moderate climb to a broad bench.

In an open flat, you will see a collection of use trails heading right toward the river. Follow these just 50 steps for a better view of Nevada Fall than is afforded along the trail. Spurred onward by the sight and sound of plummeting Nevada Fall, you climb eastward, diving into forest

OPTION: Nevada Fall Viewpoint

▶8 Just a few steps before the Nevada Fall bridge you can strike north-west to find a short spur trail that drops to a viewpoint beside the fall's brink. This viewpoint's railing is seen from the fall's bridge, thereby giving you an idea where the trail ends, although its start is rather cryptic. Don't stray along the cliff's edge and, as said earlier, respect the river—people have been swept over this fall too.

and then commencing a series of more than two dozen short switchbacks, well decorated with wildflowers in early summer. Near the top, Nevada Fall slips out of view and your attention can focus on the vertical walls of towering Liberty Cap that rise directly beside you. The climb ends at the top of a joint-controlled gully where, on brushy slopes, you once again meet the JMT, with outhouses just a few steps up the trail (2.8 miles). ▶7

From this junction you head southwest (right) along the JMT toward nearby Nevada Fall, climbing briefly to broad slabs adjoining the river-bank and soon reaching a handsome bridge (3.0 miles). ▶8 Before crossing the bridge, you can descend to a cryptic—but fenced—view over the falls, see the Option above. You now strike southwest, immediately passing more glacier polish and erratic boulders and shortly ending a gentle ascent at a junction with the Panorama Trail (Trail 41), which originates at Glacier Point (3.25 miles). ▶9 Now you begin a descent to Happy Isles, starting with a high traverse along a trail blasted into the rock. A stout rock wall protects you from the possibility of a slide, so you can instead imbibe the ever-changing panorama of domelike Liberty Cap and broad-topped Mount Broderick—both once overridden by glaciers. As you progress west, Half Dome, lying behind the just-mentioned domes, becomes prominent, its hulking mass vying for your attention. All the while, Nevada Fall decorates the foreground, its water dancing and churning down through the air. A long traverse, followed by switchbacks, leads down to Clark Point (4.2 miles), ▶10 where the JMT continues left down rocky, cobbled switchbacks, while I direct you right, to take the connector trail back toward the Mist Trail. If your knees are tired, the JMT is a slightly easier route, lacking the endless steps of the Mist Trail past Vernal Fall. However, there is often sand and gravel overlaying the rocky base, and I find it the more treacherous of the two choices. As for distance, my current estimates indicate both are the same length to within 0.01 mile—take your choice!

As you descend back toward the Silver Apron at the top of Vernal Fall, you soon come across a switchback where you will understand my

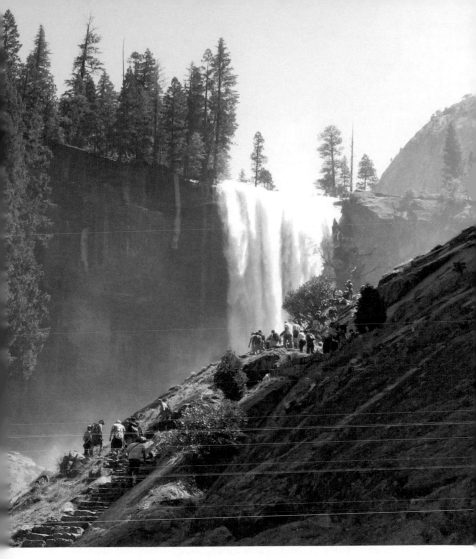

Hiking up *the Mist Trail below Vernal Fall*

attraction to this trail segment—the trail is following the top of the cliff directly atop the Mist Trail (absolutely don't throw any rocks), and you get to stare straight at Vernal Fall from a near-aerial perspective. As this lookout is not fenced, just stay a few steps back from the edge. Continuing down switchbacks, you reach the junction near Emerald Pool and the Silver Apron (4.65 miles), ▶11 and turning left, now retrace your steps down past Vernal Fall to the Happy Isles shuttle stop (6.4 miles). ▶12

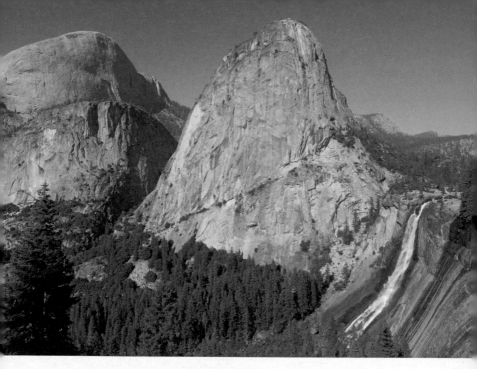

Nevada Fall *and Half Dome, Mount Broderick, and Liberty Cap*

🚶	**MILESTONES**	
▶1	0.0	Start at shuttle stop 16, Happy Isles
▶2	0.25	Sign with mileages at start of official trail
▶3	1.0	Vernal Fall bridge
▶4	1.2	Left onto Mist Trail at Mist Trail–John Muir Trail junction
▶5	1.6	Brink of Vernal Fall
▶6	1.75	Left at junction near the Silver Apron
▶7	2.8	Right onto John Muir Trail at top of Mist Trail
▶8	3.0	Nevada Fall bridge
▶9	3.25	Right at Panorama Trail–John Muir Trail junction
▶10	4.2	Right at Clark Point
▶11	4.65	Left at junction near the Silver Apron
▶12	6.4	Return to shuttle stop 16, Happy Isles

Half Dome

If I as a first-time visitor were allowed to do only one day hike in the park, I would unquestionably choose this hike—the one that I most associate with Yosemite and on whose summit I've sat countless times admiring the surrounding landscape. On a good summer day, 300 hikers attempt this summit, this number dictated by the number of permits made available by the national park, but many turn back, either from exhaustion or from fear. Indeed, Half Dome is not for acrophobes, klutzes, those out of shape, or those who have bad knees. The hike up Half Dome's shoulder and its cables is exposed and potentially life-threatening, especially when the rock is wet or thunderstorms threaten. Do not attempt to climb the dome's shoulder and its cables if weather is threatening because the exposed rock becomes very slippery and a lightning strike is possible. Remarkably few people have died on this route—almost all in bad weather—but more fall and are injured. In addition to standard hiking gear, remember to reserve your Half Dome permit (see page 21) and take a pair of gloves with good traction; this makes holding the metal cables much more pleasant—rubber gardening gloves with a sticky grip are excellent.

Most people day hike Half Dome from Yosemite Valley, but some enjoy it as a two- to three-day backpacking trip, spending one to two nights in Little Yosemite Valley. Many a Yosemite backpacker has spent his or her first night in the "wilderness" in Little Yosemite Valley. Indeed, more backpackers camp in it than in any other Yosemite backcountry area. During the summer this area is patrolled by

TRAIL USE
Day Hike, Backpack

LENGTH
14.7 miles, 6–12 hours
(over 1–3 days)

VERTICAL FEET
One-way: +5,140', −335'
Round-trip: ±5,475'

DIFFICULTY
− 1 2 3 **4** 5

TRAIL TYPE
Out-and-Back

FEATURES
Canyon
Summit
Stream
Waterfall
Wildflowers
Great Views
Camping
Steep
Granite Slabs
Geological Interest

FACILITIES
Bear Box
Campgrounds
Horse Staging
Lodging
Restrooms
Shuttle Stop
Store
Water
Visitor Center

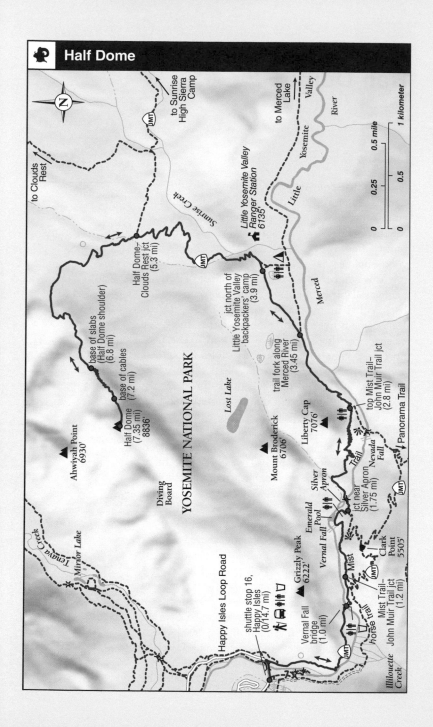

Half Dome

to Sunrise
High Sierra
Camp

to Clouds
Rest

JMT

Sunrise Creek

to Merced
Lake

Yosemite
Valley

Little
Yosemite
River

*Little Yosemite Valley
Ranger Station*
6135'

JMT

Half Dome–
Clouds Rest jct
(5.3 mi)

jct north of
Little Yosemite Valley
backpackers' camp
(3.9 mi)

base of slabs
(Half Dome shoulder)
(6.8 mi)

base of cables
(7.2 mi)

trail fork along
Merced River
(3.45 mi)

Merced

Ahwiyah Point
6930

Half Dome
(7.35 mi)
8836'

YOSEMITE NATIONAL PARK

Lost Lake

top Mist Trail–
John Muir Trail jct
(2.8 mi)

Liberty Cap
7076'

Diving
Board

Mount
Broderick
6706'

Panorama Trail

Nevada
Fall

Silver
Apron

jct near
Silver Apron
(1.75 mi)

Trail

Tenaya Creek

Mirror Lake

Emerald
Pool

Vernal Fall

JMT

Grizzly Peak
6222

shuttle stop 16,
Happy Isles
(0/14.7 mi)

Happy Isles Loop Road

Mist

Clark Point
5505'

JMT

Vernal Fall
bridge
(1.0 mi)

Mist Trail–
John Muir Trail jct
(1.2 mi)

horse trail

Illilouette Creek

JMT

0   0.25   0.5 mile

0   0.5   1 kilometer

N

rangers stationed near the backpackers' camp. If you hike only this far, not continuing to the summit of Half Dome, your route up and down the Mist Trail is 7.8 miles, increasing to 9.3 miles if you follow the John Muir Trail up and down.

Permits

Overnight visitors require a wilderness permit for the Happy Isles to Little Yosemite Valley Trailhead, issued by Yosemite National Park. Both day hike and overnight users require a special permit to climb Half Dome, issued by Yosemite National Park; see page 21 for details. Pick up your wilderness permit at the Yosemite Valley Wilderness Center. You will receive your Half Dome day-use permit by email.

Maps

This trail is covered by the Tom Harrison *Yosemite Valley* map (1:24,000 scale), the National Geographic Trails Illustrated *#306 Yosemite SW* map (1:40,000 scale), and the USGS 7.5-minute series *Half Dome* map (1:24,000 scale).

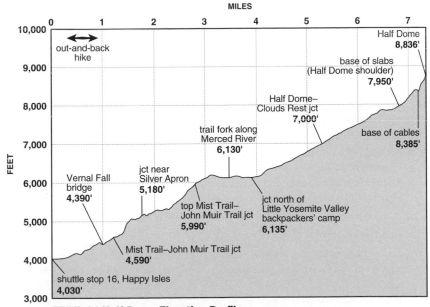

TRAIL 34 Half Dome Elevation Profile

Best Time

Half Dome's hiking season is limited to when its cables are in place, which depends a lot on the amount of snowfall and on the presence or absence of stormy weather. Cables may be placed as early as early May or as late as mid-June, and they may be removed anytime in October—typically the park accepts permit requests from Memorial Day weekend until about mid-October, but having a permit does not guarantee the cables will be up. An early start is recommended so you can complete the steep climb from Yosemite Valley with cooler temperatures, and there is less of a chance of a thunderstorm if you summit before 2 p.m. And of course, starting early is a good idea because most people won't be quite sure how long it will take them to ascend to the summit.

World-class climbers can climb the face of Half Dome in about the same time that the average hiker takes to reach the summit by trail.

Finding the Trail

The trailhead is located at Happy Isles, Yosemite Valley shuttle stop 16, along Happy Isles Loop Road. Because this road is closed to vehicular traffic, except the shuttle buses, take the shuttle bus to reach the trailhead. Note that for those staying in Upper Pines Campground, it is more efficient to walk to this trailhead than to take the shuttle—just cut through the campground to Happy Isles Loop Road. Those staying at Lower Pines and North Pines Campgrounds should walk the short distance to shuttle stop 15 to avoid a long shuttle ride back via Half Dome Village (Curry Village). Other day hikers can park their cars in either the Half Dome Village parking area or the large day-use parking area near Yosemite Village. Overnight hikers must park their cars at the backpackers' parking area, located a short distance east along Happy Isles Loop Road. From the parking area it is a 0.4-mile walk to the Happy Isles shuttle stop. There are water faucets and toilets at the shuttle stop and just beyond the Vernal Fall bridge, 1 mile into your hike.

Trail Description

From the shuttle stop ▶1 you walk briefly east across a bridge and head south, soon reaching a large wooden sign proclaiming the start of the famous John Muir Trail (JMT) (0.25 mile), which heads about 210 miles southward to the summit of Mount Whitney. After a few minutes walking along the paved track, you reach a small spring-fed cistern,

beyond which the climb south steepens. Just before bending east, note
the decimated forest at the base of Glacier Point Apron, the aftermath
of a massive rockslide in July 1996. The deposit of boulders lies close to
the cliff wall, and beyond is a ring of trees, toppled by the air blast that
accompanied the slide—the giant, largely intact rock slabs were tumbling at an astonishing 270 miles per hour by the time they reached the
valley floor. If you look at the apron, you see a series of oblique-angle
cliffs—all of them remarkably similar in orientation because they've
fractured along the same series of joint planes time and again across
geologic history. At the canyon's south end, Illilouette Fall plunges 370
feet over a vertical, also joint-controlled cliff.

   Climbing east, you head up a canyon whose floor in times past was
buried by as much as 1,800 feet of glacier ice. Hiking beneath the unstable, highly fractured south wall of Sierra Point, you cross a talus slope—
an accumulation of rockfall boulders that is likely to continue growing
over time. Entering forest shade once more, you ascend a steep stretch of
trail before making a quick drop to the Vernal Fall bridge (1.0 mile). ►2
From it you see Vernal Fall, a broad curtain of water plunging 320 feet
over a vertical cliff before cascading toward you. Looming above the fall
are two glacier-resistant masses, Mount Broderick (left) and Liberty Cap
(right). Just beyond the bridge are restrooms, a drinking fountain (including a tap for bottles), and an emergency phone.

   Climbing under forest cover alongside the river, you soon reach a
junction where the Mist Trail continues upriver (left), your route, while
the JMT starts a switchbacking ascent to the right (1.2 miles). ►3 The JMT
is the route taken by hikers not keen on the steep steps that comprise
the Mist Trail, as well as those with horses or other pack stock; the two
routes reintersect at the top of Nevada Fall. Dressed for the upcoming
mist, which can really soak you in May or June, start up the Mist Trail,
and soon, rounding a bend, receive your first spray as you're crossing
steep rocky slabs; be courteous and safe as you pass people here. If you're
climbing this trail on a sunny day, you may see one, if not two, rainbows
come alive in the fall's spray. The spray increases as you advance up the
tall, steep steps toward the fall, with just a brief respite as the trail ducks
beneath a large boulder.

   Beyond it, complete 300-plus steps, most of them wet, guiding you up
through a verdant, spray-drenched garden into a forested gully. The stairs
through this passage have been recently reengineered, but they are still
steep and tall—work your way up slowly. Then, reaching an alcove beneath
an ominous overhang, you scurry left up a last set of stairs. These, protected

by a railing, guide one to the top of a vertical cliff. Pausing here you can study your route, the nearby fall, and the river gorge. The railing leads to the brink of Vernal Fall, where peering over, you stare down at the pulsing mass of water. Unfortunately, people venture beyond it and sometimes are swept over the fall; I am fond of the analogies comparing the river's edge to a cliff face, because both are equally dangerous. At high flow the risk is more obvious, but even when dry the rock is so smooth that people have lost their footing and fallen into the current. Just above it is Emerald Pool, and due to its treacherous current, wading and swimming are forbidden.

Plunging into the upper end of chilly Emerald Pool is churning Silver Apron, and a bridge spanning its narrow gorge is your immediate goal. The trail is a little vague in this area due to use paths, but the correct route leaves the river near the pool's far (east) end and climbs south (right); outhouses are visible in the forest to the right. Ascending a few tight switchbacks, the trail soon angles east across slabs to a somewhat indistinct junction (1.75 miles). ►4 From it a view-blessed trail climbs to Clark Point, where it meets the JMT, a possible return route. For now, curve left and traverse across slabs decorated by succulent, yellow stonecrops in spring, and then cross the Silver Apron bridge. Beyond it you have a short, moderate climb to a broad bench.

In an open flat, you will see a collection of use trails heading right toward the river. Follow these just 50 steps for a better view of Nevada Fall than is afforded along the trail. Spurred onward by the sight and sound of plummeting Nevada Fall, you climb eastward, first under forest cover, but soon commence a series of more than two dozen short switchbacks, well decorated with wildflowers in early summer. Near the top, Nevada Fall slips out of view and your attention can focus on the vertical walls of towering Liberty Cap that rise directly beside you. The climb ends

OPTION: Nevada Fall Viewpoint

From the top of the Mist Trail ►5, you can detour right along the John Muir Trail (where you otherwise head left) to a vista down Nevada Fall— I suspect that this will appeal only to people hiking Half Dome as a multi-day excursion. Climbing briefly, you rapidly emerge on slabs and see a sturdy bridge ahead. Just before reaching the bridge, you can strike northwest to find a short spur trail that drops to a viewpoint beside the fall's brink. The descent to the railing is quite cryptic—the rock is too steep to descend until you are about 50 steps north of the falls.

at the top of a joint-controlled gully, where, on brushy slopes, you once again meet the JMT and turn left (2.8 miles). ►5 Outhouses are just a few steps up the trail.

From this junction you climb a rocky slope that is densely lined with scrubby huckleberry oaks, narrowing to a gully near its top. Beyond, you quickly descend into forest cover and reach the banks of the Merced River, here broad, deep, and calm enough for a brief swim on your return. Beneath lodgepole and Jeffrey pines, white firs, and incense cedars, you continue northeast along the river's azalea-lined bank, then quickly encounter a trail fork (3.45 miles). ►6

Those bound for Half Dome generally take the left fork after first obtaining enough water from the Merced River, your last reliable source. This trail traverses sandy slopes a little inland from the river, soon reaching a junction north of the backpackers' camp (3.9 miles). ►7 If you are camping in Little Yosemite Valley, the right fork at ►6 is the marginally shorter option, continuing nearly dead flat, mostly under conifer cover close to the river's shore.

From the junction north of the backpackers' camp, you've not yet expended half the energy required to reach Half Dome's summit, though you have covered half the distance. The trail continues a mostly forested ascent, with the ground bare save a few cryptic orchid species. You continue left, toward Half Dome, at a junction where the JMT bends to the right (5.3 miles). ►8 The trail bends west just before reaching a saddle, with filtered views north across Tenaya Canyon. Small, flat areas near here make a nice high campsite if you're game to carry enough water for the night from the Merced River. Much of the year, a nearby spring (shown on the map) provides water but isn't to be trusted in late summer or drought years. With increasing elevation, you've passed an important ecological transition and are now leaving the lower montane zone for the upper montane zone, the domain of red firs and Jeffrey pines instead of white firs and incense cedars. Half Dome's northeast face comes into view before the trail tops a crest, and soon you also have views backward to Clouds Rest and its satellites, the Quarter Domes. Between them and you, glaciers once spilled into Tenaya Canyon, but the shoulder of Half Dome, west of and above you, never was glaciated. Those on horseback need to end here, if not a bit sooner, under forest cover. On this ridge are the last possible campsites, ideal for those seeking a particularly early-morning or late-evening view from Half Dome—once again, you have had to carry all your water from Little Yosemite Valley.

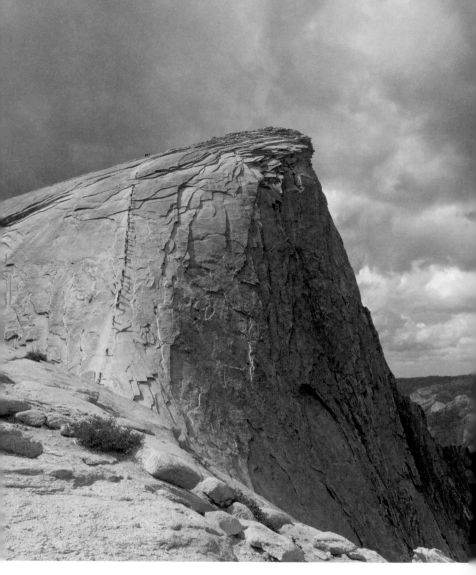

Approaching the top *of the subdome, with Half Dome's cables behind*

    This flat, relaxing traverse ends all too soon at the base of Half Dome's intimidating shoulder (6.8 miles). ▶9 Beyond here a permit is required for all people, and rangers indeed patrol throughout the day. This is also where you must stop—for your safety—if thunderstorms threaten or the rock is wet. Almost two dozen very short switchbacks guide you up the view-blessed ridge of the dome's shoulder. For too long the real danger on this steep section was loose gravel, making it far too easy to lose your footing, but now carefully constructed switchbacks make it safer. Topping the shoulder, you are confronted with the dome's intimidating pair of cables, which definitely cause some hikers to retreat (7.2 miles). ▶**10** If you stare up the cables and decide this is not for you, feel comfortable in your decision and spend a delightful hour basking in the sun on the shoulder, watching the antlike line of people work their way up and down the cables and deciding, quite accurately, that you have already completed a good, tough hike to an excellent viewpoint.

The ascent starts out gently enough, but it too quickly steepens almost to a 45-degree angle. On this stretch, first-timers often slow to a snail's pace, clenching both cables with sweaty hands—hands hopefully ensconced in gloves with a good grip. Looking down, you can see that you don't want to fall. Remember that even when thunderstorms are miles away, static electricity can build up here. If your hair starts standing on end, beat a hasty retreat. Assuming it is a bright sunny day, more frightening to me is the continual jockeying of people trying to pass or overtake each other, necessitating holding on to just one of the cables. This is best done courteously and where boards are laid between the cables in front of periodic posts. For me, one of the biggest advantages of a very early start for a day hike or night spent in Little Yosemite Valley is the ability to climb the cables before the crowds arrive.

The rarefied air certainly hinders your progress as you ascend, but eventually an easing gradient gives new incentive, and soon you are scrambling up to the broad summit of Half Dome, an area about the size of 17 football fields (7.35 miles). ▶**11** Most hikers proceed to the dome's high point (8,836'), located at the north end, from where they can cautiously view the dome's overhanging northwest point. Stouthearted souls peer over the lip of this point for an adrenaline-charged view down the dome's 2,000-foot-high northwest face, perhaps seeing climbers ascending it. Folks once liked camping on the summit to view the sunrise, but camping here was banned decades ago.

From the broad summit of this monolith, which began to form in the late days of the dinosaurs, you have a 360-degree panorama. You can look down Yosemite Valley to the bald brow of El Capitan and up Tenaya Canyon past Clouds Rest to Cathedral Peak, the Sierra Crest, and Mount Hoffmann. Mount Starr King—a dome that rises only 250 feet above you—dominates the Illilouette Creek basin to the south, while the Clark Range cuts the sky to the southeast. Looking due east across Moraine

Dome's summit, you see Mount Florence, whose broad form hides the park's highest peak, Mount Lyell, behind it. In this direction you will also see the forest charred in the 2014 Meadow Fire. Though your route has not passed through burned forest, smoke and fear of the fire spreading necessitated helicopter rescues of hikers atop Half Dome's summit one day. Much as your knees desire a helicopter today, to return you must now retrace your steps down to Happy Isles (14.7 miles). ▶12

Once you are at the top of Nevada Fall, there are alternative routes down. None reduce the total elevation descent, but they provide different views. Following the JMT all the way to the Vernal Fall bridge adds 0.75 mile to your return distance; this trail is more gradual than the Mist Trail and slightly easier on your knees, but my feet tend to hurt after pounding down the cobbled switchbacks that dominate the final mile of this route. It is described as the route for Merced Lake, Trail 35. Continuing along the JMT to the Clark Point vista and then cutting back to the Mist Trail for the descent past Vernal Fall also adds 0.75 mile. This route is outlined in the description of Trail 33, page 297.

🚶	**MILESTONES**	
▶1	0.0	Start at shuttle stop 16, Happy Isles
▶2	1.0	Vernal Fall bridge
▶3	1.2	Straight onto Mist Trail at the Mist Trail–John Muir Trail junction
▶4	1.75	Left at junction near the Silver Apron
▶5	2.8	Left onto John Muir Trail at top of Mist Trail
▶6	3.45	Left at trail fork along Merced River
▶7	3.9	Left at junction north of Little Yosemite Valley backpackers' camp
▶8	5.3	Left at Half Dome–Clouds Rest junction
▶9	6.8	Base of slabs (Half Dome shoulder)
▶10	7.2	Base of cables
▶11	7.35	Summit of Half Dome
▶12	14.7	Return to shuttle stop 16, Happy Isles

Merced Lake

Best done in three days with overnight stops at Little Yosemite Valley (on the way up) and Merced Lake, this hike is often done in two by energetic weekend hikers. Its route, up a fantastic river canyon, is one of the Sierra's best. Located at an elevation of about 7,200 feet, relatively large Merced Lake is about 2,000-plus feet lower than the popular lakes reached from Tuolumne Meadows' trailheads, and therefore it—and the route to reach it—is snow-free sooner and stays accessible into the fall. Also, autumn snowstorms are not a serious concern at these elevations, making October forays quite safe.

Permits

Overnight visitors require a wilderness permit for the Happy Isles to Little Yosemite Valley (LYV) Trailhead (first night at LYV backpackers' camp) or Happy Isles to Sunrise/Merced Lake Pass Thru (first night beyond LYV backpackers' camp), issued by Yosemite National Park. Pick up your wilderness permit at the Yosemite Valley Wilderness Center.

Maps

This trail is covered by the Tom Harrison *Yosemite High Country* map (1:63,360 scale), the National Geographic Trails Illustrated *#306 Yosemite SW* map and *#309 Yosemite SE* map (1:40,000 scale), and the USGS 7.5-minute series *Half Dome* and *Merced Peak* maps (1:24,000 scale).

TRAIL USE
Backpack, Horse
LENGTH
26.6 miles, 12–18 hours
(over 2–3 days)
VERTICAL FEET
One-way: +4,020', −550'
Round-trip: ±4,570'
DIFFICULTY
− 1 2 3 4 **5** +
TRAIL TYPE
Out-and-Back

FEATURES
Canyon
Lake
Stream
Waterfall
Wildflowers
Great Views
Camping
Swimming
Steep
Granite Slabs
Geological Interest

FACILITIES
Bear Boxes
Campgrounds
Horse Staging
Lodging
Restrooms
Shuttle Stop
Store
Visitor Center
Water

(continued on page 318)

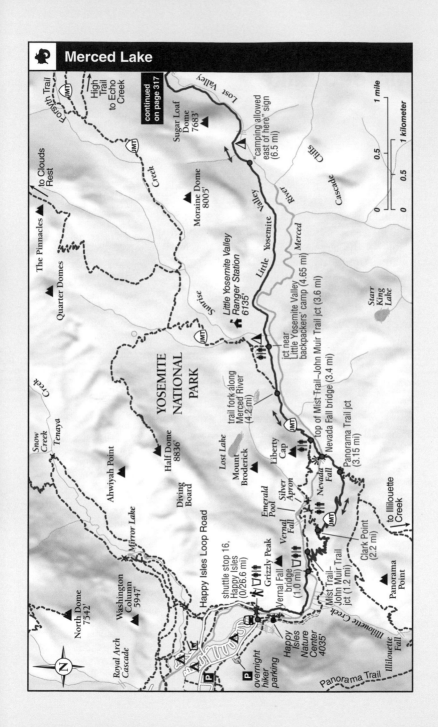

JMT

Forsyth Trail

High Trail to Echo Creek

Creek

continued on page 317

Lost Valley

JMT

Sugar Loaf Dome 7683'

to Clouds Rest

The Pinnacles

Quarter Domes

Moraine Dome 8005'

"camping allowed east of here" sign (6.5 mi)

Little Yosemite Valley

Little Yosemite Valley Ranger Station 6135'

Sunrise

YOSEMITE NATIONAL PARK

Snow Creek

Tenaya

Ahwiyah Point

Half Dome 8836'

Lost Lake

Mount Broderick

Diving Board

trail fork along Merced River (4.2 mi)

JMT

Liberty Cap

Little Yosemite Valley

Merced

Merced River

Cascade Cliffs

Starr King Lake

jct near Little Yosemite Valley backpackers' camp (4.65 mi)

Little Yosemite Valley–John Muir Trail jct (3.6 mi)

top of Mist Trail–John Muir Trail (3.4 mi)

Nevada Fall bridge (3.15 mi)

Panorama Trail jct

Washington Column 5947'

Mirror Lake

Happy Isles Loop Road

Emerald Pool

Silver Apron

Vernal Fall

Nevada Fall

JMT

to Illilouette Creek

North Dome 7542'

Royal Arch Cascade

shuttle stop 16, Happy Isles (0/26.6 mi)

Grizzly Peak

Vernal Fall bridge (1.0 mi)

Mist Trail– John Muir Trail jct (1.2 mi)

Clark Point (2.2 mi)

Panorama Point

Happy Isles Nature Center 4035'

Illilouette Creek

overnight hiker parking

P

P

Panorama Trail

Illilouette Fall

N

1 mile

1 kilometer

0.5

0.5

0

0

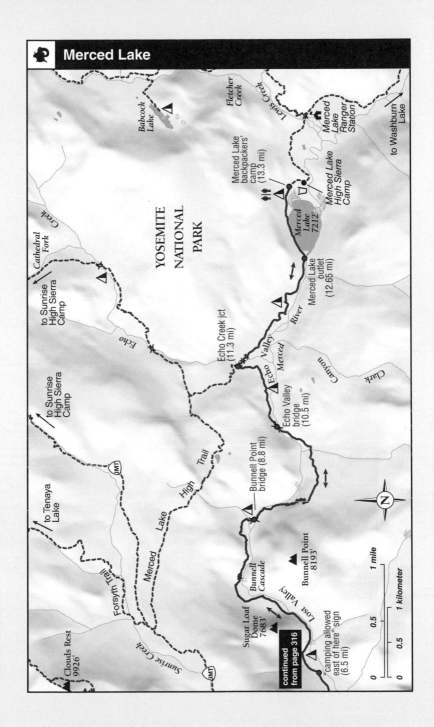

Merced Lake

Fletcher Creek

Lewis Creek

Babcock Lake

to Washburn Lake

Merced Lake Ranger Station

Merced Lake backpackers' camp (13.3 mi)

Merced Lake High Sierra Camp

Cathedral Fork Creek

YOSEMITE NATIONAL PARK

Merced Lake 7212

to Sunrise High Sierra Camp

Merced Lake outlet (12.65 mi)

Echo Creek

to Sunrise High Sierra Camp

Echo Creek jct (11.3 mi)

Merced River

Echo Valley

Clark Canyon

Echo Valley bridge (10.5 mi)

to Tenaya Lake

Merced Lake Trail

High Trail

JMT

Bunnell Point bridge (8.8 mi)

Z

Forsyth Trail

Clouds Rest 9926'

Sunrise Creek

JMT

Sugar Loaf Dome 7683'

Bunnell Cascade

Bunnell Point 8193'

Lost Valley

continued from page 316

"camping allowed east of here" sign (6.5 mi)

1 mile

1 kilometer

0.5

0.5

0

0

(continued from page 315)

Best Time

Some folks make this hike in May and June, when Vernal and Nevada Falls are spectacular, the Merced River is churning, and wildflowers are spectacular, but unfortunately that is also when mosquitoes are ubiquitous and voracious at Merced Lake, though tolerable at some of the slab-infused campsites a little below Merced Lake. Mid-July is better, but you'll still want a tent. By late July, the lake's environs are relatively mosquito free, and the lake is about as warm as it is going to get. This deep lake stays tolerably "warm" through mid-August, then begins to chill. Anglers and the relatively recluse may find September best, after the crowds have left. I have even enjoyed October walks, with the yellow hues of fall and bright blue skies. The nights and morning temperatures are nippy, but the afternoon ones are about perfect.

Finding the Trail

The trailhead is located at Happy Isles, Yosemite Valley shuttle stop 16, along Happy Isles Loop Road. Because this road is closed to vehicular traffic, except the shuttle buses, use the shuttle bus or walk to reach the trailhead. Overnight hikers should park their cars at the backpackers' parking

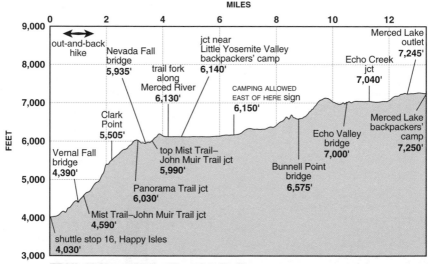

TRAIL 35 Merced Lake Elevation Profile

area, located along Happy Isles Loop Road about halfway between Half Dome Village (Curry Village) and Happy Isles. The Happy Isles shuttle stop is a 0.4-mile walk from the parking area—from here it is more efficient to walk than to take the shuttle bus. Water faucets and toilets are at the shuttle stop and just beyond the Vernal Fall bridge, 1 mile into your hike.

Logistics

There are two wilderness permit options for this walk, and you will have to select which one you prefer at the time you book your permit, eliminating the ability to be flexible based on fatigue. Those with a Happy Isles–Little Yosemite Valley permit must spend their first night at the large backpackers' campground in Little Yosemite Valley (LYV). Those with a Happy Isles pass-through permit must spend their first night at least 2 miles east of the Little Yosemite Valley backpackers' campground. However, it is at least 2 more miles before you will find the first campsite not affected by the 2014 Meadow Fire and several more miles again until there are larger sites.

Note that hikers who unsuccessfully apply for a Happy Isles permit— the most sought-after in the park—could begin this hike at Glacier Point. Again, there are pass-through and stop at Little Yosemite Valley options. If you do this, follow the instructions for the Panorama Trail (Trail 41) until it intersects the John Muir Trail, and then continue following the instructions given for this hike starting with ▶5. This adds 2.35 miles to your hike each direction but reduces the elevation gain.

Trail Description

From the Happy Isles shuttle stop ▶1 you walk briefly east across a bridge and then turn south onto a trail, soon reaching a sign proclaiming the start of the famous John Muir Trail (JMT), which heads about 210 miles southward to the summit of Mount Whitney. Winding past large boulders through a forest of oaks, California laurel, and conifers, your paved path takes you past a small spring-fed cistern whose water I wouldn't drink. Beyond it the climb south steepens, and before bending east, you get a glance back at Upper Yosemite Fall, partly blocked by the Glacier Point Apron.

Entering forest shade once more, you ascend a steep stretch of trail before making a quick drop to the Vernal Fall bridge (1.0 mile). ▶2 From it you see Vernal Fall, a broad curtain of water plunging 320 feet over a vertical cliff before cascading toward you. Looming above the fall are two glacier-resistant masses, Mount Broderick (left) and Liberty Cap (right).

Just beyond the bridge are restrooms, a drinking fountain and water faucet, and an emergency telephone.

Now you hike up to the start of the Mist Trail (1.2 miles). ►3 (The 0.8-mile shorter Mist Trail, to the brink of Vernal Fall, past Emerald Pool, and across the Silver Apron, certainly is worth taking, but the stairs ascending the steep stretch to the top of Vernal Fall are no fun with an overnight pack, especially if you are trying to race upward to avoid drenching yourself and all your gear. If you do wish to take this route, it is described in Trail 33.)

Instead you now turn right, continuing along the JMT corridor, a route yielding different rewards. One is that the miles to Clark Point are along shady, moderately graded switchbacks. Above Clark Point (2.2 miles) ►4 you have spectacular views across the canyon to Half Dome, Mount Broderick, and Liberty Cap, the last rising to the left of downward-leaping Nevada Fall. The last stretch of trail has been blasted out of the steep granite slab. A tall wall provides safe passage, except in winter when the trough with the trail is snow-filled and the trail is closed, forcing a detour from Clark Point down to the Silver Apron bridge and an ascent of the upper half of the Mist Trail. Beyond this section you intersect the end of the Panorama Trail, which started at Glacier Point (3.15 miles), ►5 and then descend to the bridge over Nevada Fall (3.4 miles). ►6 Just a few steps beyond the bridge, you can strike northwest (left) to find a short spur trail that drops to a viewpoint beside the fall's brink. This viewpoint's railing is seen from the fall's bridge, thereby giving you an idea of where the trail ends, though it starts about 50 feet farther north, curving counterclockwise down to the railings where topography permits. Back on the main trail, you descend briefly and reach the top of the Mist Trail, where hikers taking this shorter, steeper trail will rejoin this route description (3.6 miles). ►7

From the junction and its adjacent outhouses, you begin the final climb to Little Yosemite Valley, first by ascending a brushy, rocky slope and then quickly descending and reaching both forest shade and the Merced River. Beneath pines, firs, and incense cedars, you continue northeast along the river's azalea-lined bank, then quickly reach a trail fork (4.2 miles). ►8 You keep right on the main, riverside trail and continue just out of sight of the river's edge, mostly through a quite dense forest, to reach a junction at the southern edge of the Little Yosemite Valley backpackers' camp, complete with toilets, food-storage boxes, and (usually) a ranger (4.65 miles). ►9 Those bound for the JMT or Half Dome branch left, while you continue straight ahead.

With the majority of hikers heading left (north), your route is now much quieter—and wonderfully flat. Starting just a little east of the backpackers' camping area, the forests in Little Yosemite Valley and Lost Valley (the next valley east) were burned in the Meadow Fire in September 2014. Previously much of this section had been a dense forest, with abundant dead material on the ground, providing ample fuel for the fire to spread; this is a natural process and was caused by a natural lightning-strike fire, but the lack of shade and loss of beautiful dense forest stands are nonetheless unwelcome.

Trying to be optimistic, you now have a better view of the canyon's walls and admire the blackened tree trunks as artistic totems. A thick accumulation of glacial sediments covers most of the valley floor, which, like beach sand, make you work even though the trail is level. Progressing east through Little Yosemite Valley, you stay closer to the base of glacier-polished Moraine Dome than to the Merced River, though a 5-minute walk leads to the water anytime you need refreshment. Most of Little Yosemite Valley is a designated day-use area and only once you're beyond a sign (6.5 miles) ▶10 in the eastern stretches of the valley may you camp. The valley's east end is graced by the presence of a beautiful pool—the receptacle of a Merced River cascade. A cluster of popular campsites were once nestled under conifer cover to the north of this pool, but with the area badly charred and tree fall a real danger, this area will now be more popular as a midday swimming hole than a night's destination for many years to come, though some hikers are still using the once-popular campsites. Climbing slabs past the cascade, you glance back to see the east face of exfoliating Moraine Dome and the many charred trees.

Your brief cascade climb takes you closer to the 1,900-foot-high cliff dropping from Bunnell Point, which is exfoliating at an amazing rate. Rounding the base of a glacier-smoothed dome, unofficially called the Sugar Loaf, you enter Lost Valley, the next in a series of flat valleys punctuated by climbs on slabs. This valley has also been badly charred by the Meadow Fire, with barely a tree still standing. At the valley's east end, switchback up past Bunnell Cascade. The magnificent canyon scenery can easily distract one from the very real danger of this exposed section of trail.

Just beyond the V gorge, the canyon floor widens a bit, and, just before descending to the river's banks, if you trend east (right) from the trail, you will find a small camping area atop some slabs. The trail now crosses the Merced River on a bridge (8.8 miles) ▶11 and follows the south bank briefly upstream. Where the stream banks again transform into steeply sloping slabs, your upcanyon walk diverges from the water's edge and climbs a series of more than a dozen switchbacks that carry you 400 feet above the river. Your climb reaches its zenith amid a spring-fed, profuse garden bordered by aspens, which in midsummer supports a colorful array of various wildflowers and in fall is decorated with brilliant yellow aspen leaves.

Beyond this glade you soon come out onto a highly polished bedrock surface. Here you can glance west and see Clouds Rest standing on the northern horizon—a long, not terribly attractive ridge from this aspect. Now you descend back into tree cover, and among the white trunks of aspens, you continue through a forest carpet of bracken ferns and cross several creeklets before emerging on a bedrock bench above the river's inner gorge. From the bench you can study an immense arch on the broad, hulking granitic mass opposite you and watch the water churning down the bottom of the gorge. Traversing the narrow trail winding along the bench, you soon come to a bend in the river and a bridge that crosses the Merced just above the brink of its cascades (10.5 miles). ▶12 Strolling east, you soon reach the west end of spacious Echo Valley, pass a few small campsites on sandy knobs south of the trail, and proceed to a junction at its north edge with a trail ascending Echo Creek (11.3 miles). ▶13

A mile up the Echo Creek trail is a fork, where left is an alternate route back to the backpackers' camp in Little Yosemite Valley, the Merced Lake High Trail. The overall distance is 7.2 miles, versus 6.65 miles following the Merced River canyon. When the trail along the river was completed in 1931, the High Trail fell into disuse because it is almost a mile longer and climbs 750 feet more. More important, it lacks the spectacular Merced River views you've been captivated by. It does provide an alternative return route if you are curious to see some different landscape. This trail is plotted on the trail map on pages 316–317. Note that much of its length will be through forest burned in the Meadow Fire.

For now your goal is Merced Lake. Stay right, immediately crossing Echo Creek's braided river channels on three bridges, then strike southeast through boggy Echo Valley, a dense tangle of approximately 15-foot-tall lodgepole pines, regenerating after fires in 1988 and 1993; the combination of downed logs and thickets of young trees make camping implausible. After mounting a shelf at the east end of Echo Valley, you are again at the river's edge, and from here there are multiple campsites north of the trail, some in sandy flats among slabs and others in small stands of lodgepole pine. If conditions are expected to be buggy at Merced Lake, these make ideal campsites for smaller groups. Continuing on slabs

past the churning river, you reach Merced Lake's outlet (12.65 miles)
►14, at which there are no suitable campsites, and continue around Merced Lake's north shore to the designated backpackers' camping area, just
a little northeast of the lake (13.3 miles). ►15 The backpackers' campsite
is the only decent camping option along the shores of Merced Lake, with
most other flat areas being too close to the water's edge. Pit toilets and
food-storage boxes are an added bonus. Other camping options present
themselves if you continue approximately 0.3 mile upstream, past the
Merced Lake High Sierra Camp to flat forested terrain on the next shelf
up. Eighty-foot-deep Merced Lake, being a large one at a moderate elevation, supports three species of trout: brook, brown, and rainbow. After
your stay, return to the Happy Isles shuttle stop (26.6 miles) ►16.

🚶 MILESTONES

►1	0.0	Start at shuttle stop 16, Happy Isles
►2	1.0	Vernal Fall bridge
►3	1.2	Right onto John Muir Trail at Mist Trail junction
►4	2.2	Right at Clark Point junction
►5	3.15	Left at Panorama Trail junction
►6	3.4	Nevada Fall bridge
►7	3.6	Straight ahead on John Muir Trail at top of Mist Trail
►8	4.2	Right at trail fork along Merced River
►9	4.65	Straight at junction near Little Yosemite Valley backpackers' campground
►10	6.5	End of Little Yosemite Valley no-camping area (CAMPING ALLOWED EAST OF HERE sign)
►11	8.8	Bunnell Point bridge
►12	10.5	Echo Valley bridge
►13	11.3	Straight at Echo Creek junction
►14	12.65	Merced Lake outlet
►15	13.3	Merced Lake backpackers' campground
►16	26.6	Return to shuttle stop 16, Happy Isles

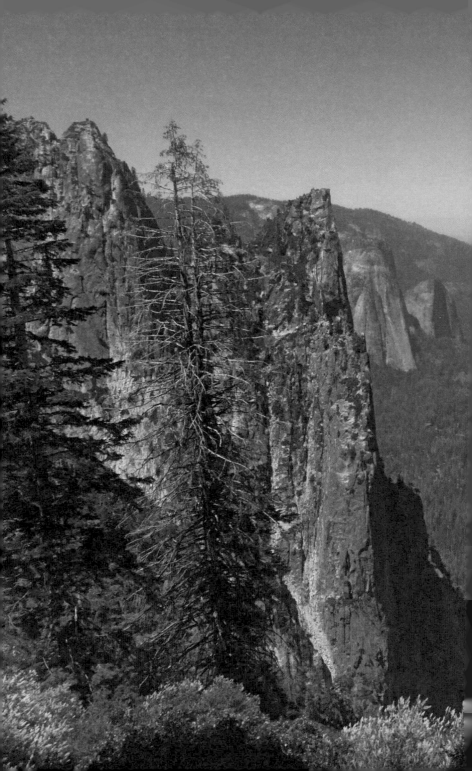

CHAPTER 6

Yosemite Valley's South Rim

This chapter is actually composed of two groups: four trails starting along Glacier Point Road and heading to extremely scenic viewpoints, and two trails starting from Glacier Point and descending several thousand feet to the floor of Yosemite Valley.

In the first group, visitor use to each viewpoint is inversely proportionate to its distance from the trailhead. Dewey Point is the farthest and may get one or two dozen visitors on a summer's day, while Glacier Point is easily the closest and receives thousands of visitors. Glacier Point is arguably the best viewpoint in the entire park, if not in the entire Sierra, because more than any other promontory it offers both an aerial view of the most spectacular part of the valley and a panorama of the high peaks behind. Whereas you can drive almost to Glacier Point (followed by just a brief walk), you'll have to make short hikes (an hour or two, round-trip) to acrophobic Taft Point or to broad-topped Sentinel Dome, which offer slightly different Kodak moments. These two walks can be combined into a single loop, described as an option in the Taft Point hike.

Of the two trails starting from Glacier Point and descending to Yosemite Valley, the Four Mile Trail is shorter, indeed half the length of the Panorama Trail. Most people would consider it the less spectacular, not passing by three waterfalls or beneath the looming presences of Mount Broderick and Liberty Cap, but I rate the view of Yosemite Falls from halfway down as one of the valley's best vistas.

Opposite: *Looking west down the length of Yosemite Valley to the Cathedral Rocks (see Trail 40, page 349)*

Yosemite Valley's South Rim

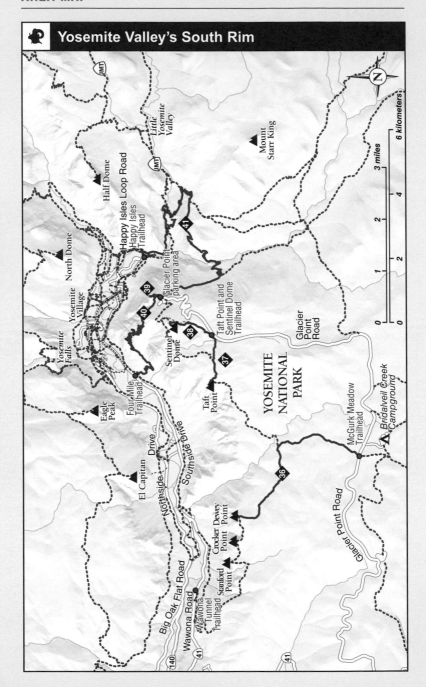

Yosemite Valley's South Rim

Trail	Difficulty	Length	Type	USES & ACCESS	TERRAIN	NATURE	OTHER
36	2	7.8					
37	1–2	2.4					
38	1–2	2.2					
39	1	0.5					
40	2	4.7					
41	3	8.65					

TYPE
- Point-to-Point
- Loop
- Out-and-Back
- Balloon

DIFFICULTY
– 1 2 3 4 5 +
less   more

USES & ACCESS
- Day Hiking
- Backpacking
- Horses
- Running
- Wheelchair Access
- Stroller Access
- Child-Friendly
- Caution

TERRAIN
- Canyon
- Summit
- Lake
- Stream
- Waterfall

NATURE
- Autumn Colors
- Wildflowers
- Giant Sequoias

FEATURES
- Great Views
- Camping
- Swimming
- Secluded
- Steep
- Granite Slabs
- Historical Interest
- Geological Interest

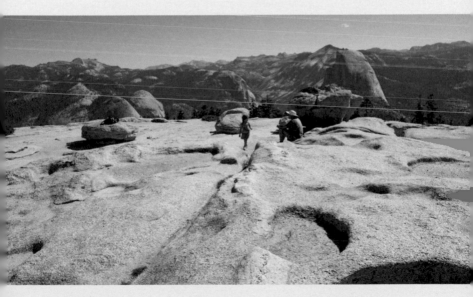

Enjoying the view up *Tenaya Canyon from Sentinel Dome (see Trail 38, page 340)*

Yosemite Valley's South Rim

Dewey Point 330

Dewey Point provides an aerial view of Yosemite Valley's landmarks from a western perch. You peer over the Cathedral Rocks as you gaze down the length of Yosemite Valley and up Tenaya Canyon. This hike from the McGurk Meadow Trailhead along Glacier Point Road is the easiest of routes to scenic Dewey Point. Unlike the rigorous, hot climb from the Wawona Tunnel, your route is a much cooler, rolling traverse confined between 6,800 feet and 7,385 feet. You have views only at the walk's terminus, but along the way you pass through flower-filled McGurk Meadow and the dense, rich conifer forests along the valley's south rim. Because of the relatively gentle nature of the trail, it is suitable for both children and runners.

Taft Point 335

The views from Taft Point down to the floor of Yosemite Valley rival those from Glacier Point. However, because Taft Point is reached by trail, it is less visited than mobbed Glacier Point, and you can sit at the lookout in near solitude. The Fissures, deep slots in the rock, are an added bonus. Generally lacking protective railings, Taft Point and The Fissures are potentially dangerous, so don't bring along children unless you can keep them under strict control. A visit to Taft Point can be combined with an ascent of Sentinel Dome, a 5-mile balloon that is described as an option.

Sentinel Dome 340

Sentinel Dome is a perfect first peak experience for a family and a must-visit destination for view seekers. While it lacks the aerial Yosemite Valley views at Dewey Point, Taft Point, and Glacier Point, its view of the Yosemite high country surpasses these other locations. For little effort you can see all the way to Yosemite's eastern boundary. An ascent of Sentinel Dome can be combined with a trip to Taft Point (see the Option on page 339).

TRAIL 38

Day Hike, Child-Friendly
2.2 miles,
Out-and-Back
Difficulty: **1** **2** 3 4 5

Glacier Point 344

This is more of a vista point than a walk, but it is included here because it is simply too phenomenal to miss. The attraction is the enormity of the view, not just the gushing waterfall in spring, making it a must-visit location anytime Glacier Point Road is open, usually mid-May–October.

TRAIL 39

Day Hike, Wheelchair
Access, Stroller Access,
Child-Friendly
0.5 mile, Balloon
Difficulty: **1** 2 3 4 5

Four Mile Trail 349

This trail provides a scenic descent to Yosemite Valley that will acquaint you with the valley's main features, with perfect views of the Yosemite Falls sequence and a feel for the valley's 3,000-foot depth. Not much energy is expended, but it is hard on the knees. You can also hike the route in reverse. Some may choose to combine an ascent of the Four Mile Trail and a descent of the Panorama Trail for a truly exhilarating day, eliminating the need for a car shuttle between Yosemite Valley and Glacier Point.

TRAIL 40

Day Hike
4.7 miles, Point-to-Point
Difficulty: 1 **2** 3 4 5

Panorama Trail 355

This is the most scenic of all trails descending to the floor of Yosemite Valley, passing three waterfalls and offering spectacular views along the way. Either take a bus up to Glacier Point or have someone drop you there and meet you at Half Dome Village. I have also ascended the Four Mile Trail in the cool morning hours and then descended via the Panorama Trail while enjoying the superior afternoon lighting on Vernal and Nevada Falls.

TRAIL 41

Day Hike
8.65 miles,
Point-to-Point
Difficulty: 1 2 **3** 4 5

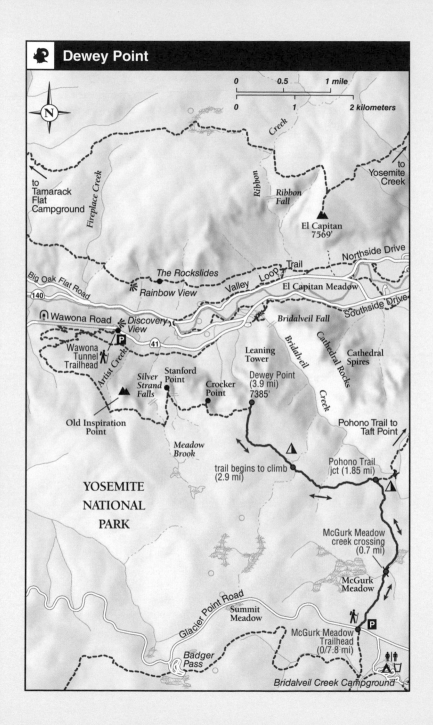

0   0.5   1 mile

0   1   2 kilometers

to
Yosemite
Creek

Creek

Ribbon

Ribbon
Fall

El Capitan
7569'

to
Tamarack
Flat
Campground

Fireplace Creek

Northside Drive

The Rockslides

Valley Loop   Trail

Big Oak Flat Road

Rainbow View

El Capitan Meadow

140

Southside Drive

Wawona Road

Discovery
View

Bridalveil Fall

41

Wawona
Tunnel
Trailhead

Leaning
Tower

Bridalveil

Cathedral
Rocks

Cathedral
Spires

Artist Creek

Silver
Strand
Falls

Stanford
Point

Crocker
Point

Dewey Point
(3.9 mi)
7385'

Creek

Old Inspiration
Point

Meadow
Brook

Pohono Trail to
Taft Point

trail begins to climb
(2.9 mi)

Pohono Trail
jct (1.85 mi)

YOSEMITE

NATIONAL

PARK

McGurk Meadow
creek crossing
(0.7 mi)

McGurk
Meadow

Glacier Point Road

Summit
Meadow

Badger
Pass

McGurk Meadow
Trailhead
(0/7.8 mi)

Bridalveil Creek Campground

Dewey Point

Dewey Point provides an aerial view of Yosemite Valley's landmarks from a western perch. You peer over the Cathedral Rocks as you gaze down the length of Yosemite Valley and up Tenaya Canyon. The hike from the McGurk Meadow Trailhead along Glacier Point Road is the easiest of routes to scenic Dewey Point. Unlike the rigorous, hot climb from the Wawona Tunnel, your route is a much cooler, rolling traverse confined between 6,800 feet and 7,385 feet. You have views only at the walk's terminus, but along the way you pass through flower-filled McGurk Meadow and the dense, rich conifer forests along the valley's south rim.

TRAIL USE
Day Hike, Backpack,
Horse, Run,
Child-Friendly

LENGTH
7.8 miles, 3–5 hours
(over 1–2 days)

VERTICAL FEET
One-way: +850', –590'
Round-trip: ±1,430'

DIFFICULTY
– 1 **2** 3 4 5 +

TRAIL TYPE
Out-and-Back

Permits

Overnight visitors require a wilderness permit for the McGurk Meadow Trailhead, issued by Yosemite National Park. Pick up your wilderness permit at the Yosemite Valley Wilderness Center, Big Oak Flat Entrance Station, or Wawona Visitor Center.

FEATURES
Summit
Wildflowers
Great Views
Camping
Secluded

Maps

This trail is covered by the Tom Harrison *Yosemite High Country* map (1:63,360 scale), the National Geographic Trails Illustrated *#306 Yosemite SW* map (1:40,000 scale), and the USGS 7.5-minute series *El Capitan* map (1:24,000 scale).

FACILITIES
Bear Boxes
Campground
Toilet

Best Time

Wildflowers in McGurk Meadow are best from about late June to mid-July, but unfortunately bloodsucking mosquitoes also thrive when the soils are still moist. Therefore, late July onward is most relaxing,

Of the three Cathedral Rocks seen from Dewey Point, the highest is the only one accessible to competent cross-country hikers—via an exposed walk up its south ridge.

and because Dewey Point's views do not change much (Ribbon Fall dries up early), the hike is a rewarding one through mid-October.

Finding the Trail

From a signed junction along Wawona Road, drive 7.4 miles up Glacier Point Road to the signed trailhead, on your left. This is 0.25 mile before the spur road to the Bridalveil Creek Campground, which is the only campground along Glacier Point Road. The closest water faucets and toilets are at the pullout at the Wawona Road junction, in the Bridalveil Creek Campground, and at Glacier Point.

Trail Description

Starting from Glacier Point Road, ▶1 the lodgepole-shaded trail drops gently to the north of largely hidden Peregoy Meadow before topping a low divide. Next it drops moderately and reaches the south edge of sedge-filled McGurk Meadow, where you cross its creek (0.7 mile). ▶2 Until late summer, the meadow will have an abundance of wildflowers, including shooting star, paintbrush, cinquefoil, and corn lily. The trail skirts the western edge of a narrow finger of McGurk Meadow; a much larger expanse of meadow lies hidden to the west of the trail. Looking east from the meadow, note the low summits of the Ostrander Rocks.

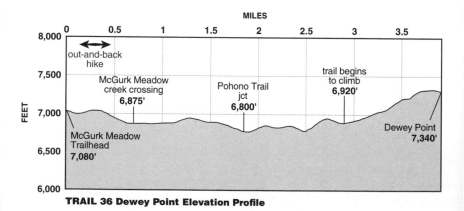

TRAIL 36 Dewey Point Elevation Profile

OPTION: **Pohono Trail**

▶4 If you can get someone to meet you at the Wawona Tunnel, then
you can turn this walk into a point-to-point hike by continuing west from
Dewey Point and descending 4.75 miles to Discovery View (Tunnel View)
along this highly scenic portion of the Pohono Trail. This route takes
you past Crocker Point (in 0.6 mile), Stanford Point (0.5 mile beyond
Crocker), and then down past Old Inspiration Point to Discovery View
on the east side of the Wawona Tunnel, a total distance of 4.75 miles;
the route is shown on the hike map on page 330. There is no permanent
water source along the route, so bring enough with you. Reversing the
walk is not recommended, as it is an arduous climb from the Wawona
Tunnel to the valley rim, and an especially hot ascent in summer.

Leaving McGurk Meadow, you first reenter a lodgepole forest; soon crest
a shallow, viewless saddle; and then descend at a reasonable gradient to a
low-crest trail junction (1.85 miles) with the Pohono Trail. ▶3 The right
(eastern) fork quickly drops to Bridalveil Creek; a collection of campsites
is along the creek's western bank, a pleasant late-summer destination for a
family trip. Day hikers, if you haven't brought along sufficient water, you
can obtain some from this perennial creek.

You turn left, heading west along the Pohono Trail, passing through
a series of sandy flats, and then crossing a broad, low divide. The fir forest here is wonderfully dense—this is one of the rare bits of Yosemite to
not yet suffer the consequences of a catastrophic forest fire, and it is well
worth enjoying the deep shade that the lichen-laden firs provide. Traipsing along you cross three Bridalveil Creek tributaries, the first two larger,
the third smaller (2.9 miles), ▶4 and then start up a fourth that drains a
curving gully. To your right (north) are some small campsites, if there is
still water in these tributaries. On the gully's upper slopes, Jeffrey pine,
huckleberry oak, and greenleaf manzanita replace the fir cover. In a few
minutes you reach highly scenic 7,385-foot Dewey Point, located at the
end of a short spur trail (3.9 miles). ▶5 If you have a head for heights,
you can look straight down the massive face that supports Leaning Tower.
Just to the right are the steep Cathedral Rocks rising on the other side of
Bridalveil Creek. Looking across Yosemite Valley, the broad, smooth face
of El Capitan rises high above the valley floor. Also intriguing is the back
side of Middle Cathedral Rock, with an iron-rich, rust-stained surface.

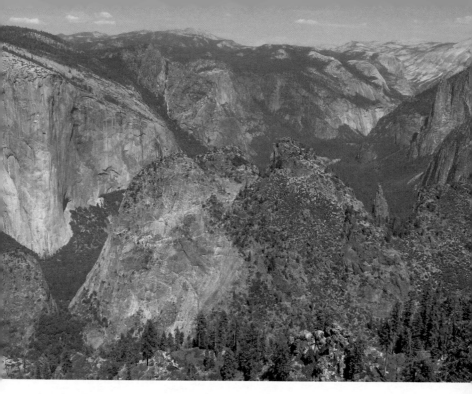

Looking across *to El Capitan and east into Yosemite Valley from Dewey Point*

Finally, you see the Cathedral Spires head-on, so they appear as one. If you are hiking before July, you're also likely to see wispy Ribbon Fall across Yosemite Valley. Bridalveil Fall, however, is blocked by the Leaning Tower. Due to transport difficulties, most people will return the way they came (7.8 miles). ▶6 However, if a generous party member is willing to return for the car, some of the group can continue west along the Pohono Trail to the Wawona Tunnel—see the Option on page 333.

🚶	MILESTONES	
▶1	0.0	Start at McGurk Meadow Trailhead
▶2	0.7	McGurk Meadow creek crossing
▶3	1.85	Left onto Pohono Trail
▶4	2.9	Trail begins to climb
▶5	3.9	Dewey Point
▶6	7.8	Return to McGurk Meadow Trailhead

Taft Point

The views from Taft Point down to the floor of Yosemite Valley rival those from Glacier Point. However, because Taft Point is reached by a longer trail, it is less visited than mobbed Glacier Point, and you can sit at the lookout in near solitude. The Fissures, deep slots in the rock, are an added bonus. Generally lacking protective railings, Taft Point and The Fissures are potentially dangerous, so don't bring along children unless you can keep them under strict control.

Maps

This trail is covered by the Tom Harrison *Yosemite Valley* map (1:24,000 scale), the National Geographic Trails Illustrated *#306 Yosemite SW* map (1:40,000 scale), and the USGS *Yosemite Valley* map (1:24,000 scale).

Best Time

Because Taft Point provides a good view of Yosemite Falls, you should visit this viewpoint while the falls are still flowing with considerable volume, which is late May–mid-July. This also is the best time for wildflowers. If you don't mind a wispy to nonexistent Yosemite Falls, then you can take the trail through October, when Glacier Point Road still is likely to be open.

Finding the Trail

From a signed junction along Wawona Road, drive 13.2 miles on Glacier Point Road to a parking area on your left; this is 2.3 miles before the Glacier Point parking lot entrance. The parking lot fills early, after

TRAIL USE
Day Hike, Run

LENGTH
2.4 miles, 1–2 hours

VERTICAL FEET
One-way: +110', −335'
Round-trip: ±445'

DIFFICULTY
− **1 2** 3 4 5 +

TRAIL TYPE
Out-and-Back

FEATURES
Summit
Wildflowers
Great Views
Geological Interest

FACILITIES
Bear Boxes
Restrooms

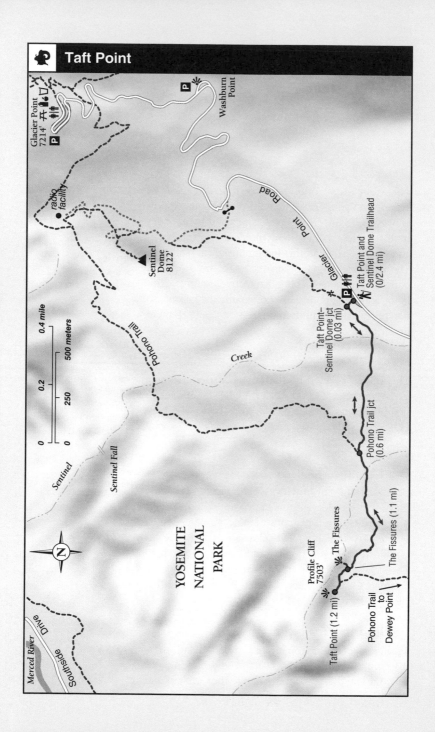

Taft Point

P Glacier Point 7214'

Washburn Point

P

radio facility

Sentinel Dome 8122'

Point Road

Glacier

Taft Point and Sentinel Dome Trailhead (0/2.4 mi)

P

Taft Point–Sentinel Dome jct (0.03 mi)

Creek

Pohono Trail

Pohono Trail jct (0.6 mi)

0.4 mile

500 meters

0.2

250

0

0

The Fissures (1.1 mi)

Sentinel Fall

Sentinel

YOSEMITE NATIONAL PARK

Profile Cliff 7503'

The Fissures

The Fissures

N

Taft Point (1.2 mi)

Pohono Trail to Dewey Point

Merced River

Southside Drive

which cars begin lining Glacier Point Road and small pullouts up to 0.5 mile before and after the main trailhead parking.

The closest water faucets are at the pullout at the Wawona Road junction, in the Bridalveil Creek Campground, and at Glacier Point.

Trail Description

From the parking area ▶1 you descend briefly to a trail (0.03 mile), ▶2 turn left, and start southwest on it; right leads to Sentinel Dome. After about 0.1 mile of easy descent, you pass a trailside outcrop that is almost entirely composed of glistening whitish-gray quartz. In a minute you come to seasonal Sentinel Creek—seasonal due to its small, low-elevation drainage area, which keeps tiny Sentinel Fall from being one of Yosemite Valley's prime attractions. After boulder-hopping the creek, your trail undulates west past pines, firs, and open sandy flats to a crest junction with the Pohono Trail (0.6 mile). ▶3

From the junction you turn left to descend the Pohono Trail to a seeping creeklet that drains through a small field of corn lilies. In this and two other nearby damp areas, you may also find bracken fern and a burst of color from an assortment of wildflowers, including green monument plant, white corn lilies, purple monkshood, and orange Sierra tiger lilies, which can all grow to head height. Descending toward the Yosemite

Taft Point was named to commemorate President William Howard Taft's October 1909 visit to Yosemite Valley, where he met aged John Muir. Taft jokingly suggested that Yosemite Valley should be dammed, as was proposed for Hetch Hetchy.

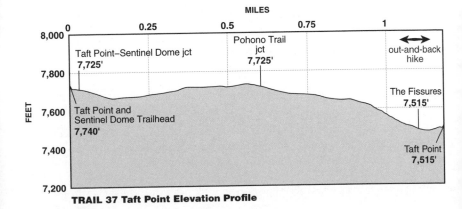

TRAIL 37 Taft Point Elevation Profile

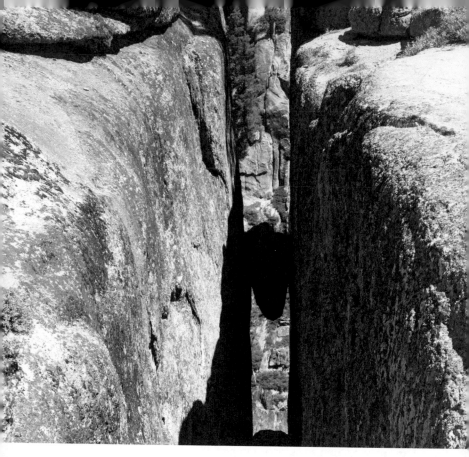

The Fissures *at Taft Point*

Valley rim, you cross drier slopes, which are covered with shrubs and drought-tolerant wildflowers, including wavyleaf Indian paintbrush and wild buckwheats. Soon you arrive at The Fissures—five vertical, parallel fractures that cut through overhanging Profile Cliff just beneath your feet (1.1 miles). ▶4 Because The Fissures area, like your entire route, is unglaciated, there is more loose rock and gravel, and a careless step could result in an easy slip—dangerous in this area. A short unsigned spur trail leads to fantastic views down the slots.

Beyond The Fissures, there is soon a junction where the Pohono Trail makes a near U-turn and continues to the left (west), while you walk briefly up a spur trail to a small railing—offering remarkably little protection—at the brink of a conspicuous point and get an acrophobia-inducing view of overhanging Profile Cliff beneath you (1.2 miles). ▶5 For even better views of Yosemite Valley and the High Sierra, walk just a few steps west to the

OPTION: **Taft Point and Sentinel Dome**

Most people retrace their steps to the car, but you could instead complete a 5.15-mile loop that combines a trip to Taft Point and to Sentinel Dome. If you wish to do this, at ▶3, instead of continuing back to the trailhead (right option on the return), continue left along the Pohono Trail, descending to Sentinel Creek and then completing an ascending traverse around the side of Sentinel Dome. At a junction in a gully, turn right on a trail signposted for Sentinel Dome. Climbing now, the trail keeps crossing paths with an old service road; stick to the steep trail, climbing a hill. Soon signs point you right toward Sentinel Dome, and you will intersect Trail 38 just 0.15 mile below the summit. The entirety of this loop is shown on the hike map on page 336.

true Taft Point, a location few visitors wander over to. From it your sight line of the valley's monuments, including the Cathedral Spires and Rocks, El Capitan, the Three Brothers, Yosemite Falls, and Sentinel Rock, is completely unobstructed. It is the view northwest to the prow of El Capitan that is showiest from here—impressive how the gentle rolling upland is abruptly truncated with the 3,000-foot-tall granite wall. When you have finished inhaling the view, retrace your steps to the car (2.4 miles) ▶6—or see the Option above for a variant that leads directly to Sentinel Dome. As you turn toward the car, make sure you return on the eastbound Pohono Trail; the trail makes a near U-turn at the Taft Point promontory, and it is easy to find yourself on the wrong path—until it occurs to you that you should be heading uphill just next to The Fissures.

 MILESTONES

▶1	0.0	Start at Taft Point and Sentinel Dome Trailhead
▶2	0.03	Left toward Taft Point (versus Sentinel Dome)
▶3	0.6	Left onto Pohono Trail
▶4	1.1	The Fissures
▶5	1.2	Taft Point
▶6	2.4	Return to Taft Point and Sentinel Dome Trailhead

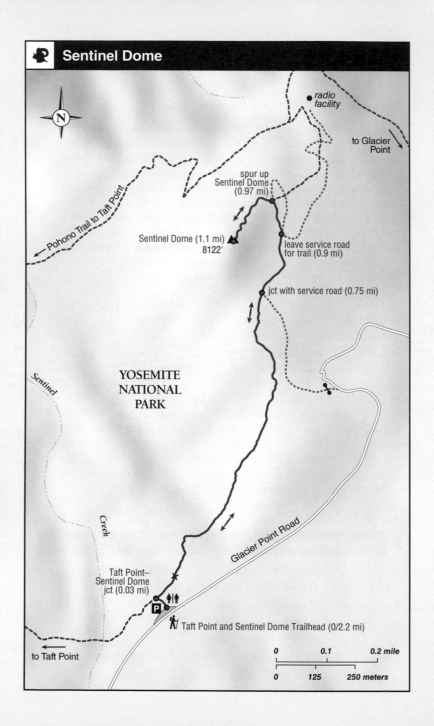

Sentinel Dome

radio facility

to Glacier Point

Pohono Trail to Taft Point

spur up Sentinel Dome (0.97 mi)

Sentinel Dome (1.1 mi) 8122'

leave service road for trail (0.9 mi)

jct with service road (0.75 mi)

YOSEMITE NATIONAL PARK

Sentinel

Creek

Glacier Point Road

Taft Point–Sentinel Dome jct (0.03 mi)

Taft Point and Sentinel Dome Trailhead (0/2.2 mi)

to Taft Point

| 0 | 0.1 | 0.2 mile |

| 0 | 125 | 250 meters |

Sentinel Dome

Sentinel Dome is a perfect first peak experience for a family, as well as a must-visit destination for every view seeker. While it lacks the aerial Yosemite Valley views available at the rim vista points (Dewey Point, Taft Point, and Glacier Point), its view of the Yosemite high country surpasses these other locations. For little effort you can see all the way to Yosemite's eastern boundary.

Maps

This trail is covered by the Tom Harrison *Yosemite Valley* map (1:24,000 scale), the National Geographic Trails Illustrated #306 *Yosemite SW* map (1:40,000 scale), and the USGS *Yosemite Valley* map (1:24,000 scale).

Best Time

Because Sentinel Dome provides a good view of Yosemite Falls, if your goal is to see the falls churning, you should visit this viewpoint while the falls are still flowing with considerable volume, which is late May–mid-July. If the expansive views of the southern and eastern reaches of the park propelled you to this destination, then you can take the trail anytime Glacier Point Road is open and the snow has melted, usually from early May through at least late October. And of course, Vernal and Nevada Falls, off to the east, will be flowing year-round—the white stripes they delineate on the panoramic landscape simply become thinner as the year progresses.

TRAIL USE
Day Hike,
Child-Friendly

LENGTH
2.2 miles, 1–2 hours

VERTICAL FEET
One-way: +470', –80'
Round-trip: ±550'

DIFFICULTY
– **1 2** 3 4 5 +

TRAIL TYPE
Out-and-Back

FEATURES
Summit
Great Views
Granite Slabs
Geological Interest

FACILITIES
Bear Boxes
Restrooms

Finding the Trail

From a signed junction along Wawona Road, drive 13.2 miles on Glacier Point Road to a parking area, on your left. This is 2.3 miles before the Glacier Point parking lot entrance. The parking lot fills early, after which cars begin lining Glacier Point Road and small pullouts up to 0.5 mile before and after the main trailhead parking. The closest water faucets are at the pullout at the Wawona Road junction, in the Bridalveil Creek Campground, and at Glacier Point.

Trail Description

From the parking area ►1 you descend briefly to a trail (0.03 mile), ►2 turn right, and begin a curving descent into a shallow gully; left leads to Taft Point. The trail now traverses north, across sandy slopes and through additional gullies, before climbing more diligently on an open sandy slope, all the while your gaze fixed on Sentinel Dome, which lies straight ahead; slabs lie just beneath the surface here and only a few shrub species can scrape out a living in the pitiful soils. Atop this slope, you meet a service road (0.75 mile) ►3 that you follow north (left). Walking through open forest cover, you soon diverge left back onto a trail (0.9 mile) ►4 and almost immediately arrive at the northern base of the dome (0.97 mile), ►5 where you meet a path ascending from Glacier Point. Turning left, you now climb southwest on quite safe, unexposed bedrock slopes—just watch your footing because though there is nowhere *far* to fall, it is remarkably easy to slip on the gravel and sand lying atop slabs of rock.

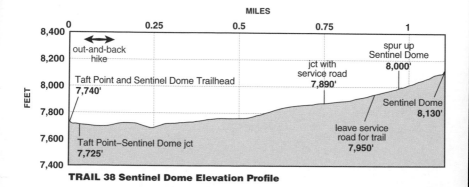

TRAIL 38 Sentinel Dome Elevation Profile

At an elevation of 8,122 feet, Sentinel Dome is the second-highest view- H
point above Yosemite Valley (1.1 miles). ►6 Only Half Dome—a strenuous
hike—is higher. Sentinel Dome was formed by the exfoliation of rock lay- △
ers, rather than by glaciation. Indeed, you will find no evidence of glacial
polish on Sentinel Dome's summit, and the rock exposed here has been ✦
weathering for hundreds of thousands of years. Exfoliation is the shedding
of thin layers of granite slab from the surface of the dome, and if you stare
closely at the steep sides of Sentinel Dome, you can, without too much ▲
imagination, see it as a giant onion slowly being peeled apart.

Seen from the summit, El Capitan, Yosemite Falls, and Half Dome
stand out as the three most prominent valley landmarks. Northwest
of Half Dome are two bald features, North and Basket Domes. On the
skyline above North Dome stands blocky Mount Hoffmann, the park's
geographic center, while to the east, above Mount Starr King (an unglaciated, true dome), stands the rugged crest of the Clark Range. A disc atop
the summit identifies these landmarks and many others—likely fueling
your desire to explore ever more of Yosemite. Note, however, that the
disc atop the peak proclaiming the names of distant peaks is not 100%
accurate—you cannot see Mount Ritter from the summit. In years past
almost everyone who climbed Sentinel Dome expected to photograph
its windswept, solitary Jeffrey pine, made famous by Ansel Adams. That
tree, unfortunately, succumbed to drought in the late 1970s, but there
are still gnarled, wind-weathered trees to satisfy your photographic
needs. After a long summit break, retrace your steps to the car or combine this excursion with a walk to Taft Point, described as an option in
Trail 37 (2.2 miles). ►7

🚶 MILESTONES

►1	0.0	Start at Taft Point and Sentinel Dome Trailhead
►2	0.03	Right toward Sentinel Dome (versus Taft Point)
►3	0.75	Left onto service road
►4	0.9	Left back onto trail
►5	0.97	Left on Sentinel Dome spur trail
►6	1.1	Sentinel Dome's summit
►7	2.2	Return to Taft Point and Sentinel Dome Trailhead

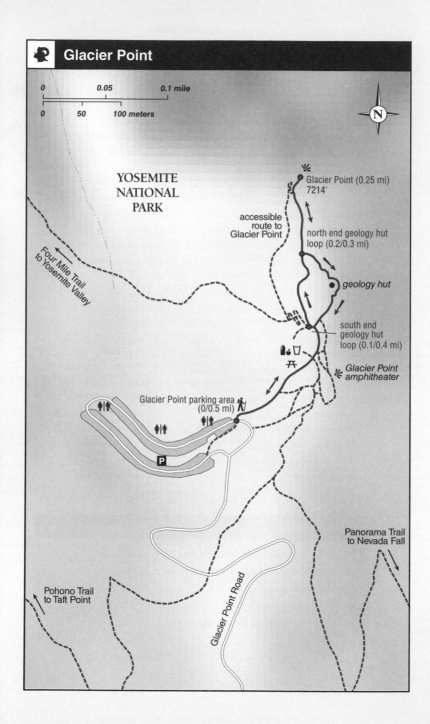

Glacier Point

0   0.05   0.1 mile

0   50   100 meters

N

YOSEMITE
NATIONAL
PARK

Glacier Point (0.25 mi)
7214'

accessible
route to
Glacier Point

north end geology hut
loop (0.2/0.3 mi)

geology hut

Four Mile Trail
to Yosemite Valley

south end
geology hut
loop (0.1/0.4 mi)

Glacier Point
amphitheater

Glacier Point parking area
(0/0.5 mi)

P

Panorama Trail
to Nevada Fall

Pohono Trail
to Taft Point

Glacier Point Road

Glacier Point

This is more of a vista point than a walk, but it is included here because it is simply too phenomenal to miss. The attraction is the enormity of the view, not just the gushing waterfalls in spring, making it a must-visit location anytime Glacier Point Road is open, usually mid-May–October. It is also a location important to Yosemite's history, from the seminal photo of President Theodore Roosevelt and John Muir to the infamous fire fall. From the early 1870s until January 1968, a large pile of embers was pushed off Glacier Point at evening darkness to create the renowned fire fall—a glowing "waterfall."

Maps

This trail is covered by the Tom Harrison *Yosemite Valley* map (1:24,000 scale), the National Geographic Trails Illustrated *#306 Yosemite SW* map (1:40,000 scale), and the USGS *Yosemite Valley* map (1:24,000 scale).

Best Time

If your goal is a panoramic view of Yosemite's falls, you should visit Glacier Point while the falls, and especially Yosemite Falls, are still flowing with considerable volume, which is mid-May–mid-July. If you are simply attracted to the aerial view of Yosemite Valley and the expansive peaks rising to the east, then head to this viewpoint anytime Glacier Point Road is open, usually from mid- to late May through at least October. But the real answer is that while the time of year doesn't matter much, the time of day is essential: You should

TRAIL USE
Day Hike, Wheelchair
Access, Stroller
Access, Child-Friendly

LENGTH
0.5 mile, 15–30 minutes

VERTICAL FEET
Round-trip: ±90'

DIFFICULTY
– **1** 2 3 4 5 +

TRAIL TYPE
Balloon

FEATURES
Waterfall
Great Views
Granite Slabs
Geological Interest

FACILITIES
Bear Boxes
Restrooms
Store
Tour Bus Stop
Water

plan to arrive before 9 a.m. or after 4 p.m., when the crowds are much diminished and the lighting on the cliffs is most engaging; late afternoon lighting is best. You will also better enjoy the drive out here with fewer people on the road and more available parking spaces.

Finding the Trail

From a signed junction along Wawona Road, drive 15.5 miles up Glacier Point Road to a large parking lot at its end. There is a water faucet next to the Glacier Point store, en route to the vista point.

Logistics

Rather than drive up to Glacier Point, whose parking lot can be overflowing on summer weekends, consider taking a Yosemite tour bus. Check the bus schedule in the *Yosemite Guide,* a newsletter presented to tourists at all park entrance stations.

Trail Description

Leaving the large parking area, ▶1 follow the broad paved path past the front of the store and continue 150 feet around the east (right) side of the store to where the trail bends left (west). Just beyond, the trail forks—follow the signs slightly left toward Glacier Point (0.1 mile). ▶2 Continue right where signs point left for the Four Mile Trail, and you will soon reach Glacier Point (0.25 mile). ▶3 Note that if you have a wheelchair or stroller, at ▶2 continue a little farther to the left, and a ramp will lead you to Glacier Point by a more gradual path. On your return trip, fork left at a small junction (0.3 mile) ▶4 to visit the geology

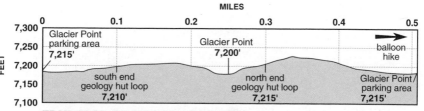

TRAIL 39 Glacier Point Elevation Profile

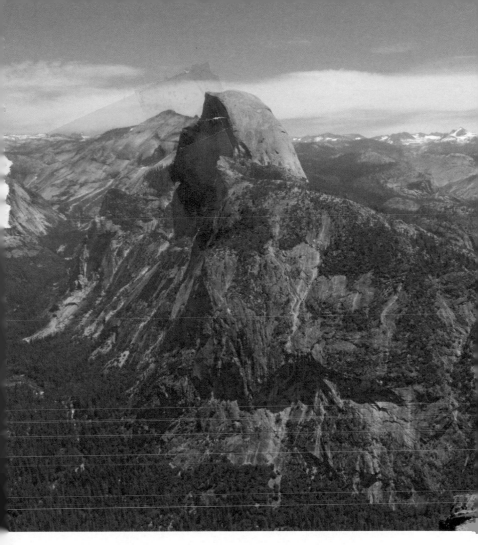

Vista *to Half Dome with Tenaya Canyon and Clouds Rest to the left*

hut, with informative panels about Yosemite's glaciation and excellent views to the east. From here, return to the parking area (0.5 mile). ▶5 You can add 0.1 mile to your return distance by detouring to a series of viewpoints along the east rim, eventually reaching an amphitheater, and then bending right on any number of small trails leading back to the parking area.

Of more interest than the nonessential route description is the breathtaking panorama visible from the railings at Glacier Point. From west-northwest, clockwise you see the following readily identifiable features: Eagle Peak, Yosemite Falls (northwest), Indian Canyon, Royal Arch Cascade (before July), Royal Arches (north), Washington Column with North Dome above, Tenaya Canyon (northeast), and Half Dome with Clouds Rest behind it. Looking east from near the geology hut or the Glacier Point amphitheater, you stare up the Merced River canyon, gazing upon Vernal and Nevada Falls with Liberty Cap rising above Nevada Falls and smaller Mount Broderick to its left. Farther east is Little Yosemite Valley, and beyond, naked Bunnell Point, from which your eyes wander south to the sharp-tipped Clark Range. Straight up the Merced drainage is Mount Florence, with the tip of Mount Lyell (the park's highest summit) just emerging to its right and Mount Maclure peering over its left shoulder. Finally, the unglaciated dome of Mount Starr King dominates the landscape to the southeast, with Illilouette Fall barely visible in the alcove below.

As I stand at these viewpoints, I cannot help but imagine what the valley looked like in times past—most notably at the various glacial maxima. While the eastern half of Yosemite Valley was likely filled to the brim with ice, ice may not have reached all the way to the top of the walls farther west in the valley. What is certain is that the glacier was thick, especially because the bedrock on the valley floor is covered in most places with more than 1,000 feet of sediment—sediment that was deposited after the glaciers retreated.

⩗	MILESTONES	
▶1	0.0	Start from the Glacier Point parking area
▶2	0.1	Left at south end geology hut loop
▶3	0.25	Glacier Point
▶4	0.3	Left at north end geology hut loop
▶5	0.5	Return to Glacier Point parking area

Four Mile Trail

This trail provides a very scenic descent to Yosemite Valley—a descent that will acquaint you with the valley's main features, giving you perfect views of the Yosemite Falls sequence and a personally experienced feel for the valley's 3,000-foot depth. This hike is rated easy because not much energy is expended, but it is hard on the knees. You can also hike the route in reverse, and those in good shape may choose to combine an ascent of the Four Mile Trail and a descent of the Panorama Trail for a truly exhilarating day.

Maps

This trail is covered by the Tom Harrison *Yosemite Valley* map (1:24,000 scale), the National Geographic Trails Illustrated *#306 Yosemite SW* map (1:40,000 scale), and the USGS *Yosemite Valley* map (1:24,000 scale).

Best Time

Because the view of Yosemite Falls is the centerpiece of this walk, the best time to visit is most certainly when Yosemite Falls are at their greatest, about late April–June. However, the road to Glacier Point may not be open before mid- to late May—make sure you know its status before planning your hike. During the month of July, the falls diminish appreciably, are wispy in August, and usually gone in September. Note as well that the Four Mile Trail is closed at its Yosemite Valley terminus in winter and early spring because it can be quite icy.

TRAIL USE
Day Hike

LENGTH
4.7 miles, 2–4 hours

VERTICAL FEET
One-way: +60', –3,290'

DIFFICULTY
– 1 **2** 3 4 5 +

TRAIL TYPE
Point-to-Point

FEATURES
Canyon
Waterfall
Great Views
Steep
Geological Interest

FACILITIES
Bear Boxes
Restrooms
Store
Tour Bus Stop
Water

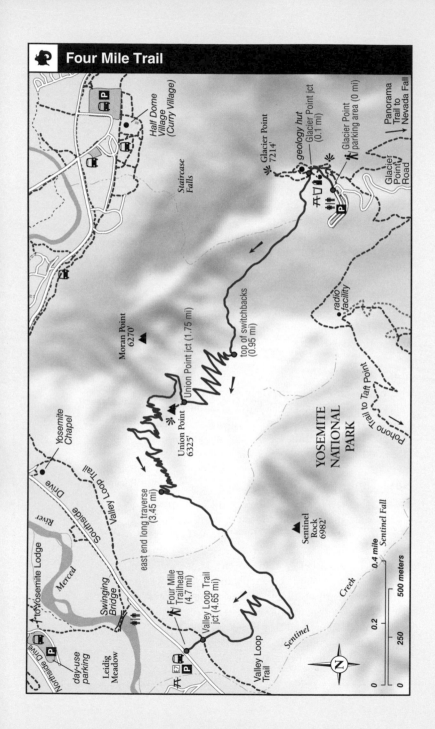

Four Mile Trail

Half Dome Village (Curry Village)

P

Staircase Falls

Glacier Point 7214'

geology hut

Glacier Point jct (0.1 mi)

Glacier Point parking area (0 mi)

Panorama Trail to Nevada Fall

Glacier Point Road

P

radio facility

top of switchbacks (0.95 mi)

Moran Point 6270'

Union Point jct (1.75 mi)

Union Point 6325'

Pohono Trail to Taft Point

YOSEMITE NATIONAL PARK

Yosemite Chapel

Valley Loop Trail

east end long traverse (3.45 mi)

Sentinel Rock 6982'

Sentinel Fall

Southside Drive

Merced River

to Yosemite Lodge

Swinging Bridge

Four Mile Trailhead (4.7 mi)

Valley Loop Trail jct (4.65 mi)

Valley Loop Trail

Sentinel Creek

Northside Drive

day-use parking

P

Leidig Meadow

N

0   0.2   0.4 mile

0   250   500 meters

Finding the Trail

From a signed junction along Wawona Road, drive 15.5 miles up Glacier Point Road to its end; the hike starts from the road-end parking area. On the Yosemite Valley end, the trailhead is located on Southside Drive just east of the Sentinel Beach Picnic area. This is 3.2 miles beyond where CA 41 (from Wawona) merges with Southside Drive. The trailhead is also served by the El Capitan shuttle route—it is stop E7. There is limited trailhead parking, so if you have a car and are hiking *up* this route, note there is additional parking just west of the Yosemite Valley Lodge in the Yosemite Falls day-use parking area, stop E2 on the El Capitan shuttle route and stop 7 on the Valley shuttle route. You can either walk 0.6 mile south to the trailhead along a bike path and then, once across the Merced River, briefly west along the Valley Loop Trail, or

Before building the Yosemite Falls Trail (Trail 30), John Conway first worked on this trail, completing it in 1872. Originally about 4 miles long, it was rebuilt and lengthened in 1929, but the trail's name stuck.

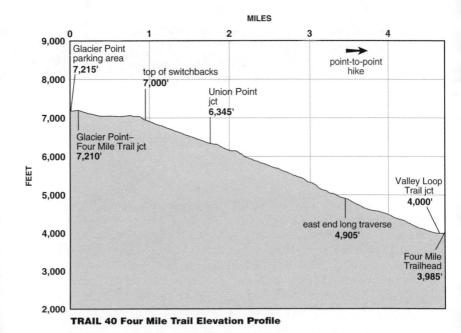

TRAIL 40 Four Mile Trail Elevation Profile

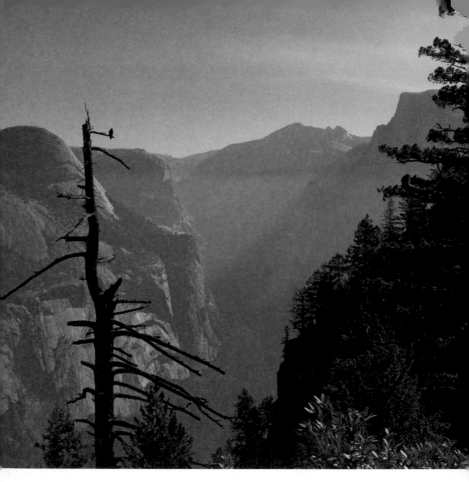

Eastern portions of Yosemite Valley *as seen near the top of the Four Mile Trail*

take the El Capitan shuttle bus. There is a water faucet next to the Glacier Point store, near the start of the walk.

Logistics

Because most people do this hike in one direction, you have a transport problem to solve. Rather than roping a friend into driving you to Glacier Point, it is better to take a Yosemite tour bus up to Glacier Point. In the past it has made two morning trips up to the point, giving you ample time to complete your hike. Check the bus schedule in the *Yosemite Guide,* a free newsletter presented to tourists at all park entrance stations. An alternative is to hike up and down this route (doubling the distance) or pair an ascent of the Four Mile Trail with a descent of the Panorama Trail (Trail 41).

Trail Description

Our trail starts at the northeastern corner of the large Glacier Point parking lot ▶1 and then trends past the northeastern (right) side of a concession-aire's shop, which, along with other minor structures, replaced the grand Glacier Point Hotel. This three-story hotel, together with the adjacent historic Mountain House—built in 1873—burned to the ground in July 1969. If this is your first time to Glacier Point, you will most certainly want to head to the vista point first (Trail 39)—I still do—but then take a left turn (0.1 mile) ▶2 that takes you down a staircase to the marked start of the Four Mile Trail.

If you had been on this trail on some early morning from the 1970s until 1990, when hang gliders were banned, you could have seen pilots land in meadows below you, taking sky trails from Glacier Point to the valley floor.

Beyond, you enter a shady bowl whose white firs and sugar pines usually harbor snow patches into late May or June. You then contour northwest, eventually emerging from forest shade and, looking east, see unglaciated Glacier Point's two overhanging rocks capping a vertical wall.

Soon you curve northwest, veer in and out of a cool gully, and continue along the nearly flat view-rich route. As the trail sidles in and out of gullies, adjusting its aspect, you exchange more easterly views of Royal Arches, Washington Column, and North Dome for those of Yosemite Falls, the Three Brothers, El Capitan, and Sentinel Rock. Indeed your valley views evolve continually on this walk because you are sidling west-ward as well as descending; use the changing height and shape of Sentinel Rock to gauge your downward progress.

Skirting around a descending ridge, the switchbacks then begin (0.95 mile), ▶3 and where gravel lies on hard tread, you can easily take a minor spill if you're not careful. Chinquapin, greenleaf manzanita, and huckleberry oak dominate the first dozen switchback legs, thereby giving you unobstructed panoramas, though making the hike a hot one for anyone ascending from the valley floor on a summer afternoon. The switchbacks end at a junction (1.75 miles) ▶4 with a short spur trail to Union Point. It is a beautiful viewpoint and the 0.1 mile to its ter-minus is worth the effort—though I'll admit you will see similar views along the main trail. On the main trail, bear right and duck east into a gully shaded by conifers that censor your views. Two long switchbacks through the shaded bowl lead back to rockier, drier terrain—and more tight switchbacks.

About midway down the series of switchbacks, canyon live oaks begin to compete with white firs and Douglas-firs, and your view is occasionally obstructed by their dense, opaque canopy. After descending two-thirds of the vertical distance to the valley floor, the switchbacks temporarily end (3.45 miles). ►5 A long, steady descent now ensues, mostly past canyon live oaks, whose curved-upward trunks are their response to creeping talus, deposits of rockfall from above.

Gaps in the vegetation continue to provide views of Yosemite Valley. At this elevation, about 1,000 feet above the valley floor, are, in my opinion, the Goldilocks views; they are just right. You aren't so high that you are looking straight down, flattening the landscape, and you aren't so low that you simply stare up, similarly lacking in perspective. Instead, you are effectively floating in the middle of the valley and simultaneously appreciate the enormity of the granite walls and the shapes of the individual features. To the west are Cathedral Rocks (on the left) and El Capitan (on the right), and straight ahead is the alcove holding Yosemite Falls. Looking down to Leidig Meadow and the surrounding forests, those towering conifers continue to look remarkably tiny.

Soon black oaks and incense cedars appear, and beyond, you cross a creeklet that usually flows until early July. Your steady descent again enters oak cover, and you skirt below the base of imposing but now largely hidden Sentinel Rock. At last a final group of switchbacks guides you down to a straightaway that soon intersects the valley floor's Valley Loop Trail (4.65 miles), ►6 and just beyond you reach your endpoint, the Four Mile Trailhead on Southside Drive (4.7 miles). ►7

🚶 MILESTONES

►1	0.0	Start from Glacier Point parking area
►2	0.1	Left at Glacier Point–Four Mile Trail junction
►3	0.95	Top of switchbacks
►4	1.75	Right at Union Point junction
►5	3.45	Eastern end of long traverse
►6	4.65	Straight ahead at Valley Loop Trail junction
►7	4.7	Finish at Four Mile Trailhead in Yosemite Valley

Panorama Trail

This is the most scenic of all trails descending to the floor of Yosemite Valley, passing three waterfalls and offering spectacular views along the way. Either take a bus up to Glacier Point or have someone drop you there and meet you down at Half Dome Village (Curry Village). I have also combined this walk with the Four Mile Trail many times, ascending the Four Mile Trail in the cool morning hours and then descending via the Panorama Trail.

Maps

This trail is covered by the Tom Harrison *Yosemite Valley* map (1:24,000 scale), the National Geographic Trails Illustrated *#306 Yosemite SW* map (1:40,000 scale), and the USGS *Yosemite Valley* map (1:24,000 scale).

Best Time

All of the trail is usually snow-free by early June and can be walked anytime until Glacier Point Road closes, usually in late October. While the granite walls look similarly colossal all year—maybe even becoming more fabulous in the lower-elevation sunlight of early fall—the volume of water spilling down Nevada and Vernal Falls peaks in June, remains impressive through July, and then diminishes notably through August.

Finding the Trail

From a signed junction along Wawona Road, drive 15.5 miles up Glacier Point Road to its end; the hike starts from the road-end parking area. The

TRAIL USE
Day Hike
LENGTH
8.65 miles, 4–6 hours
VERTICAL FEET
One-way:
+1,000', –4,190'
DIFFICULTY
– 1 2 **3** 4 5 +
TRAIL TYPE
Point-to-Point

FEATURES
Canyon
Stream
Waterfall
Wildflowers
Great Views
Steep

FACILITIES
Bear Boxes
Restrooms
Store
Tour Bus Stop
Water

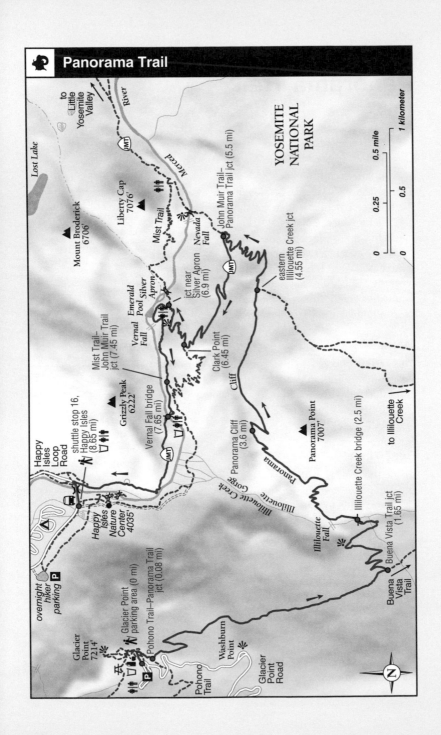

Panorama Trail

to Little Yosemite Valley

Lost Lake

River

Merced

JMT

YOSEMITE NATIONAL PARK

Liberty Cap 7076'

Mount Broderick 6706'

Mist Trail

Nevada Fall

John Muir Trail– Panorama Trail jct (5.5 mi)

eastern Illilouette Creek jct (4.55 mi)

Emerald Pool   Silver Apron

jct near Silver Apron (6.9 mi)

JMT

Vernal Fall

Mist Trail– John Muir Trail jct (7.45 mi)

Clark Point (6.45 mi)

Panorama Cliff

Grizzly Peak 6222'

shuttle stop 16, Happy Isles (8.65 mi)

Vernal Fall bridge (7.65 mi)

Panorama Cliff (3.6 mi)

Panorama Point 7007'

JMT

Panorama

Happy Isles Loop Road

Illilouette Creek bridge (2.5 mi)

Happy Isles Nature Center 4035'

Illilouette Creek Gorge

Illilouette Fall

to Illilouette Creek

overnight hiker parking P

Glacier Point parking area (0 mi)

Pohono Trail–Panorama Trail jct (0.08 mi)

Buena Vista Trail jct (1.65 mi)

Buena Vista Trail

Washburn Point

Glacier Point 7214'

Pohono Trail

Glacier Point Road

N

1 kilometer

0.5 mile

0.5

0.25

0.5

0

0

trail's end is located at Happy Isles, Yosemite Valley shuttle stop 16, along Happy Isles Loop Road. Because this road is closed to vehicular traffic, except the shuttle buses, you must take the shuttle bus back to your car, campsite, or other Yosemite Valley lodging at the end of the walk.

Gravels just above the brink of Illilouette Fall are remnants of a thick accumulation created when the last glacier formed a low ice dam across the creek's mouth.

Logistics

Because most people do this hike in one direction, you have a transport problem to solve. Rather than roping a friend into driving you to Glacier Point, it is better to take a Yosemite tour bus up to Glacier Point. In the past it has made two morning trips up to the point, giving you ample time to complete your hike. Check the bus schedule in the *Yosemite Guide,* a newsletter presented to tourists at all park entrance stations. An alternative is, of course, to hike up and down this route (doubling the distance) or to combine an ascent of the Four Mile Trail (Trail 40) with a descent of the Panorama Trail. There is a water faucet next to the Glacier Point store, near the start of the walk.

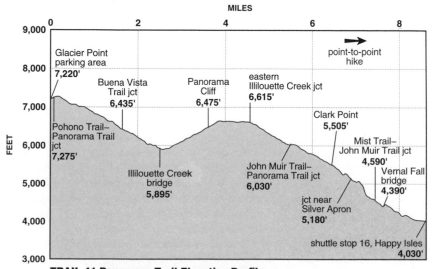

TRAIL 41 Panorama Trail Elevation Profile

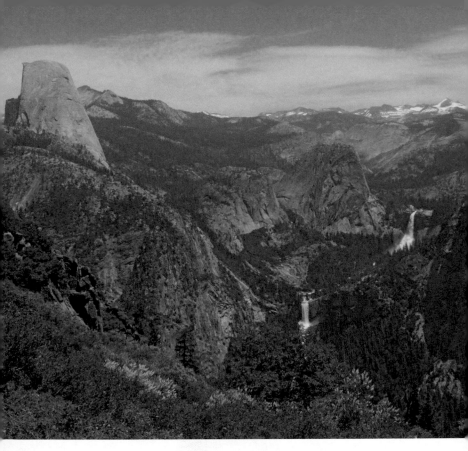

The scene east *to Half Dome, Vernal Fall, Nevada Fall, and up the Merced River canyon*

Trail Description

Just east of the entrance to the Glacier Point parking lot, ▶1 you take a trail that starts south to an amphitheater pointing east toward Vernal and Nevada Falls and, continuing south, quickly reaches a fork (0.08 mile). ▶2 The Pohono Trail veers right, but you trend left, on the Panorama Trail, climbing a bit more before starting a moderate descent, mostly with grand views to the east. A 1986 natural fire blackened most of the forest from near the trailhead to just beyond the upcoming Buena Vista Trail junction, with only patches of trees surviving. In the open areas, black oaks are thriving, and shrubs have regenerated with a vengeance. Between charred trunks are occasional great views of Half Dome, Mount Broderick, Liberty Cap, Nevada Fall, and Mount Starr King. Views become more restricted as you descend, and eventually you meet the Buena Vista Trail (1.65 miles). ▶3

Your trail branches left and switchbacks down. At the northern end of the third zigzag, this one a little longer than the first two, an indistinct spur trail goes a few steps below the trail to a viewpoint. Here, from atop an overhanging cliff, you have an unobstructed view of 370-foot-high Illilouette Fall, which splashes just 600 feet away over a low point on the rim of massive Panorama Cliff. Behind it Half Dome rises boldly, while above Illilouette Creek, Mount Starr King rises even higher. This is not a vista point to be missed, for Illilouette Fall, nestled in a narrow alcove, mostly hides itself from view. The trail makes one final switchback, ducks back into conifer cover alongside Illilouette Creek, and then crosses the creek on a wide bridge, wisely placed upstream of the fall (2.5 miles). ►4 Illilouette Creek looks tempting for cooling your feet or for wading, but be forewarned that it could carry you swiftly downstream and over the fall.

Now sidling north just above the creek's banks, your trail climbs gradually, soon passes above the brink of Illilouette Fall, and then starts a major climb of the slopes above the extensive Panorama Cliff. Various other spur trails trend toward the lip of the cliff, but none provides much view in return. The trail first climbs briefly along the rim, then switchbacks away from the cliff edge, once again returning to the rim as you round Panorama Point. A former viewpoint at this location was undermined, in part, by a monstrous rockfall that broke loose during the winter of 1968–69; it is wise to remain a few steps back from the edge. Where the trail cuts quite close to the cliff is a superlative panorama extending from Upper Yosemite Fall east past Royal Arches, Washington Column, and North Dome to Half Dome (3.6 miles). ►5

Your moderate climb ends after 200 more feet of elevation gain, and then you descend gently to the rim for some more views, now dominated by the monuments to the east: Half Dome, Mount Broderick, Liberty Cap, Clouds Rest, and Nevada Fall. As a word of caution, the John Muir Trail (JMT) near Vernal Fall is exactly at the bottom of this cliff; I have been aghast to watch people throw rocks and sticks off the edge here, unaware either of the trail beneath them or of the standard etiquette that you never launch anything off a cliff because you don't know what is beneath you. Your contour ends at a junction with a trail up Illilouette Creek, leading to locations including the Merced Pass lakes; you turn left toward Nevada Fall (4.55 miles). ►6

Beyond the trail junction you make a mile-long, switchbacking, generally viewless descent through conifer forest—soft underfoot in comparison to the gravelly trail cover so far. In spring, patches of western azaleas with large, light pink flowers delight your senses. You pass slabs on which is a low rock wall, once built to divert runoff away from the unseen JMT located at the base of the cliff face. Beyond is a trail split, each branch descending a few steps to the JMT (5.5 miles). ▶7 Your route is to the left, but I suggest that you first take an extra detour right and walk over to the nearby brink of roaring Nevada Fall, a round-trip distance of about 0.4 mile. Just a few steps beyond the Nevada Fall bridge, you can strike northwest to find a short spur trail that drops to a viewpoint beside the fall's brink. This viewpoint's railing is seen from the fall's bridge, thereby giving you an idea of where the trail ends. Note that the round-trip distance for this detour is not included in the total trip distance.

From the Panorama Trail–JMT junction, you now turn west (left) and begin a descent to Happy Isles, starting with a high traverse along a trail blasted into the rock. A stout rock wall protects you from the possibility of a slide, so you can instead imbibe the ever-changing panorama of domelike Liberty Cap and broad-topped Mount Broderick—both once overridden by glaciers. As you progress west, Half Dome becomes prominent. All the while, Nevada Fall decorates the foreground, its water dancing and churning down through the air. Eventually you descend to Clark Point (6.45 miles), ▶8 where the JMT continues left down rocky, cobbled switchbacks, while I direct you right, to take the connector trail toward the Mist Trail. If your knees are tired, the JMT is a slightly easier route, lacking the endless steps of the Mist Trail past Vernal Fall. However, there is often sand and gravel overlaying the rocky base, and I find it the more treacherous of the two choices. As for distance, my current estimate indicates that both are the same length to the nearest 0.01 mile—take your choice!

As you descend toward the top of Vernal Fall, you soon come across a switchback where you will understand my attraction to this trail segment—this trail is following the top of the cliff directly atop the Mist Trail (absolutely don't throw any rocks) and you get to stare straight at Vernal Fall from a near-aerial perspective. As this lookout is not fenced, just stay a few steps back from the edge. Continuing down switchbacks, you reach a T-junction with the Mist Trail near the rock slabs termed the Silver Apron (6.9 miles); ▶9 turn left, soon passing Emerald Pool and finding yourself at the brink of Vernal Fall.

Following the crowds, you trend left, climb briefly, and are funneled into a fenced passageway leading you to a gully south of Vernal Fall. Now begin the infamous Mist Trail stairs. Down, down, down, much

of the time on big blocky stairs. The first few flights of stairs are under
conifer cover, emerging on a flatter traverse where it is mandatory to
stop, admire, and photograph Vernal Fall. In spring and early summer
this is the last location you can safely take out a nonwaterproof camera,
and oglers are often treated to a double rainbow in Vernal Fall's spray.
The stairs continue down this verdant route, the spray soaking until you
cross an exposed stretch of slab and reenter forest cover. Continuing
along the banks of the Merced River, you reach another junction with the
JMT (7.45 miles), ▶10 where you continue straight ahead, soon reaching
a bridge across the Merced with yet another stupendous view of Vernal
Fall (7.65 miles). ▶11

With the density of people increasing with proximity to Happy Isles,
you now descend a paved trail around unseen Sierra Point. Passing
through scrub oak forest, you soon round a corner with views back to
Illilouette Fall and Glacier Point—what a different perspective than you
had many miles ago when you were looking straight down. Before long
you reach Happy Isles Loop Road, turn left, and follow it to the shuttle
stop at Happy Isles (8.65 miles). ▶12

🚶	MILESTONES	
▶1	0.0	Start at Glacier Point parking area
▶2	0.08	Left at Pohono Trail–Panorama Trail junction
▶3	1.65	Left at Buena Vista Trail junction
▶4	2.5	Illilouette Creek bridge
▶5	3.6	Panorama Cliff
▶6	4.55	Left at eastern Illilouette Creek junction
▶7	5.5	Left at Panorama Trail–John Muir Trail junction
▶8	6.45	Right at Clark Point junction
▶9	6.9	Left at junction near the Silver Apron
▶10	7.45	Right at Mist Trail–John Muir Trail junction
▶11	7.65	Vernal Fall bridge
▶12	8.65	Finish at shuttle stop 16, Happy Isles

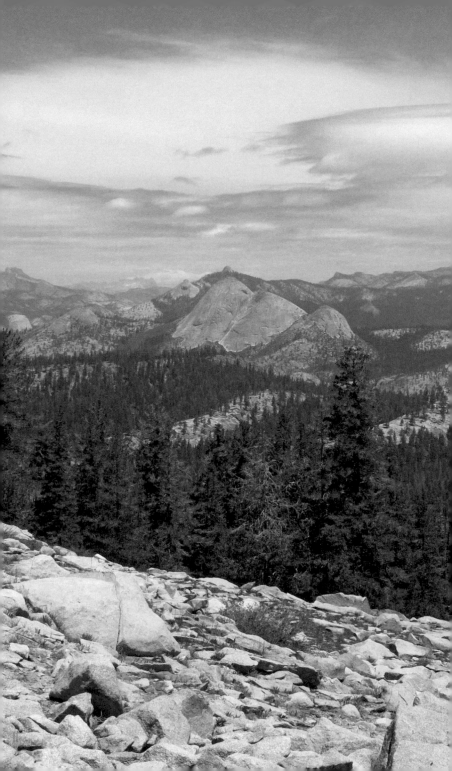

CHAPTER 7

South Yosemite

South Yosemite, as covered in this book, includes the region bounded to the north by Glacier Point Road, to the west by Wawona Road (CA 41), to the south by Beasore Road in Sierra National Forest, and to the east by steep mountainous terrain, a broad swath of land. South Yosemite mirrors chapter 4's Northwest Yosemite in its relative solitude, except for a few very popular destinations (covered in this book of course). Like Northwest Yosemite, this area has a smattering of lakes, some waterfalls, and a grove of giant sequoias. The trails between Glacier Point Road and the Wawona area are mostly quite forested—being less ostentatiously showy, they appeal more to hikers keen on a quiet forest walk. Several loops take in this scenery but are not included here. If this landscape appeals to you, consider a walk from Wawona up Chilnualna Fall to Royal Arch and Buena Vista Lake; it is described in the companion book, *Yosemite National Park: A Complete Hiker's Guide.*

Instead, included in the book are a collection of lake destinations and the unmissable Mariposa Grove of Big Trees. Ostrander Lake is a favorite destination because a quite moderate walk leads to a stunning subalpine lake setting that is much less crowded than those in the Tuolumne Meadows area. The two walks starting just outside the park in a western part of Ansel Adams Wilderness traverse stunning scenery, but the long drive up lengthy forest service roads to the trailhead diminishes their popularity. They are the Lillian Lakes loop and a long loop over Isberg Pass into the southeastern reaches of Yosemite National Park. It is the Mariposa Grove of Big Trees, however, that is the prime attraction in this region, located just south of the South Fork Merced River canyon. This grove is unique in that it has a network of trails among the giant sequoias; no such trail system exists at the park's two other groves, the Tuolumne and Merced. Until 2015 most visitors here rode trams on a road that wound through the grove. Now discontinued, the grove's trails have just been restored and rebuilt, providing better-built trails for visiting the lower grove and enhancing everyone's experience in the upper grove—and most important, reducing the impact on sequoias.

Opposite: *From Horizon Ridge, look east to see Mount Starr King and the Clark Range (see Trail 42, page 368).*

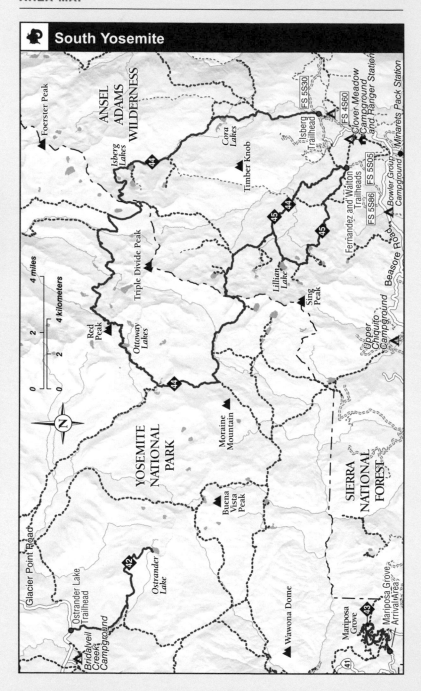

South Yosemite

ANSEL
ADAMS
WILDERNESS

Foerster Peak

Isberg
Lakes

Cora
Lakes

Timber Knob

FS 5S30

FS 4S60

Isberg
Trailhead

Clover Meadow
Campground
and Ranger Station

Minarets Pack Station

44

Fernandez and Walton
Trailheads

FS 5S05

Bowler Group
Campground

FS 5S86

Beasore Road

44

45

45

Triple Divide Peak

Lillian
Lake

Sing
Peak

Red
Peak

Ottoway
Lakes

Upper
Chiquito
Campground

44

4 miles

4 kilometers

2

2

0

0

N

YOSEMITE
NATIONAL
PARK

Moraine
Mountain

SIERRA
NATIONAL
FOREST

Buena
Vista
Peak

Glacier Point Road

42

Ostrander
Lake

Ostrander Lake
Trailhead

Wawona Dome

Mariposa
Grove

43

Mariposa Grove
Arrival Area

Bridalveil
Creek
Campground

41

South Yosemite

Trail	Difficulty	Length	Type	USES & ACCESS	TERRAIN	NATURE	OTHER
42	3	12.5	Point-to-Point	Day Hiking, Backpacking, Horses, Running, Child-Friendly	Lake		Great Views, Camping, Geological Interest
43	2	5.8	Loop	Day Hiking, Child-Friendly		Wildflowers, Giant Sequoias	Historical Interest
44	5	44.1	Point-to-Point	Backpacking, Horses, Running	Canyon, Lake, Stream	Wildflowers	Great Views, Camping, Secluded, Granite Slabs, Geological Interest
45	3–4	12.2	Loop	Day Hiking, Backpacking, Horses, Running, Child-Friendly	Lake	Wildflowers	Great Views, Camping, Swimming, Secluded, Granite Slabs, Geological Interest

TYPE
- Point-to-Point
- Loop
- Out-and-Back
- Balloon

DIFFICULTY
– 1 2 3 4 5 +
less   more

USES & ACCESS
- Day Hiking
- Backpacking
- Horses
- Running
- Wheelchair Access
- Stroller Access
- Child-Friendly
- Caution

TERRAIN
- Canyon
- Summit
- Lake
- Stream
- Waterfall

NATURE
- Autumn Colors
- Wildflowers
- Giant Sequoias

FEATURES
- Great Views
- Camping
- Swimming
- Secluded
- Steep
- Granite Slabs
- Historical Interest
- Geological Interest

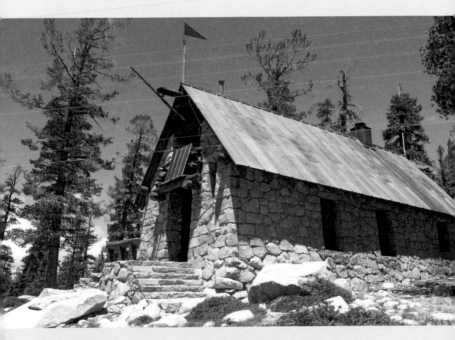

Ostrander Lake ski hut *(see Trail 42, page 368)*

South Yosemite

Ostrander Lake, one of Yosemite's most easily reached high-elevation lakes at which camping is permitted, is a popular destination for backpackers. It is a similarly popular day hike objective because it is achievable as a long day's excursion for the many people staying in Yosemite Valley. It is also popular in winter and spring with cross-country skiers due to the ski hut at the lake.

Mariposa Grove is Yosemite's largest grove of giant sequoias, or *Wawona,* as the American Indians called them, and this loop winds past all the grove's highlights. In the past, hikers kept crossing paths with a road carrying ubiquitous green trams that ferried the majority of visitors around on guided tours. The tours were discontinued in 2015, so all visitors now admire these majestic giants on foot, providing a quieter ambience to absorb the trees' grandeur. This loop follows a trail that is in part the route of the old tram road (pavement now removed for more pleasant walking) and elsewhere the so-called perimeter loop. Signs at the start describe many other variants of this loop, if you'd prefer a longer or shorter alternative.

All cars, save those with a handicap placard, now park in a large lot near Yosemite's south entrance station, the Mariposa Grove Welcome Plaza. From there a free shuttle bus ferries visitors to the Grove Arrival Area, near the location of the old tram departure kiosk and parking.

Isberg–Red Peak– Fernandez Passes Loop 381

TRAIL 44

Backpack, Horse
44.1 miles,
Point-to-Point
Difficulty: 1 2 3 4 **5**

Crossing four passes over 44 miles, this loop introduces you to many of southern Yosemite's highlights. Though well traveled during the summer months, these trails will never be crowded because they are a long drive up a small road and are not part of any of the popular long-distance trails running the length of the Sierra; everyone you will see on the trail has planned a trip explicitly to visit this location. With permits relatively easy to come by, endless lakes for swimming or relaxing, superb views from the passes, and some beautiful rocks, this is a perfect loop for someone wishing to delve a little deeper into Yosemite's backcountry.

Vanderburgh–Lillian Lakes Loop . . . 402

TRAIL 45

Day Hike, Backpack,
Horse, Run,
Child-Friendly
12.2 miles, Loop
Difficulty: 1 2 **3 4** 5

If you are in shape, you could hike this entire circuit in one day without overexerting yourself. However, it is so scenic that three days are recommended—sufficient time to visit the lakes not lying on the main circuit, Lady and Chittenden Lakes. Visiting both of these desirable lakes and exploring the trailside gems, Vanderburgh, Staniford, and Lillian, lengthens your route to about 16 miles, adds about 700 feet of ascent and descent, and changes its classification to a moderate three-day hike. Alternatively, for some folks a trip just to Vanderburgh Lake—the first lake you'll encounter—is a worthy goal in itself, ideal for novice backpackers, day hikers, or those with children.

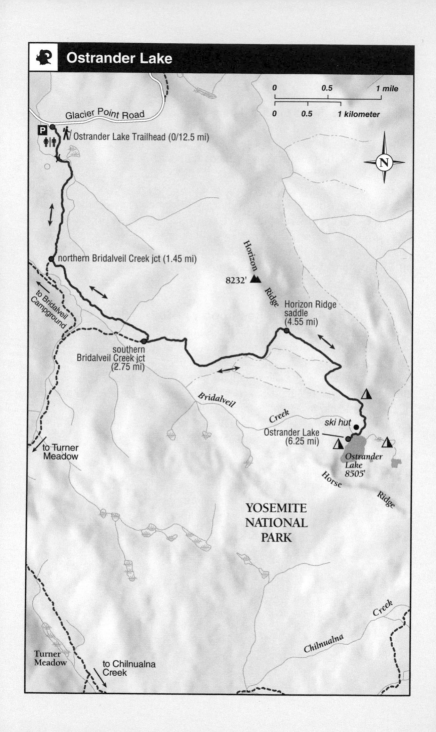

Ostrander Lake

0   0.5   1 mile

0   0.5   1 kilometer

N

Glacier Point Road

Ostrander Lake Trailhead (0/12.5 mi)

Horizon Ridge

8232'

Horizon Ridge saddle (4.55 mi)

northern Bridalveil Creek jct (1.45 mi)

to Bridalveil Campground

southern Bridalveil Creek jct (2.75 mi)

Bridalveil

Creek

ski hut

Ostrander Lake (6.25 mi)

to Turner Meadow

Ostrander Lake 8505'

Horse

Ridge

YOSEMITE NATIONAL PARK

Turner Meadow

to Chilnualna Creek

Chilnualna   Creek

Ostrander Lake

Ostrander Lake, one of Yosemite's most easily reached high-elevation lakes at which camping is permitted, is a popular destination for backpackers. It is a similarly popular day hike objective because it is achievable as a long day's excursion for the many people staying in Yosemite Valley. It is also popular in winter and spring with cross-country skiers due to the ski hut at the lake.

Permits

Overnight visitors require a wilderness permit for the Ostrander Lake Trailhead, issued by Yosemite National Park. Pick up your wilderness permit at the Yosemite Valley Wilderness Center, Big Oak Flat Entrance Station, or Wawona Visitor Center.

Maps

This trail is covered by the Tom Harrison *Yosemite High Country* map (1:63,360 scale), the National Geographic Trails Illustrated #306 *Yosemite SW* map (1:40,000 scale), and the USGS 7.5-minute series *Half Dome* map (1:24,000 scale).

Best Time

All of the trail is usually snow-free by late June. It is not a trail particularly distinguished by its wildflower display, so it is best to wait until mid-July or August to avoid mosquitoes. By September, Ostrander Lake is too cool for pleasant swimming, but it is still a very desirable destination through early October. Major storms aren't likely in this period, but if one hit, you could get out in 2 or 3 hours.

TRAIL USE
Day Hike, Backpack, Horse, Run, Child-Friendly

LENGTH
12.5 miles, 6–9 hours (over 1–2 days)

VERTICAL FEET
One-way: +1,710', –200'
Round-trip: ±1,910'

DIFFICULTY
– 1 2 **3** 4 5 +

TRAIL TYPE
Out-and-Back

FEATURES
Lake
Great Views
Camping
Geological Interest

FACILITIES
Bear Boxes
Campground
Toilets

369

Ostranger Lake is at the headwaters of Bridalveil Creek, which produces Bridalveil Fall. In early days, the fall was known as Pohono, and its source, Pohono Lake.

Finding the Trail

Turn onto Glacier Point Road (from Wawona Road, CA 41) at a well-signed junction. There is a large pullout with water and toilets at this junction. Drive 8.9 miles up Glacier Point Road to a turnoff on your right. This parking area is 1.2 miles past the spur road to Bridalveil Creek Campground, the only campground along Glacier Point Road. The closest water faucet is at the Bridalveil Creek Campground.

Trail Description

From Glacier Point Road ▶1 you start along the route of a former jeep road and soon encounter the first of several thickets of lodgepole pines. This area was badly burned in the 1987 Lost Bear Fire, making these trees about 30 years old as of my writing. The first trees are now producing cones, and the stand will slowly thin in the coming decade—except where the Empire Fire, burning patches in this area in late 2017, has reset the clock. Along the east side of the trail, more of the young lodgepole cover survives, and in time, red fir will begin to emerge, replacing the lodgepole over a century. Passing through these thickets of trees, you cross a sluggish creek on a small bridge and then amble an easy mile, passing in and out of an assortment of meadows, to

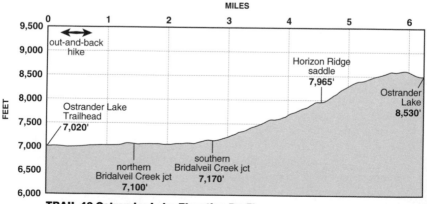

TRAIL 42 Ostrander Lake Elevation Profile

reach a ridge junction (1.45 miles). ▶2 From it a short lateral right drops to Bridalveil Creek—possibly a difficult June crossing—then climbs equally briefly to the Bridalveil Creek Trail. You turn left, continuing on the main trail.

Your route now contours southeast past unseen Lost Bear Meadow and after a mile makes a short ascent east along a trickling creek to its crossing. You are now back in burned territory, and if you're wondering why the young trees are somewhat different heights from those you passed earlier, it is because you've just passed through landscape burned in a 1985 fire. The trail next crosses an area burned in 1999, and at the creek crossing it is in a patch burned in the 1988 Horizon Fire. And once again, the Empire Fire left an additional footprint in 2017, here burning more intensively on the east side of the trail. The areas burned by each fire sometimes interfinger and overlay each other, creating a remarkable mosaic of tree ages. Just beyond the ford your route curves west to a junction (2.75 miles) ▶3 with a second lateral that branches right to Bridalveil Creek and then to the Bridalveil Creek Trail; you stay left. Though you are now about halfway to Ostrander Lake, you've climbed very little, and from this junction you face 1,500 feet of vertical gain, continuing through a mixture of burned and mature forest.

The steepening trail climbs east in places through patches of intact forest, over open slabs with views of the Bridalveil Creek basin, and in long stretches through more severely burnt territory. The culverts diverting water beneath the trail are a giveaway that this trail wasn't just constructed for foot traffic. You then curve southeast into a Jeffrey pine stand before climbing east through a white-fir forest, dotted with bright-red snow plants, should you be making a late-June excursion. As you climb to the top of a saddle that bisects Horizon Ridge, red firs largely supplant the white fir forests that dominate at lower elevations (4.55 miles). ▶4

Climbing southeast, your track ascends straight up the not-too-steep nose of Horizon Ridge on broken slabs. You now enjoy your first expansive views of the walk, staring north to Mount Hoffmann and northeast to Half Dome. Partway up, it quite surprisingly passes through patches of sagebrush and elsewhere through the more common pine-mat manzanita. About 400 feet above your first saddle is a second one, and the trail first switchbacks and then curves up to a third. From it the trail makes a momentary descent southeast before bending to start a short, final ascent south into unburned forest surrounding Ostrander Lake. Near this bend you get far-ranging views across the Illilouette Creek basin. You can see the tops of Royal Arches and Washington Column and, above and east of them, North, Basket, and Half Domes. Behind Half Dome stands the park's geographic center, broad-topped Mount Hoffmann. Reigning over the Illilouette Creek basin is Mount Starr King and its entourage of lesser domes. To the east and northeast the jagged crest of the Clark Range cuts the sky. If you wanted to carry water up from the lake, sandy patches east of the trail would make stunning campsites—and likely be virtually mosquito free at all times.

Beyond is a short, final ascent south, and then you drop quickly to Ostrander Hut, on the north shore of Ostrander Lake (6.25 miles). ▶5 When it is snowbound, cross-country skiers can stay in it with prior reservations, by lottery. The hut is on a rocky moraine left by a glacier that retreated perhaps 16,000 years ago. Behind it, lying in a bedrock basin, is 25-acre, trout-populated Ostrander Lake. The jointed escarpment of Horse Ridge drops precipitously into the lake. Camping is good along the west shore or on a shelf a bit east of the lake. After a restful stay, return the same way to the Ostrander Lake Trailhead (12.5 miles). ▶6

🚶	**MILESTONES**	
▶1	0.0	Start at Ostrander Lake Trailhead
▶2	1.45	Left at northern Bridalveil Creek junction
▶3	2.75	Left at southern Bridalveil Creek junction
▶4	4.55	Reach saddle on Horizon Ridge
▶5	6.25	Ostrander Lake
▶6	12.5	Return to Ostrander Lake Trailhead

Mariposa Grove of Big Trees

The Mariposa Grove is Yosemite's largest grove of giant sequoias, or *Wawona*, as the American Indians called them, and this loop winds past all the grove's highlights. In the past, hikers kept crossing paths with a road carrying ubiquitous green trams that ferried the majority of visitors around on guided tours. The tours were discontinued in 2014, so all visitors now admire these majestic giants on foot, providing a quieter ambience to absorb the trees' grandeur. This loop follows a trail that is in part the route of the old tram road (the pavement has been removed for more pleasant walking) and elsewhere the Perimeter Trail. Signs at the start describe many other variants of this route, if you prefer a longer or shorter alternative.

All cars, save those with a handicap placard, now park in a large lot near Yosemite's south entrance station, the Mariposa Grove Welcome Plaza. From there a free, seasonal shuttle bus ferries visitors to the Mariposa Grove Arrival Area, near the location of the old tram departure kiosk and parking.

TRAIL USE
Day Hike,
Child-Friendly

LENGTH
5.8 miles, 3–4 hours

VERTICAL FEET
Round-trip: ±1,090'

DIFFICULTY
– 1 **2** 3 4 5 +

TRAIL TYPE
Balloon

FEATURES
Wildflowers
Giant Sequoias
Historical Interest

FACILITIES
Bear Boxes
Restrooms
Shuttle Stop
Water

Maps

This trail is covered by the Tom Harrison *Yosemite High Country* map (1:63,360 scale), the National Geographic Trails Illustrated #306 *Yosemite SW* map (1:40,000 scale), and the USGS 7.5-minute series *Mariposa Grove* map (1:24,000 scale). Also pick up a copy of the National Park Service brochure for the area, titled "Visiting the Mariposa Grove," before beginning your walk.

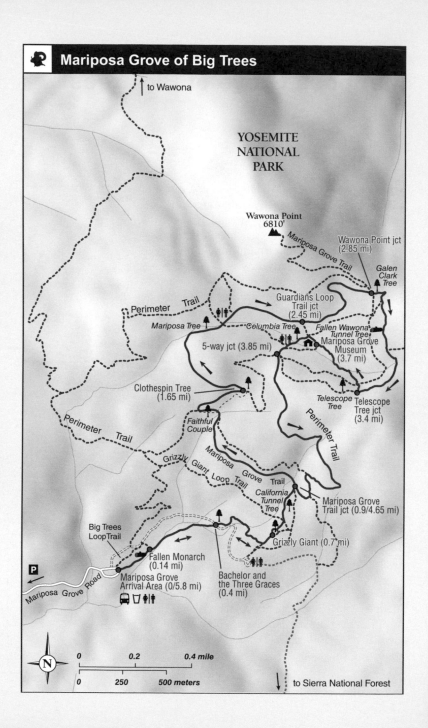

Mariposa Grove of Big Trees

to Wawona

YOSEMITE
NATIONAL
PARK

Wawona Point
6810'

Wawona Point jct
(2.85 mi)

Mariposa Grove Trail

Galen
Clark
Tree

Guardians Loop
Trail jct
(2.45 mi)

Perimeter Trail

Mariposa Tree

Columbia Tree

Fallen Wawona
Tunnel Tree

Mariposa Grove
Museum
(3.7 mi)

5-way jct (3.85 mi)

Clothespin Tree
(1.65 mi)

Telescope
Tree

Telescope
Tree jct
(3.4 mi)

Faithful
Couple

Perimeter Trail

Perimeter Trail

Grizzly Giant Loop Trail

Mariposa Grove Trail

California
Tunnel
Tree

Mariposa Grove
Trail jct (0.9/4.65 mi)

Big Trees
Loop Trail

Grizzly Giant (0.7 mi)

P

Fallen Monarch
(0.14 mi)

Mariposa Grove
Arrival Area (0/5.8 mi)

Bachelor and
the Three Graces
(0.4 mi)

Mariposa Grove Road

N

0   0.2   0.4 mile

0   250   500 meters

to Sierra National Forest

Best Time

Unless you are on skis or snowshoes, the Mariposa Grove is best visited no sooner than late May, when the snow has melted and grasses, wildflowers, and deciduous trees and shrubs have awoken from their long winter's slumber. Visitors in June and early July will be treated to a colorful wildflower display in the moister upper grove. As this is Yosemite's most-visited sequoia grove, expect crowds of people unless you visit early or late in the day. For a quieter experience, visit on a weekday, preferably not in June–August.

Giant sequoias grow in shallow soil because bedrock lies only a couple of feet down.

Finding the Trail

From the park's south entrance station along CA 41, drive north 400 feet to a junction with Mariposa Grove Road. Turn right, and almost immediately turn right again into the Mariposa Grove Welcome Plaza, where you park your car. From here, take a free shuttle bus to the trailhead. People with handicap placards can continue along the bus route to the Mariposa Grove Arrival Area; stop at the Welcome Plaza to receive more information about the regulations for handicap access. There are toilets and a water faucet in the parking area.

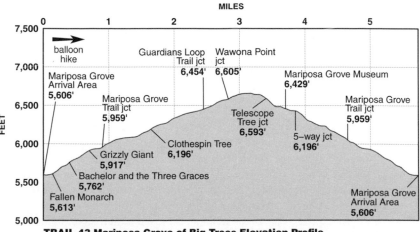

TRAIL 43 Mariposa Grove of Big Trees Elevation Profile

The Grizzly Giant has enough timber to build about 20 homes, but fortunately sequoia wood is very brittle, shattering when a tree falls— a feature that saved it from being logged into oblivion.

Trail Description

Two trails, a northern and a southern one, leave from the eastern, upper end of the Mariposa Grove parking lot. The northern (left) one leads to the Perimeter Trail, which leads to a junction with a trail that winds 4.75 miles down to Wawona.

Your route is instead the southern (right) trail, the Mariposa Grove Trail ▶1 (as well as the route of the Big Trees Loop and Grizzly Giant Loop Trails) toward the Fallen Monarch. The signs along the first stretch of this trail not only identify the notable sequoias but also educate you on their natural history, including bark, cones, fire, reproduction, and associated plants and animals.

Walking along a stretch of boardwalk installed to prevent countless feet from trampling the sequoias' shallow, sensitive roots, you reach the Fallen Monarch, which is largely intact, including its roots, despite having toppled more than 300 years ago. Near the Fallen Monarch is a junction (0.14 mile) ▶2 where the quite short Big Trees Loop Trail turns left, while you continue right, still following the Mariposa Grove Trail. The trail climbs to a crossing of the old tram road (0.4 mile). ▶3 At this spot stand the Bachelor and the Three Graces. Continuing up the winding trail, mostly following alongside a moist drainage, you reach the Grizzly Giant (0.7 mile). ▶4 Like the Leaning Tower of Pisa, this still-growing giant seems ready to fall any second, and one wonders how such a top-heavy, shallow-rooted specimen could have survived as long as it has. Though it's the largest tree in the park—and probably the oldest at between 1,900 and 2,400 years—there are at least 25 that are larger, mostly growing to the south in Sequoia National Park. It has a trunk volume of about 34,000 cubic feet, compared to about 52,500 cubic feet for the largest, the General Sherman, in Sequoia National Park's Giant Forest Grove.

Heading north from the east end of the enclosure circling the Grizzly Giant, leave the Mariposa Grove Trail, turning left to follow the Grizzly Giant Loop Trail for just 250 feet. Now branch right, and in a few steps reach the California Tunnel Tree, the only still-living tree through which a path was cut. It once had a deep burn, which was cut away in 1895 so that tourists could ride a stagecoach through it. Beyond this tree, head along the path to reach the broad trail that is the old tram road (0.9 mile),

▶5 and then turn left to follow it upward; signs indicate that you are back on the Mariposa Grove Trail.

Your upward route climbs diligently, but the wide, flat surface makes for pleasant walking. The northwest-trending trail quickly leaves the lower grove and climbs across a more exposed, hot slope not suitable for sequoias; quickly the conifer cover thins and shrubs dominate the surrounding slopes. Entering a small draw, you again reach a small cluster of giant trees, including the Faithful Couple, a pair of sequoias growing so close together that their trunks have merged at the base. Continuing on the old tram route, you pass a trail cutting in from the left and then switchback to the east, the path winding up the draw among scattered, mostly smaller sequoias. The next named waypoint is the Clothespin Tree, which bears a remarkable resemblance to its namesake due to severe fire damage (1.65 miles). ▶6 From here the old road switchbacks back to the left (your route), while a steeper route to the upper grove branches off to the right.

Completing a broad arc, you climb to the Mariposa Tree, marking the start of the upper grove; you will immediately notice that the trail's gradient subsides as you walk alongside a small rivulet and enjoy a cooler, more shaded environment. Just beyond is an X-junction, where left leads to the Perimeter Trail (and the trail to Wawona), right heads to the Mariposa Grove Cabin (a small museum), and you continue straight ahead. Passing a toilet, your route continues past additional small spurs to a junction where it merges with the Guardians Loop Trail (2.45 miles). ▶7 Do not be tempted to detour right to the Mariposa Grove Cabin, as your return route leads past it. Instead, continue up the Mariposa Grove Trail to another X-junction (2.85 miles). ▶8 Turning left leads 0.55 mile northwest to the summit of Wawona Point (the route of the Mariposa Grove Trail), a possible detour if you have spare time. No sequoias grow along this route, probably because of insufficient groundwater. From the point, you see the large, partly human-constructed meadow at Wawona to the northwest and the long, curving cliff of Wawona Dome, breaking a sea of green, to the north. Turning right is the Guardians Loop Trail, the continued route of the old tram trail that loops through the upper grove but misses all the "important" trees. Instead, cross the tram road

A giant sequoia can live more than 2,000 years, producing more than half a billion seeds in this time. Only one seed is required to replace the parent.

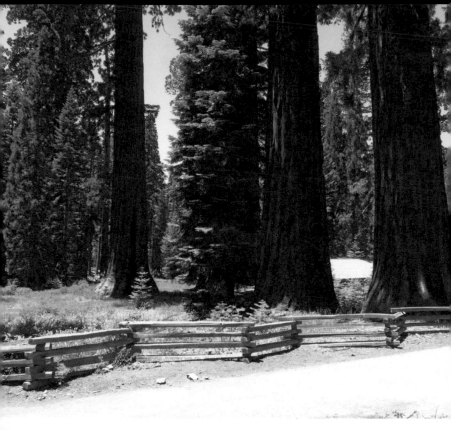

A grove of giant trees *near the Mariposa Grove museum*

and continue along a much smaller trail, the Perimeter Trail, signposted
to the Galen Clark Tree.

Walk just 120 feet east to reach the Galen Clark Tree, a fine specimen
named for the man who first publicized this grove and later became its first
guardian. From here, turn right to follow the Perimeter Trail south, now
paralleling the old road a little to its east. Your next noteworthy stop is the
Fallen Wawona Tunnel Tree. This tree, which in 1881 was the first giant
sequoia to have a tunnel carved through it, toppled during the late winter
or spring of 1969 and now makes a fine backdrop for photos. Continuing
clockwise, you pass a junction with a minor trail that branches left, leading to Biledo Meadow in Sierra National Forest, and continue skirting the
upper edge of the upper grove. This trail provides a wonderful vantage
point of the upper grove, for you are looking down a relatively steep slope,
making it possible to gaze at both the bases and the middles of the trees,
albeit not the tops. The next junction is just shy of the Telescope Tree,

where you turn right to descend toward the museum (3.4 miles). ▶9 But first take just a few more steps along the Perimeter Trail, and duck into the Telescope Tree, which has been hollowed out by fire. Inside it you can look straight up to the heavens. This tree is still very much alive, despite having lost much of its internal structure, because water and dissolved nutrients are conducted in the sapwood, the layer immediately beneath the thick bark, just as in all trees. The heartwood—the material at the center of the tree—is just dead sapwood whose function is support.

After the requisite silhouetted photos up through the center of the Telescope Tree, you return the few steps to ▶9 and descend the steep forested slope. This is one of my favorite slopes in the Mariposa Grove, boldly decorated with flowers in early summer and an engaging mixture of young and mature sequoias. Contemplate just how much the shape of the trees shifts as they mature, from densely branched conical conifers to tall, bare trunks and massive aerial branches. The reasonably steep trail quickly leads to a tangle of junctions near the Mariposa Grove Cabin, a museum (3.7 miles). ▶10 In the museum you will find information and displays on the giant sequoia, its related plants and animals, and the area's history. After your foray inside, the most pleasant route to continue along is a collection of small trails just north of the old tram road that lead to the Columbia Tree, at 285 feet the tallest tree in the grove and towering above a lovely moist glade that's usually colorful with flowers.

A few steps take you past a toilet and back to the old road. Following it a few more steps west, you reach a five-way junction—and some choices (3.85 miles). ▶11 You have come from the northeast; we'll call this option trail 1. Facing the way you came and turning clockwise, trail 2 is the continuation of the old road (Guardians Loop Trail) heading back up, trail 3 is the Perimeter Trail leading back to the Telescope Tree, and trails 4 and 5 lead down to the lower grove and shuttle stop. Trail 4 follows the Perimeter Trail down, reintersecting the Mariposa Grove Trail ▶5 near the California Tunnel Tree, while trail 5 drops to reach the Mariposa Grove Trail at the Clothespin Tree. Here I describe trail 4 because it is consider-

The 2,200-year-old Wawona Tunnel Tree, like many others, had a fire-scarred base and was enlarged first in 1881 for stagecoaches and much later for automobiles to pass through it.

ably shorter, but if you prefer a gentler grade on a broader trail, take the fifth spoke, which is directly on your right when facing downhill. It leads

0.5 mile straight down to the Clothespin Tree, ►6 from which you can retrace your route from earlier to the shuttle stop.

Following the fourth trail option, you take the Perimeter Trail south down an open slope 0.85 mile to reach a junction with a minor trail, where you turn left; soon thereafter, at a second bigger junction, you head right. Just a few more steps lead you to the Mariposa Grove Trail near the California Tunnel Tree (4.65 miles). ►12 From here, retrace your route to the shuttle stop (5.8 miles). ►13 If you reach the California Tunnel Tree with spare time and energy, consider taking the Grizzly Giant Loop Trail northwest to the Mariposa Grove Arrival Area; it adds about 0.35 mile but lets you walk through different forest patches.

	MILESTONES	
►1	0.0	Start at the Mariposa Grove Arrival Area
►2	0.14	Right at Fallen Monarch
►3	0.4	Cross road at Bachelor and the Three Graces
►4	0.7	Grizzly Giant
►5	0.9	Left back onto Mariposa Grove Trail beyond the California Tunnel Tree
►6	1.65	Clothespin Tree
►7	2.45	Straight at Guardians Loop Trail junction
►8	2.85	Straight onto Perimeter Trail where Mariposa Grove Trail turns left to Wawona Point
►9	3.4	Right near Telescope Tree, turning off Perimeter Trail
►10	3.7	Right near Mariposa Grove Museum
►11	3.85	Southwest at five-way junction to descend Perimeter Trail
►12	4.65	Left onto Mariposa Grove Trail near California Tunnel Tree
►13	5.8	Return to the Mariposa Grove Arrival Area

Isberg–Red Peak–
Fernandez Passes Loop

Crossing four passes over 44 miles, this loop introduces you to many of southern Yosemite's highlights. Though well traveled during the summer months, these trails will never be crowded because they are a long drive up a small road and are not part of any of the popular long-distance trails running the length of the Sierra; everyone you will see on the trail has planned a trip explicitly to visit this location. With permits relatively easy to come by, endless lakes for swimming or relaxing, superb views from the passes, and some beautiful rocks, this is a perfect loop for someone wishing to delve a little deeper into Yosemite's backcountry.

Permits

Overnight visitors require a wilderness permit for the Isberg Trailhead (loop as described) or Walton Trailhead (loop in reverse), issued by Sierra National Forest. Pick up your wilderness permit at the Clover Meadow Ranger Station or other Sierra National Forest permit-issuing stations (see "Permits," page 21).

Maps

This trail is covered by the Tom Harrison *Ansel Adams Wilderness* map (1:79,200 scale), the National Geographic Trails Illustrated *#309 Yosemite SE* map (1:40,000 scale), and the USGS 7.5-minute series *Timber Knob, Mount Lyell, Merced Peak,* and *Sing Peak* maps (1:24,000 scale).

TRAIL USE
Backpack, Horse
LENGTH
44.1 miles, over 4–7 days
VERTICAL FEET
Round-trip:
+9,130', –8,710'
DIFFICULTY
– 1 2 3 4 **5** +
TRAIL TYPE
Point-to-Point (or loop with an extra 3.5 miles of walking)

FEATURES
Canyon
Lake
Stream
Wildflowers
Great Views
Camping
Secluded
Steep
Granite Slabs
Geological Interest

FACILITIES
Bear Boxes
Campgrounds
Horse Staging
Ranger Station
Toilets
Water

(continued on page 385)

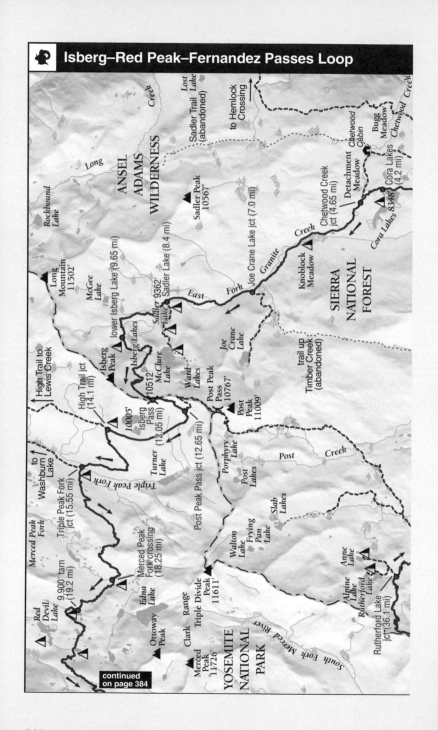

Isberg–Red Peak–Fernandez Passes Loop

Creek

Lost Lake

Sadler Trail (abandoned)

to Hemlock Crossing

Chetwood Cabin

Bugg Meadow

Chetwood Creek

ANSEL ADAMS WILDERNESS

Long

Rockbound Lake

Sadler Peak 10567'

Detachment Meadow

Chetwood Creek jct (4.65 mi)

Cora Lakes (4.2 mi)

Cora Lakes 8348'

McGee Lake

Long Mountain 11502'

Sadler Lake (8.4 mi)

Joe Crane Lake jct (7.0 mi)

Granite

Creek

Knoblock Meadow

SIERRA NATIONAL FOREST

lower Isberg Lake (9.65 mi)

Sadler 9362 Lake

East Fork

High Trail to Lewis Creek

Isberg Lakes

Isberg Peak

High Trail jct (14.1 mi)

10512'

McClure Lake

Ward Lakes

Joe Crane Lake

trail up Timber Creek (abandoned)

10005'

Isberg Pass (12.05 mi)

Post Peak Pass 10767'

Post Peak 11009'

to Washburn Lake

Turner Lake

Porphyry Lake

Post

Creek

Triple Peak Fork jct (15.55 mi)

Post Peak Pass jct (12.65 mi)

Post Lakes

Triple Peak Fork

Merced Peak Fork

Merced Peak Fork crossing (18.25 mi)

Slab Lakes

Walton Lake

Frying Pan Lake

9,900' tarn (19.2 mi)

Red Devil Lake

Edna Lake

Anne Lake

Ottoway Peak

Triple Divide Peak 11611'

Alpine Lake

Rutherford Lake

Clark Range

Rutherford Lake jct (36.1 mi)

South Fork Merced River

Merced Peak 11726'

YOSEMITE NATIONAL PARK

continued on page 384

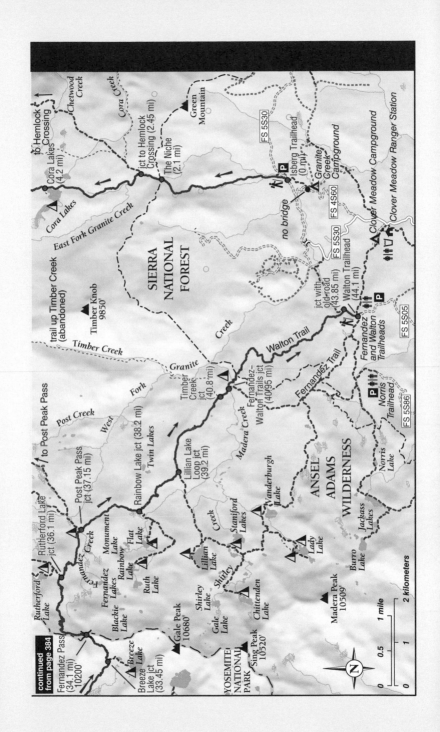

continued from page 384

Fernandez Pass (34.1 mi) 10200'

to Post Peak Pass

Post Creek

West

Fork

Granite

Timber

Creek

trail up Timber Creek (abandoned)

Timber Creek

Timber Knob 9850'

SIERRA NATIONAL FOREST

East Fork Granite Creek

Cora Lakes (4.2 mi)

Cora Lakes

to Hemlock Crossing

Chetwood Creek

Cora Creek

Cora Creek

jct to Hemlock Crossing (2.45 mi)

The Niche (2.1 mi)

Green Mountain

FS 5S30

Isberg Trailhead (0 mi)

Granite Creek Campground

FS 4S60

no bridge

FS 5S30

Clover Meadow Campground

Clover Meadow Ranger Station

Walton Trailhead (44.1 mi)

jct with old road (43.85 mi)

FS 5S05

Walton Trail

Fernandez and Walton Trailheads

Fernandez Trail

Fernandez– Walton Trails jct (40.95 mi)

Timber Creek jct (40.8 mi)

Lillian Lake Loop jct (39.2 mi)

Rainbow Lake jct (38.2 mi)

Twin Lakes

Rutherford Lake jct (36.1 mi)

Rutherford Lake

Post Peak Pass jct (37.15 mi)

Monument Lake

Flat Lake

Rainbow Lake

Fernandez Lakes

Ruh Lake

Fernandez Creek

Blackie Lake

Breeze Lake

Breeze Lake jct (33.45 mi)

Gale Peak 10680'

Gale Lake

Shirley Lake

Lillian Lake

Shirley Creek

Shirley Lake

Chittenden Lake

Stanford Lakes

Madera Creek

Vanderburgh Lake

Lady Lake

Norris Trailhead

FS 5S86

Norris Lake

ANSEL ADAMS WILDERNESS

Burro Lake

Jackass Lakes

Madera Peak 10509'

Sing Peak 10520'

YOSEMITE NATIONAL PARK

N

0   0.5   1 mile

0   1   2 kilometers

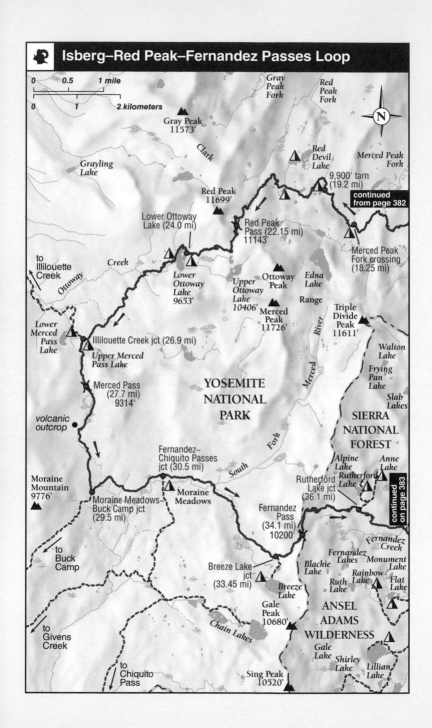

Isberg–Red Peak–Fernandez Passes Loop

0   0.5   1 mile

0   1   2 kilometers

Gray
Peak
Fork

Red
Peak
Fork

N

Gray Peak
11573'

Grayling
Lake

Red Devil
Lake

Merced Peak
Fork

Clark

9,900' tarn
(19.2 mi)

continued
from page 382

Red Peak
11699'

Lower Ottoway
Lake (24.0 mi)

Red Peak
Pass (22.15 mi)
11143'

Merced Peak
Fork crossing
(18.25 mi)

to
Illilouette
Creek

Creek

Lower
Ottoway
Lake
9653'

Upper
Ottoway
Lake
10406'

Ottoway
Peak

Edna
Lake

Ottoway

Merced
Peak
11726'

Range

Triple
Divide
Peak
11611'

Lower
Merced
Pass
Lake

Illilouette Creek jct (26.9 mi)

Upper Merced
Pass Lake

Walton
Lake

Frying
Pan
Lake

Slab
Lakes

River

Merced Pass
(27.7 mi)
9314'

YOSEMITE
NATIONAL
PARK

SIERRA
NATIONAL
FOREST

volcanic
outcrop

Merced

Fork

Alpine
Lake

Anne
Lake

Fernandez–
Chiquito Passes
jct (30.5 mi)

South

Rutherford
Lake jct
(36.1 mi)

Rutherford
Lake

continued
on page 383

Moraine
Mountain
9776'

Moraine Meadows–
Buck Camp jct
(29.5 mi)

Moraine
Meadows

Fernandez
Pass
(34.1 mi)
10200'

Fernandez
Creek

to
Buck
Camp

Breeze Lake
jct
(33.45 mi)

Fernandez
Lakes

Blackie
Lake

Monument
Lake

Rainbow
Lake

Flat
Lake

to
Givens
Creek

Breeze
Lake

Ruth
Lake

Gale
Peak
10680'

Chain Lakes

ANSEL
ADAMS
WILDERNESS

to
Chiquito
Pass

Gale
Lake

Shirley
Lake

Lillian
Lake

Sing Peak
10520'

(continued from page 381)

Best Time

In most years these trails will be snow-free by early July, with snow lingering until the middle of July in higher snowfall years. Abundant wildflowers are in peak bloom during July, but because mosquitoes will plague July visitors along this loop's lower elevations, many hikers will select August as the best month for a visit. Lakes tend to reach their highest temperatures in late July– early August. September is still pleasant along this loop, but be prepared for cooler nighttime temperatures and the possibility of the year's first minor snowfall. By October, larger storms are possible and visitors should only disappear this deep into the wilderness if the weather forecast is for sun.

Finding the Trail

From the CA 49–CA 41 junction in Oakhurst, drive north on CA 41 (toward Yosemite) 3.5 miles up to a junction with Forest Service Road 222, signposted for Bass Lake. Follow FS 222 east 3.4 miles. Beyond, continue straight ahead, but your road is now called Malum Ridge Road (FS 274). Continue east 2.4 miles to a left (north) junction with FS 7 (5S07), Beasore Road.

Paved but windy Beasore Road climbs north, passing Chilkoot Campground at the 4.0-mile mark, followed by a series of dirt roads departing westward. At 7.6 miles beyond the campground, you reach a four-way intersection at Cold Spring Summit, where Sky Ranch Road (FS 6S10X) departs to the left, while turning right leads to a parking area with toilets. Continuing straight ahead, Beasore Road winds another 8.5 miles, going past Beasore Meadows, Jones Store, Mugler Meadow, and Long Meadow before coming to a junction with FS 5S04, opposite Globe Rock, a total of 20.1 miles from the start of FS 7. (FS 5S04 leads north to the Chiquito Lake Trailhead.)

Beyond Globe Rock the road's condition begins to deteriorate—though hopefully funding will have appeared to resurface it before you drive it. As of mid-2018, numerous giant potholes slowed your progress. Passing a spur to Upper Chiquito Campground, the impressive granite domes named the Balls, and the Jackass Lake Trailhead, you reach the Bowler Campground after 6.6 miles. Ahead is a series of spur roads leading to trailheads to the right: first the Norris Trailhead (FS 5S86) and just beyond the Fernandez and Walton Trailheads (FS 5S05), where you will finish your walk. Next you pass FS 5S88, which branches south 0.4 mile to Minarets Pack Station. Here you meet the end of paved Minarets Road (FS 4S81), which has ascended 52 paved miles north from the community of North Fork. Though a longer route, it is in better condition than Beasore Road and is a possible return route if you found the Beasore Road potholes too jarring. From this junction, continuing straight ahead, drive northeast 1.8 miles, now on FS 5S30 to a junction at the Clover Meadow Ranger Station, a grand total of 31.1 miles since you turned onto Beasore Road. Here is the small cabin where you will pick up your wilderness permit. The entrance to the Clover Meadow Campground is just beyond it, a pleasant campground with piped water, vault toilets, and—amazingly—cell reception!

You still have a short distance to reach your trailhead, however. Staying on FS 5S30, you first stay left at a junction with FS 4S60 (bound for primitive Granite Creek Campground), descend to cross the West Fork of Granite Creek, then immediately turn right and parallel the creek east, now on a truly unpaved road. At a Y-junction, bear left (right descends back to the Granite Creek Campground), briefly drive up a steep hill (yes, it is two-wheel drive), level out, and almost immediately turn right into the quite large Isberg Trailhead parking area, 3.1 miles past the Clover Meadow Ranger Station.

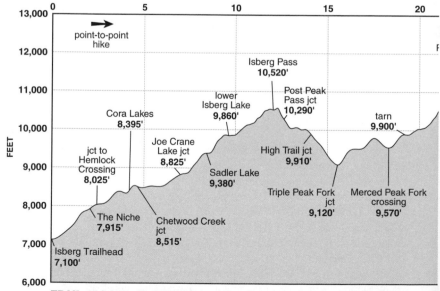

TRAIL 44 Isberg–Red Peak–Fernandez Passes Loop Elevation Profile

If you have two cars in your group, you may choose to complete a car shuttle to the Fernandez and Walton Trailheads before heading out; otherwise, on your return there is a combination of tracks and roads that make it a 3.5-mile walk back to your car (versus more than twice that along the roads). The route is described at the end of the trail description. If you have a single car, you may choose to park it at the Clover Meadow Ranger Station and walk the first 2.15 miles to the trailhead now—this will minimize your total driving time and have no effect on your walking distance.

A water faucet and outhouse are near the Clover Meadow Ranger Station.

Trail Description

After the long drive to the Isberg Trailhead, ►1 walking, even with a full pack on, probably feels good. The trail takes you north, approximately paralleling the mostly unseen East Fork Granite Creek. You plod upward along the rather dusty trail through a red fir–and–lodgepole pine forest. The first and last miles of this trail receive heavy horse traffic, hence the

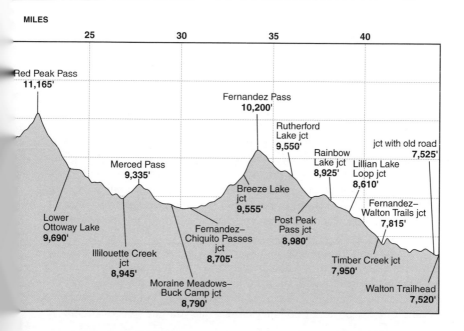

MILES

dust, but the walking is pleasant and the trail mostly in good shape. Reaching the head of the draw you've been following, the trail slowly begins an ascending traverse across a brushy slope. First north-facing and then trending more northeasterly, you make your way toward a passageway known as The Niche (2.1 miles). ▶2 You will be forgiven for imagining that you are crossing a pass because your senses tell you that you've just climbed a slope to a narrow slot between two taller ridges. Stop and look more closely and you will realize that there is a creek, the East Fork Granite Creek, flowing straight through The Niche and then dropping steeply on its journey south. Indeed, you are continuing uphill, and the creek's power has eroded only this narrow channel through the remarkably resistant rocks.

Now in a quite flat lodgepole pine forest beside the creek, the vegetation is lusher with abundant color in early summer. At full flow the creek tumbles rapidly, with the base of rounded cobble and boulders revealed as flows are reduced. Passing a signed junction with the trail to Hemlock Crossing (2.45 miles), ▶3 you stay left, continuing along the creek's western bank for a few more steps. Soon your trail too fords the East Fork Granite Creek, a broad crossing that will mean wet feet early summer and a rock hop later on. With the main river channel diverging west away from the trail, you follow a smaller tributary upward. The forests here are generally lush—purple-flowered wandering fleabane can occupy large swaths of forest floor. Climbing more steeply, the trail sidles around the east side of a small dome, crossing slabs and entering barren forest. Beyond a shallow saddle, a brief descent leads to the triplet of Cora Lakes, though only the center one, Lake 8,348 (also known as middle Cora), is visible from the trail. This grassy-shored lake offers ample camping opportunities, with use trails departing west along both its south and north shores. Camping is prohibited, however, within 400 feet of its eastern shore, the corridor through which the trail passes (4.2 miles). ▶4 The lake is shallow, making it warm and excellent for swimming yet deep enough to support trout. Upper Cora Lake, though depicted as large on maps, is a very shallow lake, with only about one-fourth of its surface still covered by water by September.

Climbing briefly over a small knob, you may note some volcanic rocks mixed in with the dominant granite, and indeed Timber Knob to the west is composed of metavolcanic rocks. You next reach a junction where a little-used trail departs east (right) toward Detachment Meadow and Chetwood Creek (4.65 miles), ▶5 while you stay straight ahead and descend back into the East Fork Granite Creek drainage. Abundant tarns and marshy meadows make the ensuing miles a mosquito factory in July, but this stretch is also resplendent with water-loving wildflowers. Reaching Knoblock Meadow at the 5.5-mile mark, you skirt its eastern edge, pass a few small campsites, and recross the creek, again a ford at high flows. The gradient increases as you continue beside the creek, admiring the flowers and crossing a series of often-dry side channels. Just beyond some small springs, noteworthy mainly for the tiny, red-streaked channels in the soil that develop downslope of them, you reach a junction with the left-trending spur trail to Joe Crane Lake (7.0 miles). ▶6 This undervisited lake lies 1.5 trail miles to the west, nestled in a steep-walled basin east of Post Peak. The trail once also led down Timber Creek, but the trail has unfortunately been abandoned along this beautiful route, and it is now difficult to navigate.

Bearing right and continuing along the creek's bank, you note that, with increasing elevation, the forest is slowly thinning and the red firs have all but disappeared, replaced by a mixture of hemlocks and lodgepole pines, as you slowly transition from the upper montane to subalpine zones. Moreover, instead of continuous forest walking, you now wander repeatedly onto broken slabs. Crossing the East Fork Granite Creek a final time at a location with grand clumps of clasping arnica, water flows are now lower and you can rock-hop across under all but the highest runoff. Switchbacks up a dry lodgepole slope lead to the next shelf, this one holding Sadler Lake. With the lake still out of view, you reach a small junction signposted for McClure Lake (8.4 miles), ▶7 but this trail also leads to fine campsites around the southern and western shores of Sadler Lake. In particular, seek out the flat, sandy locales nestled between the similarly flat slabs that ring its southern shores. However, camping is prohibited within 400 feet of the north shore of Sadler Lake—this is a seasonally marshy area. McClure Lake, 0.9 mile to the west, offers fewer camping options but one spectacular site on a hemlock bench southwest of the lake. If you wish to camp under the shelter of trees, stop here because it will be nearly 6 miles, up and over Isberg Pass, before you again have the option for a truly forested campsite.

As you round the north shore of Sadler Lake, you will notice the near-vertical walls to your north—it is atop these that the Isberg Lakes are perched. So off you head, climbing again, now on slopes even more sparsely covered with lodgepole pines. Crossing a shallow rib, the trail descends to the lowest of the Isberg Lakes (9.65 miles). ▶8 Those

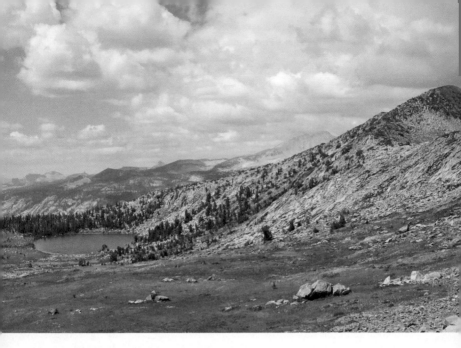

Expansive bench *to the west of Isberg Pass*

attracted to an alpine perch will look down on the landscape of slabs, sandy patches, and small stands of stunted pines and declare it the ideal campsite, but be forewarned that this broad shelf offers little protection against wind or a storm. In addition the scattered campsites over the next mile are mostly tiny, with space for only a single tent in each sandy patch. Keeping with the moist forests you have been walking through since the trailhead, the landscape surrounding the Isberg Lakes is quite vegetated; sedge meadows, expanses of dwarf bilberry, and red mountain heather creeping along the edge of boulders all add color but make it more difficult to locate an appropriate campsite.

A 300-foot slope separates the lower—and largest—Isberg Lake from the higher cluster, and to reach them you wind up slabs, strips of sand, and verdant slopes irrigated by endless trickles until you are unknowingly standing just 150 feet north of the cliff overtopping McClure Lake. The views are tremendous and the rocks engaging, here dotted with inclusions, blobs of a darker igneous rock embedded in the lighter-colored granite. Passing the last trees, the trail continues winding up through broken granite slabs. The trail is much slower walking now: narrow, in places incised, and because it is following little strips of vegetation between the rocks or winding between fractured slabs, it is almost never straight. Gazing up toward the pass, you see that the granite on the slope above has fractured

into big smooth platters—a beautiful example of exfoliation. Skirting high
around the upper Isberg Lake and its accompanying tarn, the trail makes
26 tight, but relatively gentle, switchbacks up a south-facing rib—that is,
a location where the snow melts early—and then cuts southwest beneath
Isberg Peak to Isberg Pass, continually passing little patches of color—red
mountain heather and yellow frosted buckwheat among the most common. The rock here is also colorful—admire the red-and-gray-striped
summit of Isberg Peak—because you are near the contact boundary of granitic and metamorphic rock, and many of the rocks were partially altered
during the geologic skirmishes in this zone.

Reaching the pass (12.05 miles), ▶**9** position yourself atop one of the
pleasantly flat boulders adorning the ridge and enjoy the view east to the
ridge between Sadler Peak and Long Mountain with the Ritter Range peek-
ing out behind, southeast across the expansive San Joaquin River drainage, and west and northwest into Yosemite. Procrastinating on top—who
wouldn't?—you pull yourself away and begin a surprisingly slow descent
of the west side of the pass—slow because steep slabs and broken blocks
cover the slope below. The trail traverses south to avoid the steepest terrain, but it is cumbersome walking, as on many occasions you climb a
few steps upward to bypass a small obstacle. Indeed, this stretch has the
feel of being a well-used use trail. Where the trail's gradient steepens,
you find yourself descending a steep, loose trail to the meadow below,
soon reaching the junction with a trail to Post Peak Pass (12.65), ▶**10** an
alternate route back to the Fernandez and Walton Trailheads. Springs
irrigate the landscape here, allowing a dense cover of alpine species to
establish on the slope. Continuing your descent, soon after you step across
a trickle, you leave the darker-colored diorite band and find yourself on
a fine, light-colored, coarse-grained granite that erodes easily into gullies.
Turning slowly north you are staring at a broad meadow and beyond to
oval-shaped Lake 10,005. Reaching almost a mile in length, this nearly flat
shelf is an unusual landscape feature in high-elevation Yosemite, seen just
a few places in the park, including here and a few miles north at the west
base of Long Mountain, where Harriet Lake is situated.

The trail is now flat and broader, allowing an unbroken stride, so
you can properly stretch your legs for the first time in many miles as you
tramp across this impressive expanse of meadow. Purple dots among the
grasses are diminutive lupines, while young twisted lodgepoles attest to
the weight of the winter snows. Most of the southern and western shores of
Lake 10,005 are too grassy to provide camping opportunities, but there are

many choices in the open lodgepole forest at the lake's northern end, and the sandy northern beach is an enticing extra. And of course, there are the views encompassing the entire headwaters of the Triple Peak Fork of the Merced River. Skirting past the lake, you round a corner, steep outcrops rising above you, and suddenly the landscape drops away, and you're staring north down the length of the Triple Peak Fork. A few more steps and you reach a junction, where right is the so-called High Trail or the Lyell Fork Merced Trail leading to Lewis Creek, while you turn left to drop to the Triple Peak Fork (14.1 miles). ▶11

The consuming views disappear almost immediately as you descend along a southerly trajectory through dense forest. Big hemlock trees instead garner your attention, as perhaps does the near absence of ground cover, so different from the wet forests you passed through on the southeast side of Isberg Pass. Lower, the slopes are drier yet and lodgepoles dominate, the two trees alternating in abundance as you drop toward the valley. Bending back north, the trail slowly drops to the broad, flat river corridor, a wonderful landscape of polished slabs. Crossing the Triple Peak Fork on a convenient log—hopefully still present—you reach a junction, where your route to Red Peak Pass leads left, while right descends the Triple Peak Fork to Washburn and Merced Lakes (15.55 miles). ▶12 Multiple campsites exist in this vicinity, some forested ones on lodgepole-pine shaded shelves to the west of the river and others in open sandy patches among the polished slabs well south of the trail.

Now commencing a 2,000-foot climb to the summit of Red Peak Pass, note that there are limited sheltered campsites until you reach Lower Ottoway Lake, nearly 9 miles distant. Instead, you will be traversing a landscape of subalpine meadows, slab-ringed lakes, tarns, and vistas. Leaving the bright white slabs of the river corridor behind, the trail climbs through broken rock, with small bluffs constraining the trail's route, forcing it to wind up the passageways between them. Brief lodgepole-covered shelves break the ascent, some with magnificently large trees. At 0.8 mile above the Triple Peak Fork, the trail bends northward to follow a long bench, the beautiful form of Triple Divide Peak visible straight ahead. Soon a forest strip provides an easy path upward again, and you climb along a seasonal trickle in a forest now comprised of hemlock, western white pine, and, of course, lodgepoles. The trail's location is well placed, leading toward Red Peak Pass with the least extra elevation gain as you weave your way westward along the base of the Clark Range. Crossing a small saddle cradling two small tarns, the view seeker will find the smallest of campsites, and the trail then winds down 250 feet to cross the Merced Peak Fork. At first on granite, the trail crosses into gray metamorphic rock near the bottom of the slope, hosting a drier plant community, before reaching the lush, green valley floor. Though wonderfully flat, the meadow-filled stream corridor holds only a few small campsites, most on the west side of the step-across creek crossing (18.25 miles). ▶13 You could alternatively strike south before the creek crossing, heading to a collection of tarns upstream in search of campsites.

With views to the northeast, stretching from Florence to Forester Peaks, the trail resumes an upward trajectory, skirting right along the base of the escarpment. Note that the cliffs overhead are all grayish metamorphic rock, while you are on the other side of the geologic contact, walking among the most beautifully polished granite slabs, with trees now growing only in strips of deeper soil between the ribs of rocks. The trail winds ever upward to reach a tarn at 9,900 feet, perched atop a shelf (19.2 miles). ▶14 Almost entirely surrounded by superbly smooth slabs, this lake features wonderful views across the Merced River to the Cathedral Range. Campsites are again small, but many a sandy patch lies nestled between the rolling slabs. Below and west of you is Red Devil Lake, ringed by exceptionally large expanses of flat granite slabs—and as expected, numerous campsites. The easiest way to access this lake is to initiate a left-trending descent just before you begin the climb above Lake 9,900. Skirting briefly to the north, the trail bypasses the lakeshore and then ascends granite slabs on a rib to its west. The gradient lessens where you cross again onto the gray metamorphic rock, soon reaching another flat, tarn-dotted shelf. Trees are now virtually absent and, for the most part, so are campsites because the metamorphic rocks break down into rather sharp-cornered gravel, and the sandy patches so welcome among granite slabs are absent. The tread leads to a larger tarn, the westernmost of the cluster, that you bypass near its outlet; this is the main stream flowing to Red Devil Lake (20.3 miles).

Passing around this final tarn, you walk a few more steps across the wonderfully flat shelf, continuing to absorb the views of the Cathedral Range, before beginning the switchbacking climb of the final 1,000 feet to the summit of Red Peak Pass. The flats you just passed and the ensuing climb are often densely covered with alpine wildflowers because the higher nutrient concentration and water-holding capacity of the metamorphic rocks support a greater density of plants. First you walk a little north and then surmount a rib extending northeast from near the summit. Turning

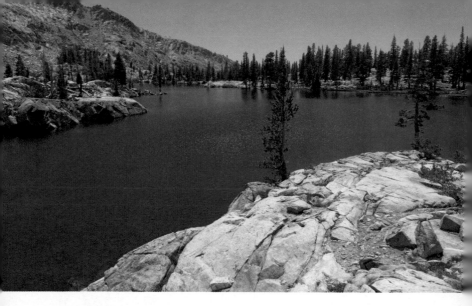

Lower Ottoway Lake

toward the pass, the trail now switchbacks steadily up this slope, slowly sidling into a drainage where a cluster of tarns marks the headwaters of the Red Peak Fork. The final headwall is ascended via tight switchbacks up a steep talus slope; fortunately the trail is in good shape, having been reworked to minimize summer snow cover and rockfall damage. Atop the pass at last, massive Red Peak blocks your view to the northwest, but Upper Ottoway Lake is visible at the base of a long set of switchbacks. The Cathedral Range, all the way from near Cathedral Peak to Mount Lyell, is laid out before you, while the Ritter Range is partially visible to the east. As you stand on your second pass of the trip, you are at almost exactly the midpoint in your excursion (22.15 miles). ▶15

Sandy, gravelly switchbacks take you down the west side of Red Peak Pass. Once around the base of the talus fans emanating from Red Peak, you walk through a grassy meadow strip and soon reach the point where you would cut south to Upper Ottoway Lake (22.9 miles). Though the beautiful lake tightly cupped by steep summits is well worth a detour for a look-see, take note that camping options are very limited. Continuing down the trail, Lower Ottoway Lake looks quite close and is indeed only 0.7 mile in a straight line, but this descent is never fast. Perhaps the trickles of water to step across, the narrow rocky trail, or the near 800-foot descent in just over a mile are to blame, though I suspect I am simply too easily distracted by the incessant bursts of color as the trail leads from one wet vegetated shelf to another, endlessly crossing little flower-filled drainages. Even lower, where the trail sidles onto a drier slope, flowering shrubs are numerous and robust. Continuing to oscillate between meta-morphic and granite rock, you transition permanently onto the granite slabs just above Lower Ottoway Lake—indeed, the geologic boundary almost certainly dictated why this lovely slab-ringed lake formed just here. Reaching Lower Ottoway Lake (24.0 miles), ▶16 campsites exist both along the lake's eastern shore in a lodgepole pine glade and on a shallow rib to the northwest of the lake.

Encircling heath-fringed Lower Ottoway Lake, the trail's descent continues down slabs along Ottoway Creek's north shore. The creek soon drops far below the trail level, plunging down its granite channel. With decreasing elevation, the slab cover is slowly more interrupted by forest glades, some with room for a campsite. Beyond one such flat, the trail crosses Ottoway Creek; a fallen log currently provides easy passage, but otherwise expect wet feet until late summer. You alternate between drier slab environments and moister forested ones where dwarf bilberry carpets much of the forest floor and one-sided wintergreen emerges next to fallen logs. Continuing generally downward, the trail rises and falls over a pair of spurs emanating from a spur west of Merced Peak and now remains mostly under a conifer canopy until nearly the summit of Fernandez Pass, some 9 miles ahead. As you approach the junction with the trail down Illilouette Creek (26.9 miles), ▶17 red firs rejoin the mix of conifers in moister draws. Our route turns left at this junction, toward Merced Pass, but if it is late in the day, consider seeking out the beautiful campsites by the shores of Upper Merced Pass Lake, a short distance up the drain-age to your left. Lower Merced Pass Lake, along the trail down Illilouette Creek, also offers camping. If you are hiking in late summer or autumn, it is advisable to fetch water from these lakes, as the small creeks along the next many miles often run dry.

Turning toward Merced Pass, you wind briefly up between some slabs and through open lodgepole forest. In comparison to your past two efforts, Merced Pass requires remarkably little exertion, and you soon reach the summit of this viewless high point, the drainage divide between the Yosemite Valley–bound main Merced River drainage and the Wawona-bound South Fork Merced River drainage (27.7 miles). ▶18 Descending gently to the south of the pass, you soon pass through a long meadow corridor bisected by a small seasonal creek. Of greatest note through here is a prominent outcrop of volcanic rock, indeed columnar basalt, that you skirt on its eastern side. If you have 10 spare minutes, it is well worth a detour to its flat top. Descending through a flower-filled gully, the trail steps across the creek a third time, then diverges from the watercourse, trending south along a shelf through a moist red fir forest. This delightful stretch leads to another junction, where right is signposted to Buck Camp and your route leads left toward Moraine Meadows and Fernandez Pass (29.5 miles). ▶19

The walk east to Moraine Meadows is almost continuously through lush vegetation, passing marshy reed-encircled tarns, crossing multiple tributaries, and rambling through densely vegetated lodgepole forest. If you are walking in July, you may unfortunately not notice any of these features as you try to outrun the swarms of mosquitoes often cohabiting this moist territory. By late summer, you may encounter no water at all, reaching the yellowing grass of Moraine Meadows and declaring it a pleasant forest walk. At the indistinct T-junction in Moraine Meadows, your route continues straight ahead, while right leads to destinations including the Chain Lakes and Chiquito Pass (30.5 miles). ▶20 If water is still flowing the South Fork Merced River—not guaranteed at the very end of summer in dry years—a few campsites exist to its south at the perimeter of the meadows.

Now following the northern bank of the South Fork Merced River eastward, you continue walking through verdant meadow strips and past small tarns. In July, flowers are everywhere—shooting stars, violets (most commonly white or yellow in color), lupines, buttercups, and so much more. You cross the South Fork Merced, either a long boulder hop or sometimes a wade, almost immediately followed by a smaller tributary. Turning farther south, the trail now continues up a draw to the side of this often-dry creek. First through lodgepoles and then into dense stands of hemlocks, you climb, soon crossing the river channel (32.35 miles). Though there might not be water present, you are unlikely to walk past without noticing this channel because it is deeply eroded and filled with some remarkably large boulders, the aftermath of a major flood a few decades back. It is especially noteworthy given the upstream catchment is a mere 1.2 square miles! A continued climb leads to a shallow lake in the middle of a broad, wet meadow and, beyond, a spur trail leading to Breeze Lake (33.45 miles). ▶21 Breeze Lake lies 0.4 mile south of the trail in a bowl ringed by steep granitic summits, including Gale Peak. There are campsites shaded by a mixture of hemlocks and lodgepole pines at both a small tarn and at the main lake, the best options located near the southwest corner of the lake. Cool water temperatures—and the eponymous breezy conditions—don't encourage swimming in this lake, but it should hold a healthy fish population.

Beyond the Breeze Lake junction, the trail gradient increases as it pushes toward the summit of 10,200-foot Fernandez Pass. Emerging from the continuous forest cover, you climb short, steep switchbacks on an open gravelly slope. Slabs and rock outcrops are again pervasive as you wind between scattered—and ever shorter—lodgepole pines and hemlocks. You top out on the broad, sandy summit and almost certainly gaze at the sawtooth profile of the Minarets, though I'll mention the view is even better as you traverse north from the pass (34.1 miles). ►22 If you've carried water from below, it would be possible to camp right atop this pass, even partially wind-sheltered by clusters of wind-blasted trees, a pleasant mixture of whitebark pines, hemlocks, and lodgepole.

In contrast to the steep trail that led you up the pass on the Yosemite side, the trail on the eastern side of the pass, now back in Ansel Adams Wilderness, is less severely inclined. Trending north, you ascend slightly along the sandy ridge before following a series of grassy passageways north, all the while admiring the evolving skyline, as the Ritter Range slowly disappears from view, replaced with an expansive vista of the peaks ringing the South Fork San Joaquin drainage. The trail traverses the shelves to bypass first a long-lasting snowfield directly east of the pass and then some steeper bluffs. Where the slabs are more broken, the trail makes a quite gradual switchbacking descent to the large meadow below. In July both the ridgetop traverse and descent will be brightly colored with flowers, the magenta mountain pride penstemon stealing center stage on the rocks. Skirting the meadow's northern border, the trail climbs just slightly to surmount a modest ridge, then descends a short steep slope to reach a spur trail leading to Rutherford and Anne Lakes (36.1 miles). ►23 Rutherford Lake, lying approximately 0.6 mile to the north, is a slab-encrusted lake offering multiple camping options along its southern and eastern shores. Anne Lake, also requiring a 0.6-mile detour, lies on a lower shelf farther east and is ringed by lodgepole forest and grassy shores. For- est campsites are present near its southeastern edge.

Turning right and continuing your descent on the main trail, you execute a few switchbacks down an open slope of red fractured granite before entering a moister, flatter forest. Passing alongside a lush, mead-owy corridor, colorful with early summer flowers, you cross Fernandez Creek on rocks and reach the junction with the trail leading to Post Peak Pass (37.15 miles). ►24 There are campsites on both sides of the creek in flat forest openings. The remaining 7 miles to the trailhead are, with few exceptions, not themselves terribly captivating. There are no lakes,

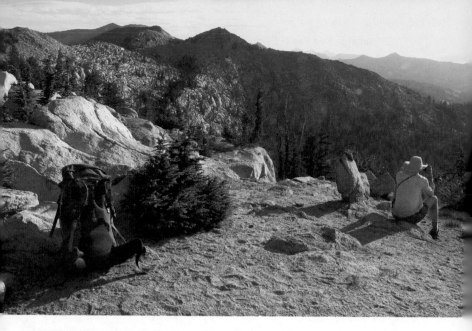

View east *from atop Fernandez Pass*

few streams, and limited views, though the walking is easy and innocuous. However, if you wish to spend another night along the way or even find a special spot for lunch, you will pass additional spur trails to not-too-far-away lake basins. For now you continue your descent, the next stretch mostly open and sandy with slabs not far beneath the surface, only entering brief stands of trees where fracture systems in the bedrock have resulted in the accumulation of deeper soils. Indeed, if you were to admire your route on a satellite photo, you would note that the distinct bend that the trail makes occurs to continue following forested benches downward, leading to a small junction beside a tarn (38.2 miles). ▶25 The Fernandez Trail, the left branch, now turns farther east again, trending back onto a rocky rib, while right leads to Flat, Rainbow, and Ruth Lakes. If you choose to detour in this direction, Flat Lake, a 0.8-mile detour each way, is forest ringed, while Rainbow (1.6 miles each way) and Ruth are slightly higher-elevation lakes surrounded by open lodgepole pine forest and slabs. Camping is prohibited within 0.25 mile of Rainbow Lake's shores, but some beautiful ridgetop campsites exist just southwest of the lake. Note that the trail leading to Flat Lake is more distinct than the one steeply climbing a ridge toward Rainbow Lake, so keep your eyes peeled for the fork.

Your descent along the Fernandez Trail continues through an open landscape of dark-colored rock and intermittent trees, always with broken views to the south and east. It soon reaches the next junction, where the right option leads 1.15 miles to lovely Lillian Lake, while the Fernandez Trail continues to the left (39.2 miles). ►**26** This point marks the end of the open slabs, as the landscape becomes more forested and moister. Red firs join the mix of trees, and soon the trail runs through a dense forest glade situated in a shallow trough before being routed back onto a ridgeline, an old moraine. Drier and sandier again, with pine-mat manzanita and juniper along the moraine crest, the trail proceeds to its end before switchbacking back to the drainage below. The next junction you reach is that with the trail up Timber Creek (40.8 miles). ►**27** Though the junction itself is signposted and obvious, the unmaintained trail rapidly deteriorates, helped on its path to oblivion by abundant uncleared tree falls.

Continuing the downward trajectory beneath forest cover, you next reach a junction in a broad sandy flat, where the Fernandez Trail forks right and the Walton Trail leads to the left (40.95 miles). ►**28** Given that these two trails lead to the same parking area and both are 3.15 miles in length, it is up to you which one you take, though the Walton Trail requires less elevation gain and has more open views—thus, it is the route described here. Continuing left through the open flat, along which there are many camping options, you soon cross Madera Creek. A possible wade under the highest of flows, this crossing quickly becomes a rock hop and will dry out in late summer. To your left (north) is an interesting geologic feature, a dark plug of olivine basalt, which was once part of the throat of a cinder cone. Glaciers removed the cinders but were too feeble to erode the lava. This dark monument is most obvious if you look north after you climb a few short, steep switchbacks to an open slope.

The open views as you cross this slabby slope are a wonderful way to end your trip, with a vista north to the ridge you've circumnavigated, as well as a vista south to the Silver Divide in the South Fork San Joaquin drainage. Dropping off the bare slabs into open lodgepole forest, the trail trends south, continuing its descending traverse across a slope. Stretches are in dry lodgepole pine forest, but interspersed are wetter glades where red firs dominate and drier rocky knobs where manzanita and huckleberry oak replace the trees. Turning right at an old road junction (43.85 miles), ►**29** you quickly reach the trailhead and a large parking area (44.1 miles). ►**30**

If your car is located here, your day is complete. Otherwise, walk to a trailhead located in the far northeastern corner of the parking area (just a little east of where you emerged) that is signposted to Clover

Meadow. This trail leads a pleasant 1.5 miles to the Clover Meadow Ranger Station, passing through beautiful mature fir forests, across open sandy flats, and eventually skirting the edge of the Clover Meadow Campground. From the ranger station, the most direct way to your car is to follow Forest Service Road 5S30 (the road on which you drove to the trailhead on the first day) 0.5 mile east, then turn onto FS 4S60, signposted for the Granite Creek Campground. This road leads 1.1 miles to the campground. Crossing Granite Creek, you will locate an old Isberg Trailhead marker beside the road and follow a short trail segment back to the parking lot, an additional 0.4 mile.

🚶 MILESTONES

▶1	0.0	Start at the Isberg Trailhead (along FS 5S30)
▶2	2.1	The Niche
▶3	2.45	Left at junction to Hemlock Crossing
▶4	4.2	Cora Lakes
▶5	4.65	Left at Chetwood Creek junction
▶6	7.0	Right at Joe Crane Lake junction
▶7	8.4	Sadler Lake
▶8	9.65	Lower Isberg Lake
▶9	12.05	Isberg Pass
▶10	12.65	Right at Post Peak Pass junction
▶11	14.1	Left at High Trail junction
▶12	15.55	Triple Peak Fork Merced River junction
▶13	18.25	Merced Peak Fork crossing
▶14	19.2	9,900-foot tarn
▶15	22.15	Red Peak Pass
▶16	24.0	Lower Ottoway Lake
▶17	26.9	Left at Illilouette Creek junction
▶18	27.7	Merced Pass
▶19	29.5	Left at Moraine Meadows–Buck Camp junction
▶20	30.5	Left at Fernandez–Chiquito Passes junction (in Moraine Meadows)
▶21	33.45	Left at Breeze Lake junction

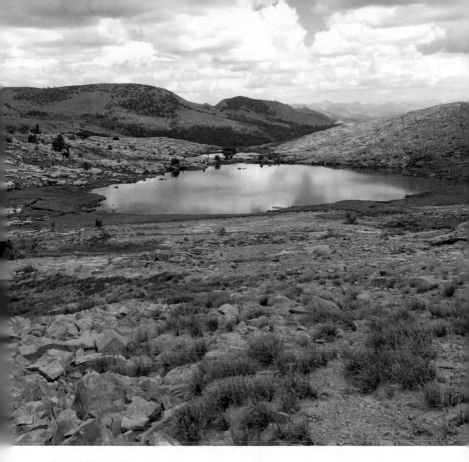

Upper *Isberg Lake*

🚶	**MILESTONES** *(continued)*	

►22	34.1	Fernandez Pass
►23	36.1	Right at Rutherford Lake junction
►24	37.15	Right at Post Peak Pass junction
►25	38.2	Left at Rainbow Lake junction
►26	39.2	Left at Lillian Lake Loop junction
►27	40.8	Right at junction with trail up Timber Creek
►28	40.95	Left at Fernandez–Walton Trails junction
►29	43.85	Right at junction with old road
►30	44.1	Finish at the Walton Trailhead (at end of FS 5S05)

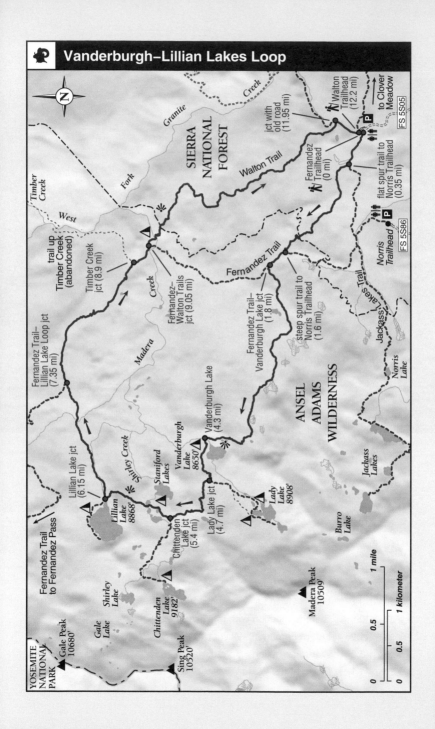

Vanderburgh–Lillian Lakes Loop

N

SIERRA NATIONAL FOREST

Granite Creek

Timber Creek

West Fork

Madera Creek

Shirley Creek

Walton Trail

Walton Trailhead (12.2 mi)

jct with old road (11.95 mi)

to Clover Meadow

FS 5S05

Fernandez Trailhead (0 mi)

flat spur trail to Norris Trailhead (0.35 mi)

Fernandez Trail

FS 5S86

Norris Trailhead

trail up Timber Creek (abandoned)

Timber Creek jct (8.9 mi)

Fernandez–Walton Trails jct (9.05 mi)

Fernandez Trail–Lillian Lake Loop jct (7.35 mi)

Fernandez Trail–Vanderburgh Lake jct (1.8 mi)

steep spur trail to Norris Trailhead (1.6 mi)

ANSEL ADAMS WILDERNESS

Norris Lake

Jackass Trail

Lillian Lake jct (6.15 mi)

Vanderburgh Lake (4.3 mi)

Vanderburgh Lake 8650'

Lady Lake jct (4.7 mi)

Lady Lake 8908'

Jackass Lakes

Burro Lake

Fernandez Trail to Fernandez Pass

Lillian Lake 8868'

Shirley Creek

Stanford Lakes

Chittenden Lake jct (5.4 mi)

Shirley Lake

Gale Lake

Chittenden Lake 9182'

Madera Peak 10509

Gale Peak 10680'

Sing Peak 10520'

YOSEMITE NATIONAL PARK

1 mile

0.5

1 kilometer

0.5

0

Vanderburgh–Lillian Lakes Loop

If you are in shape, you could hike this entire circuit in one day without overexerting yourself, sufficient time to visit the lakes not lying on the main circuit, Lady and Chittenden Lakes. Visiting both of these desirable lakes *and* exploring the trailside gems— Vanderburgh, Staniford, and Lillian—lengthens your route to about 16 miles, adds about 700 feet of ascent and descent, and changes its classification to a moderate three-day hike. Alternatively, for some folks, a trip just to Vanderburgh Lake, the first lake you'll encounter, is a worthy goal in itself, ideal for novice backpackers, day hikers, or those with children.

Permits

Overnight visitors require a wilderness permit for the Fernandez Trailhead (as described), Walton Trailhead (reverse of loop described), or Norris Trailhead (alternative starting point), issued by Sierra National Forest. Pick up your wilderness permit at the Clover Meadow Ranger Station, Yosemite Sierra Visitors Bureau in Oakhurst, or other Sierra National Forest permit-issuing stations (see "Permits," page 21).

Maps

This trail is covered by the Tom Harrison *Ansel Adams Wilderness* map (1:79,200 scale), the National Geographic Trails Illustrated *#309 Yosemite SE* map (1:40,000 scale), and the USGS 7.5-minute series *Timber Knob* map (1:24,000 scale).

TRAIL USE
Day Hike, Backpack,
Horse, Run,
Child-Friendly

LENGTH
12.2 miles, 6–12 hours
(over 1–3 days)

VERTICAL FEET
±2,310'

DIFFICULTY
– 1 2 **3 4** 5 +

TRAIL TYPE
Loop

FEATURES
Lake
Wildflowers
Great Views
Camping
Swimming
Secluded
Granite Slabs
Geological Interest

FACILITIES
Bear Boxes
Campgrounds
Horse Staging
Restrooms

Before glaciers advanced across higher Sierran lands, the Madera Creek basin may have had a large population of giant sequoias.

Best Time

This is classic subalpine Sierran country, and as elsewhere, the trails are mostly snow-free by late June, but mosquitoes keep most visitors away until late July. From then through mid-August, the lakes are optimal for swimming. To avoid crowds and find solitude, try hiking mid-September–mid-October.

Finding the Trail

From the CA 49–CA 41 junction in Oakhurst, drive 3.5 miles north on CA 41 (toward Yosemite) to a junction with Forest Service Road 222, signposted for Bass Lake. Follow FS 222 east 3.4 miles. Beyond, continue straight ahead, but your road is now called Malum Ridge Road (FS 274). Continue east 2.4 miles to a left (north) junction with FS 7 (5S07), Beasore Road.

Paved but windy Beasore Road climbs north, passing Chilkoot Campground at the 4.0-mile mark, followed by a series of dirt roads departing westward. At 7.6 miles beyond the campground, you reach a four-way intersection at Cold Spring Summit, where Sky Ranch Road (FS 6S10X) departs to the left, while turning right leads to a parking area with toilets. Continuing straight ahead, Beasore Road winds another 8.5 miles, going past Beasore Meadows, Jones Store, Mugler Meadow, and Long Meadow before coming to a junction with FS 5S04, opposite Globe Rock, a total

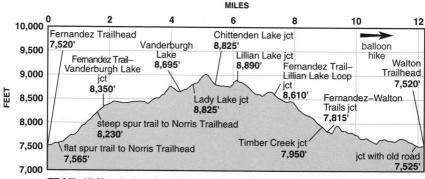

TRAIL 45 Vanderburgh–Lillian Lakes Loop Elevation Profile

of 20.1 miles from the start of FS 7. (FS 5S04 leads north to the Chiquito Lake Trailhead.)

Beyond Globe Rock the road's condition begins to deteriorate—though hopefully funding will have appeared to resurface it before you drive it. As of mid-2018, numerous giant potholes slowed your progress. Passing a spur to Upper Chiquito Campground, the impressive granite domes named the Balls, and the Jackass Lakes Trailhead, you reach the Bowler Campground after 6.6 miles. Ahead is a series of spur roads leading to trailheads to the right: first the Norris Trailhead (FS 5S86) and just beyond the Fernandez and Walton Trailheads (FS 5S05).

If you have retrieved your wilderness permit in Oakhurst, you should now turn up FS 5S05 and follow it 2.35 miles to its terminus in the large parking area. If you instead need to pick up your permit at the Clover Meadow Ranger Station, you must continue a short distance, passing FS 5S88, which branches south 0.4 mile to Minarets Pack Station. Here you meet the end of paved Minarets Road (FS 4S81), which has ascended 52 paved miles north from the community of North Fork. Though a longer route, it is in better condition than Beasore Road and is a possible return route if you found the Beasore Road potholes too jarring. From this junction, staying left, drive northeast 1.8 miles, now on FS 5S30 to a junction at the Clover Meadow Ranger Station, a grand total of 31.1 miles since you turned onto Beasore Road. Here is the small building where you will pick up your wilderness permit. The entrance to the Clover Meadow Campground is just beyond it, a pleasant campground with piped water, vault toilets, and—amazingly—cell reception! There are also toilets at the trailhead.

There is much confusion—and probably sloppiness—in the spelling of *Vanderburgh* Lake in both official and unofficial sources. For years the name was spelled *Vandeberg* on maps, but the most recent USGS topo maps are using *Vanderburgh*, matching the spelling of its namesake. However, alternative spellings, including *Vandenberg*, abound online.

Trail Description

Two trails depart from the parking area at the end of FS 5S05, the Walton Trail and the Fernandez Trail. You will be departing along the Fernandez Trail, located along the western side of the parking area, and returning along the Walton Trail, located at the northern tip of the parking area. Both are signposted with their respective names. Departing west

OPTION: Lady Lake

▶6 A spur trail takes off south (left) and climbs gently to moderately 0.6 mile to Lady Lake. As you walk along the outlet creek, about halfway to the lake, you will note an unsigned trail departing right away from the creek. From here, right leads to a large campsite above the north shore of the lake, while left leads to the east-shore moraine that juts into the lake, with an even better campsite. If you miss this cryptic junction, don't worry because you will most certainly realize when you've reached the shore of granite-rimmed, 8,908-foot-high Lady Lake. Both of these campsites are ideal for large groups—one of the few subalpine lakes that accommodates many tents without environmental concerns.

This lake's irregular form, speckled with several boulder islands, makes it a particularly attractive lake to camp at or to visit, especially because it is backdropped by hulking, metamorphic Madera Peak. Like all the lakes you might visit along this hike, Lady Lake has trout. Because it is shallow, it is a good lake for swimming late July–mid-August. Note that some online maps currently assign the name *Lady Lake* to the smaller lake to the southwest. This is incorrect; Lady Lake is the larger of the two lakes. In addition, the words *Madera Lakes* now appear across Lady Lake on some online maps. The Madera Lakes, as marked on the 1953 Merced Peak topo map, was a joint term for Lady and Vanderburgh Lakes.

along the Fernandez Trail, ▶1 you pass through a typical midelevation Sierran forest: white fir, Jeffrey pine, and lodgepole pine in the flats and draws and scrubby huckleberry oak on open slabs. A gentle ascent across morainal slopes leads to the lower end of a small meadow and meets a junction with an easily missed and little-used trail that meanders 1.15 miles to the Norris Trailhead, while your route bends to the right (0.35 mile). ▶2 Beyond the junction your trail's gradient becomes a moderate one, and red firs quickly begin to replace white firs. The forest temporarily yields to brush as you struggle up short, steep gravelly switchbacks below a small, exfoliating "dome." Now entering Ansel Adams Wilderness, you have a steady pull up to a near-crest junction (1.6 miles). ▶3 Merging from the left is steep trail that leads 1.35 miles to the Norris Trailhead. You continue a moderate ascent of the Fernandez Trail for only a few more minutes, then reach a crest junction (1.8 miles). ▶4

Here the Fernandez Trail continues right, but you branch left toward Vanderburgh Lake, along the start of the Lillian Lake Loop Trail. Heading west toward peaks and lakes, this trail's next 2 miles are generally easy. Conifers shade your way first past a waist-deep pond, on your right, then later past two often-wet, moraine-dammed, flower-filled meadows; then   the trail climbs to a bedrock notch in a granitic crest. Here are your first views of the San Joaquin drainage, including dark-colored, pyramidal-shaped Mount Goddard, nearly 50 miles southeast. On the crest you arc around a stagnant pond, then make a short descent to Madera Creek.

If you plan to camp at very popular Vanderburgh Lake (4.3 miles), ▶5 at 8,650 feet, you could leave the trail here and descend southwest to find some campsites along its east shore. The trail meanwhile curves west above good to excellent campsites along the lake's north shore. From them, steep, granitic Peak 9,852, on Madera Peak's northeast ridge, is reflected in the lake's placid early-morning waters. If you are trying to decide which of the many lakes to camp at, this is the lowest elevation and most forested of the choices, making it more or less appealing based on your predilection. At the west end of the lake, you climb bedrock to the edge of a lodgepole flat that has a junction with a trail to Lady Lake, well worth the easy detour (4.7 miles). ▶6 (See the Option on page 406.)

Beyond the Lady Lake Trail junction, your Lillian Lake Loop Trail crosses a lodgepole flat, then climbs a couple of hundred feet on fairly open granitic slabs to a ridge. Here you can stop and appreciate the skyline panorama from the Minarets south to the Mount Goddard area in Kings Canyon National Park. Descending northwest on a moderate to steep gradient, you reach an easily missed junction, where a small sign indicates that you turn left to reach Chittenden Lake (5.4 miles). ▶7 The junction is soon after the gradient has lessened and right where the trail bends farther to the east. The detour to Chittenden Lake will take you 1–2 hours round-trip, but as the highest of the lakes in the vicinity, it is well worth a diversion if you have time; see the Option on page 409.

Continuing to the northeast on the Lillian Lake Loop Trail, you go north only about 0.1 mile past the Chittenden Lake Trail junction before you see a Staniford lake. A waist-deep, grass-lined lakelet, this water body is not the Staniford Lake that attracts attention. Instead, continue until you come to a trailside pond atop a broad granitic crest. In this vicinity you can leave the trail and descend southeast briefly cross-country on low-angle slabs to the largest of the Staniford Lakes, lying at 8,708 feet. This is certainly the best lake to swim in, and if any sizable lake along this route will warm up to the low 70s in early August, it will be this one. The great bulk of the lake is less than 5 feet deep, its only deep spot being at a diving area along the west shore. Among the slabs you can find sandy camp spots.

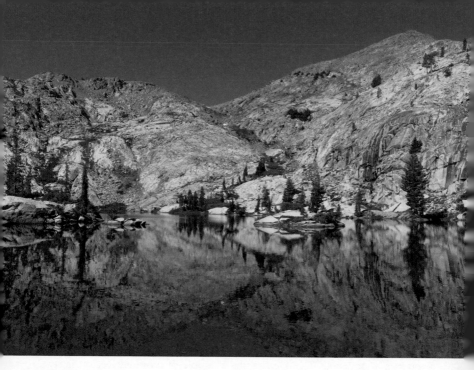

Chittenden Lake

More ponds, still part of the Staniford Lakes cluster, are seen along the northbound Lillian Lake Loop Trail before it dips into a usually dry gully. It then traverses diagonally up along a ridge with many glacier-polished slabs and with outstanding views to the Ritter Range and the entire San Joaquin drainage. You soon cross the ridge, then quickly descend to Lillian Lake's outlet creek and just beyond a junction to the spur trail around Lillian Lake's eastern and northern shores (6.15 miles). ▶8

Myriad use trails dive into the beautiful, dense hemlock forest ringing Lillian Lake's northeastern shore. Camping is prohibited within 400 feet of the northeastern shoreline, but if you continue about 0.25 mile to the north, you will encounter a series of well-used, beautiful sites set a little back from the lake. Because it's the largest and deepest lake you'll see along this hike, Lillian Lake is also the coldest, and its large population of trout does attract anglers.

Lillian Lake is the last of the lakes along this loop, and from the lake's outlet, the trail descends a forested mile east to a two-branched creek with easy fords. After a short, stiff climb over a gravelly knoll, the trail descends to a junction on a fairly open slope. Here the Lillian Lake Loop Trail ends and you rejoin the Fernandez Trail, on which you will turn right, heading south (7.35 miles). ▶9

The forest cover quickly thickens, and the trail soon enters a dense forest glade situated in a shallow trough. You are next routed back onto a ridgeline, an old moraine. Drier and sandier again, pine-mat manzanita and juniper dominate along the moraine crest, which the trail follows to its end before switchbacking back to the drainage below. The next junction you reach is that with the trail up Timber Creek (8.9 miles). ▶10 Though the junction itself is signposted and obvious, the unmaintained trail rapidly deteriorates, helped on its path to oblivion by abundant uncleared tree falls.

Continuing the downward trajectory beneath forest cover, you next reach a junction in a broad sandy flat, where the Fernandez Trail forks right and the Walton Trail leads to the left (9.05 miles). ▶11 Given these two trails lead to the same parking area and both are 3.15 miles in length, it is up to you which you take, though the Walton Trail requires less elevation gain, has more open views, and takes you through all new terrain—hence it is the route described here. Continuing through the open flat, along which there are many camping options, you soon cross Madera Creek. A possible wade under the highest of flows, this crossing quickly becomes a rock hop and will dry out in late summer. To your left (north) is an interesting geologic feature, a dark plug of olivine basalt, which was once part of the throat of a cinder cone. Glaciers removed the cinders but were too feeble to erode

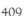

OPTION: Chittenden Lake

▶7 Beginning the 1.0-mile-long climb to 9,182-foot-high Chittenden Lake, the trail leads west then northwest from the shelf holding the Staniford Lakes. After climbing open slabs, the trail sidles up to the eastern bank of Shirley Creek. Stepping across the creek, the trail turns sharply south (left), continues briefly under forest cover, and then traverses open slabs. Across here there is no indication of a trail—just continue due south, and before long the lake comes into view.

Chittenden may be the most beautiful of all the lakes in this part of Ansel Adams Wilderness, though Lady and Lillian Lakes offer competition. Though Chittenden's water temperature does not usually rise above the low 60s, the lake's three bedrock islands will certainly tempt some swimmers. If there are more than two backpackers in your group, don't plan to camp at this lake because flat space is really at a premium. The best site is on the ridge east of the lake, boasting absolutely stunning views.

the lava. This dark monument is most obvious if you look north after you climb a few short steep switchbacks to an open slope.

The open views gleaned as you cross this slabby slope are a wonderful way to end your trip, with a vista north to the Yosemite boundary near Post Peak Pass and south to the Silver Divide in the South Fork San Joaquin drainage. Dropping off the bare slabs into open lodgepole forest, the trail trends south, continuing its descending traverse. Stretches are in dry lodgepole pine forest, but interspersed are wetter glades where red fir dominates and drier rocky knobs where manzanita and huckleberry oak replace the trees. Turning right at an old road junction (11.95 miles), ►12 you quickly reach the trailhead (12.2 miles). ►13

MILESTONES		
►1	0.0	Start at the Fernandez Trailhead (at end of FS 5S05)
►2	0.35	Right at flat spur trail to Norris Trailhead
►3	1.6	Right at steep spur trail to Norris Trailhead
►4	1.8	Left at Fernandez Trail–Vanderburgh Lake junction
►5	4.3	Vanderburgh Lake
►6	4.7	Right at Lady Lake junction
►7	5.4	Right at Chittenden Lake junction
►8	6.15	Right at Lillian Lake junction
►9	7.35	Right at Fernandez Trail–Lillian Lake Loop junction
►10	8.9	Right at junction with trail up Timber Creek
►11	9.05	Left onto Walton Trail at Fernandez–Walton Trails junction
►12	11.95	Right at old road junction
►13	12.2	Finish at the Walton Trailhead (at end of FS 5S05)

Top-Rated Trails

Appendix A

Campgrounds and RV Parks

On the introductory maps for each area, campgrounds close to the trailhead are shown. However, these are often full, so you may have to stay in a campground that is farther from your trailhead. Below is a list of campgrounds for both Yosemite National Park and each of the four bordering national forests. For each jurisdiction, a website with additional information about the campsites is given; the site will provide information on how to make campground reservations and information about facilities at each campsite. For Yosemite campground reservations, additional information is available on page 20. As for the lists of campsites, for Yosemite, campsites are clustered by access road. For national forests, campsites are listed in the order you will encounter them as you drive toward the park or its adjacent U.S. Forest Service lands. For the east side (US 395), campgrounds in the Humboldt-Toiyabe and Inyo National Forests are listed from north to south. *R* means that you can reserve a campsite in advance.

Yosemite National Park Campgrounds
nps.gov/yose/planyourvisit/camping.htm

Hetch Hetchy

Hetch Hetchy Backpacker

Big Oak Flat Road, eastward

Hodgdon Meadow (R)
Crane Flat (R)

Tioga Road, eastward

Tamarack Flat
White Wolf
Yosemite Creek

Porcupine Flat
Tuolumne Meadows (R)
Tuolumne Meadows Backpacker

Yosemite Valley

North Pines (R)
Upper Pines (R)
Lower Pines (R)
Sunnyside Walk-In
Yosemite Valley Backpacker

Glacier Point Road

Bridalveil Creek

Wawona

Wawona (R)

National Forest Campgrounds

For the four national forests bordering Yosemite, websites containing detailed campground information are as follows:

Humboldt-Toiyabe National Forest: www.fs.usda.gov/activity/htnf /recreation/camping-cabins

Inyo National Forest: www.fs.usda.gov/activity/inyo/recreation/camping -cabins

Sierra National Forest: www.fs.usda.gov/activity/sierra/recreation/camping -cabins

Stanislaus National Forest: www.fs.usda.gov/activity/stanislaus/recreation /camping-cabins

Reservations for all reservable campsites in the national forests can be made at recreation.gov.

Sierra National Forest (CA 41)

East of Fish Camp on National Forest Roads
Nelder Grove Campground
Big Sandy Campground
Soquel Campground
Greys Mountain Campground
Fresno Dome Campground
Texas Flat Group Campground

North of Fish Camp Along CA 41
Summerdale Campground (R)

Bass Lake
Crane Valley Group Campground (R)
Recreation Point Group Campground (R)
Forks Campground (R)
Lupine/Cedar Campground (R)
Spring Cove Campground (R)
Wishon Point Campground (R)

Beasore Road (Forest Service Road 7 Northeast from Bass Lake)
Chilkoot Campground (R)
Upper Chiquito Campground
Bowler Campground
Clover Meadow Campground
Granite Creek Campground

Minarets Road (FS 81 North from North Fork)
Fish Creek Campground (R)
Rock Creek Campground (R)
Soda Springs Campground
Lower Chiquito Campground
Placer Campground
Little Jackass Campground

CA 108: Humboldt–Toiyabe National Forest

East of Sonora Pass
Sonora Bridge
Leavitt Meadow

CA 120: Stanislaus National Forest

CA 120 Corridor West of Yosemite National Park
The Pines
Lost Claim (R)
Sweetwater

Cherry Road
Cherry Valley (R)

Evergreen Road
Dimond O (R)

CA 120: Inyo National Forest

East of Yosemite National Park
Lower Lee Vining
Moraine
Aspen Grove
Big Bend
Ellery
Junction
Sawmill Walk-In
Tioga Lake
Saddlebag Lake

US 395: Humboldt–Toiyabe National Forest

South of CA 108–US 395 Junction
Obsidian

Twin Lakes Road and Environs (Southwest and West from Bridgeport)
Honeymoon Flat (R)
Robinson Creek (R)
Paha (R)
Crags (R)
Lower Twin Lakes (R)
Buckeye (Along FS 017)

Green Creek Road/FS 142 (South of Bridgeport)
Green Creek
Green Creek Group (R)

Virginia Lakes Road/FS 21 (South from Conway Summit)
Trumbull Lake (R)

US 395: Inyo National Forest

North of Lee Vining
Lundy Canyon

South of Lee Vining

    June Lake Loop
    Oh! Ridge (R)
    June Lake (R)
    Reversed Creek (R)
    Gull Lake
    Silver Lake (R)

Obsidian Dome Road
Hartley Springs

Glass Creek Road
Glass Creek

Deadman Creek Road
Deadman

Mammoth Lakes and Vicinity
Shady Rest
Pine Glen (R)
Sherwin Creek (R)
Coldwater (R)
Lake George
Lake Mary (R)
Pine City
Twin Lakes (R)
Convict Lake (R)
Devils Postpile
Agnew Meadows
Upper Soda Springs
Pumice Flat
Minaret Falls
Devils Postpile
Reds Meadow

Private Campgrounds and RV Parks Outside Yosemite National Park

The following is a list of private facilities for camping. Most of these are RV parks, which cater more to those with motor homes, camper vans, and trailers than to those with tents. For each of the western Sierra highways below, the facilities are listed by their distance to the park, starting with those in the closest sites or towns. For the eastside US 395, the facilities are listed from north to south. A good website to garner others' reviews of these campsites is rvparkreviews.com.

CA 41

Bass Lake
Bass Lake Recreational Resort (Bass Lake RV Resort), 559-642-3148

Oakhurst

Elks Lodge, 559-683-2717
High Sierra RV and Mobile Park, 559-683-7662
Sierra Meadows RV Park, 559-642-1343
KOA Yosemite South–Coarsegold, 559-683-7855

CA 120

East of Buck Meadows

Yosemite Lakes RV Park, 209-962-0121
Yosemite Ridge Resort, 209-962-6877

Groveland

Pine Mountain Lake Campground, Groveland, 209-962-8615, -8625
Yosemite Pines RV Resort, just east of Groveland, 877-962-7690

Midpines

KOA Yosemite–Mariposa, 209-966-2201

CA 140

Mariposa

Mariposa Fairgrounds (south on CA 49), 209-966-2432
Indian Flat RV Park, 209-379-2339

US 395

Bridgeport

Annett's Mono Village (at Upper Twin Lake), 760-932-7071
Bridgeport Reservoir Marina and RV Park, 760-932-7001
Paradise Shores RV Park, 2399 CA 182, Bridgeport
Twin Lakes RV Resort, 877-932-7751

Between Bridgeport and Lee Vining

Lundy Lake Resort, 626-309-0415

Lee Vining

Mono Vista RV Park, Lee Vining, 760-647-6401

June Lake and Silver Lake

Golden Pine RV Park, 760-648-7473
June Lake RV and Lodge, 760-648-7967
Pine Cliff RV Resort, 760-648-7558
Silver Lake Resort and RV Park, 760-648-7525

Appendix B

Hotels, Lodges, Motels, and Resorts

Lodging within Yosemite National Park is quite limited. In Yosemite Valley there is a collection of accommodation options managed by the concessionaire Aramark. These range from the exquisite—the Majestic Yosemite Hotel (formerly the Ahwahnee Hotel)—to quite simple options, like Housekeeping Camp. There are also a number of private accommodations in Yosemite West, inholdings within the park just west of the Wawona Road, near the Glacier Point Road junction. Once outside the national park boundaries there are, not surprisingly, endless choices. The list below and the map on page v show the names of the surrounding communities, and an online search will yield the names of hotels, motels, and bed-and-breakfasts accompanied by travelers' latest reviews. Note that, among the options, the farther-afield options—Oakhurst, Mariposa, Mammoth Lakes—have the largest range but of course enormously increase your driving time to Yosemite trailheads.

Yosemite National Park: Concessionaire

Aramark, 888-413-8869 or 602-278-8888, travelyosemite.com

Yosemite Valley

The Majestic Yosemite Hotel (formerly the Ahwahnee Hotel)
Half Dome Village (formerly Curry Village)
Housekeeping Camp
Yosemite Valley Lodge

Wawona

Big Trees Lodge (formerly Wawona Hotel)

Tioga Road

Tuolumne Meadows Lodge
White Wolf Lodge

Yosemite National Park: Private

The Redwoods in Yosemite, 877-753-8566, redwoodsinyosemite.com, located at Wawona

Yosemite West, 559-642-2211, yosemitewestreservations.com, located at Yosemite West near the Glacier Point Road

Locales with Private Lodging Outside Yosemite National Park

CA 41

Fish Camp
Bass Lake
Oakhurst

CA 120

Buck Meadows
Groveland
El Portal

CA 140

Midpines
Mariposa

US 395

Bridgeport
Lee Vining
June Lake and Silver Lake
Mammoth Lakes

Appendix C

Useful Books and Maps

Backpacking and Mountaineering

Beck, Steve. *Yosemite Trout Fishing Guide*. Portland, OR: Frank Amato Publications, 1995.

Beffort, Brian. *Joy of Backpacking: Your Complete Guide to Attaining Pure Happiness in the Outdoors*. Berkeley, CA: Wilderness Press, 2007.

Berger, Karen. *Hiking Light Handbook: Carry Less, Enjoy More*. Seattle, WA: Mountaineers Books, 2004.

Clelland, Mike. *Ultralight Backpackin' Tips: 153 Amazing & Inexpensive Tips for Extremely Lightweight Camping*. Guilford, CT: Falcon Guides, 2011.

Forgey, William W., M.D. *Wilderness Medicine: Beyond First Aid,* 7th ed. Guilford, CT: Falcon Guides, 2017.

Ghiglieri, Michael Patrick, and Charles R. Farabee Jr. *Off the Wall: Death in Yosemite: Gripping Accounts of All Known Fatal Mishaps in America's First Protected Land of Scenic Wonders*. Flagstaff, AZ: Puma Press, 2007.

Ladigin, Don. *Lighten Up!: A Complete Handbook for Light and Ultralight Backpacking*. Guilford, CT: Falcon Guides, 2005.

Wilkerson, James A., M.D. *Medicine for Mountaineering & Other Wilderness Activities,* 6th ed. Seattle, WA: Mountaineers Books, 2010.

Guidebooks

Medley, Steven P. *The Complete Guidebook to Yosemite National Park*. El Portal, CA: Yosemite Conservancy, 2018.

Wenk, Elizabeth and Jeffrey P. Schaffer. *Yosemite National Park: A Complete Hiker's Guide*, 6th ed. Birmingham, AL: Wilderness Press, 2020.

Wenk, Elizabeth. *50 Best Short Hikes: Yosemite National Park and Vicinity,* 2nd ed. Birmingham, AL: Wilderness Press, 2012.

———. *John Muir Trail: The Essential Guide to Hiking America's Most Famous Trail,* 5th ed. Birmingham, AL: Wilderness Press, 2014.

History and Literature

Arnold, Daniel. *Early Days in the Range of Light: Encounters with Legendary Mountaineers.* Berkeley, CA: Counterpoint Press, 2011.

Brewer, William H. *Up and Down California in 1860–1864,* 4th ed. Berkeley: University of California Press, (1930) 2003.

Brewer, William Henry. *Such a Landscape!: A Narrative of the 1864 California Geological Survey Exploration of Yosemite, Sequoia & Kings Canyon from the Diary, Field Notes, Letters & Reports of William Henry Brewer.* El Portal, CA: Yosemite Association, 1999.

Browning, Peter. *Yosemite Place Names: The Historic Background of Geographic Names in Yosemite National Park.* Lafayette, CA: Great West Books, 2005.

Bunnell, Lafayette Houghton. *Discovery of the Yosemite.* El Portal, CA: Yosemite Association, 1991 (1880).

Farquhar, Francis P. *History of the Sierra Nevada.* Berkeley: University of California Press, (1946) 2007.

Johnson, Shelton. *Gloryland: A Novel.* San Francisco, CA: Sierra Club Books, 2009.

Johnston, Hank. *The Yosemite Grant, 1864–1906: A Pictorial History.* El Portal, CA: Yosemite Association, 1995.

King, Clarence. *Mountaineering in the Sierra Nevada.* Lincoln: University of Nebraska Press, 1997 (1872).

Muir, John. *The Mountains of California.* Berkeley, CA: Ten Speed Press, 1977 (1894).

———. *My First Summer in the Sierra.* San Francisco, CA: Sierra Club, 1988 (1911).

Righter, Robert W. *The Battle Over Hetch Hetchy: America's Most Controversial Dam and the Birth of Modern Environmentalism.* New York: Oxford University Press, 2005.

Rose, Gene. *Yosemite's Tioga Country: A History and Appreciation.* Berkeley, CA: Heyday Books, 2006.

Russell, Carl Parcher. *One Hundred Years in Yosemite: The Story of a Great Park and Its Friends*. Berkeley: University of California Press, 1947.

Sanborn, Margaret. *Yosemite: Its Discovery, Its Wonders, and Its People*. El Portal, CA: Yosemite Association, 1989.

Geology

Glazner, Allen F., and Greg M. Stock. *Geology Underfoot in Yosemite National Park*. Missoula, MT: Mountain Press, 2010.

Guyton, Bill. *Glaciers of California: Modern Glaciers, Ice Age Glaciers, the Origin of Yosemite Valley, and a Glacier Tour in the Sierra Nevada*. Berkeley: University of California Press, 1998.

Huber, N. King. *The Geologic Story of Yosemite National Park*. El Portal, CA: Yosemite Conservancy, 2014.

———. *Geological Ramblings in Yosemite*. Berkeley, CA: Heyday Books, 2007.

Matthes, François E. *Geologic History of the Yosemite Valley: Geological Survey Professional Paper 160*. Washington, D.C.: United States Government Printing Office, 1930.

———. *The Incomparable Valley: A Geologic Interpretation of the Yosemite*. Berkeley: University of California Press, 1950.

Schaffer, Jeffrey P. *The Geomorphic Evolution of the Yosemite Valley and Sierra Nevada Landscapes: Solving the Riddles in the Rocks*. Berkeley, CA: Wilderness Press, 1997.

———. *Seeing the Elephant: How Perceived Evidence in the Sierra Nevada Biased Global Geomorphology* (unpublished manuscript, 2006). [Volume 2 of the previous entry.]

Biology

Beedy, Edward C., and Edward R. Pandolfino. *Birds of the Sierra Nevada: Their Natural History, Status, and Distribution*. Berkeley: University of California Press, 2013.

Botti, Stephen J., and Walter Sydoriak. *An Illustrated Flora of Yosemite National Park*. Berkeley, CA: Heyday Books, 2001.

Gaines, David. *Birds of Yosemite and the East Slope*. Lee Vining, CA: Artemisia Press, 1992.

Horn, Elizabeth L. *Sierra Nevada Wildflowers*. Missoula, MT: Mountain Press, 1998.

Johnston, Verna R. *Sierra Nevada: The Naturalist's Companion*. Berkeley: University of California Press, 1998.

Laws, John Muir. *The Laws Field Guide to the Sierra Nevada*. Berkeley, CA: Heyday Books, 2007.

Sibley, David. *Sibley Birds West: Field Guide to Birds of Western North America,* 2nd ed. New York: Alfred A. Knopf, 2013.

Storer, Tracy I., Robert L. Usinger, and David Lukas. *Sierra Nevada Natural History,* revised ed. Berkeley: University of California Press, 2004.

Weeden, Norman F. *A Sierra Nevada Flora,* 4th ed. Berkeley, CA: Wilderness Press, 1996.

Wiese, Karen. *Sierra Nevada Wildflowers,* 2nd ed. Guilford, CT: Falcon Guides, 2013.

Wenk, Elizabeth. *Wildflowers of the High Sierra and John Muir Trail*. Birmingham, AL: Wilderness Press, 2015.

Willard, Dwight. *A Guide to the Sequoia Groves of California*. El Portal, CA: Yosemite Conservancy, 2000.

Index

Note: *Italicized* page numbers represent photographic material. Page numbers followed by *m* indicate a map.

About the Authors

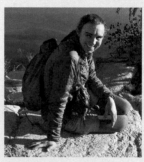

photographed by Douglas Bock

Since childhood, **Lizzy Wenk** has hiked and climbed in the Sierra Nevada and continues the tradition with her husband, Douglas Bock, and daughters, Eleanor and Sophia. As she obtained a PhD in Sierran alpine plant ecology from the University of California, Berkeley, her love of the mountain range morphed into a profession. But writing guidebooks has become her way to share her love and knowledge of the Sierra Nevada with others. Lizzy continues to obsessively explore every bit of the Sierra, spending summers hiking on- and off-trail throughout the range, but she currently lives in Sydney, Australia, during the "off-season." Other Wilderness Press titles she has authored include *John Muir Trail, One Best Hike: Mount Whitney, One Best Hike: Grand Canyon, 50 Best Short Hikes: Yosemite,* and *Wildflowers of the High Sierra and John Muir Trail,* the latter a perfect companion book for all naturalists.

Jeffrey P. Schaffer has been hiking and climbing in Yosemite National Park since 1964. He's logged thousands of miles on-trail in the park and has completed some 70 different roped ascents, including several first ascents. In 1972 he began work on his first book for Wilderness Press, *The Pacific Crest Trail.* Since then, he has written and contributed to more than a dozen Wilderness Press guidebooks, including *Yosemite National Park: A Complete Hiker's Guide.* Today, he teaches a variety of natural sciences courses at San Francisco Bay Area community colleges, does Sierran geomorphic research, leads climbs both outdoors and in climbing gyms, and lives with his wife in the Napa Valley.

Joe Walowski conceived of the Top Trails series in 2003 and was series editor of the first three titles: *Top Trails: Los Angeles, Top Trails: San Francisco Bay Area,* and *Top Trails: Lake Tahoe.* He currently lives in Seattle.